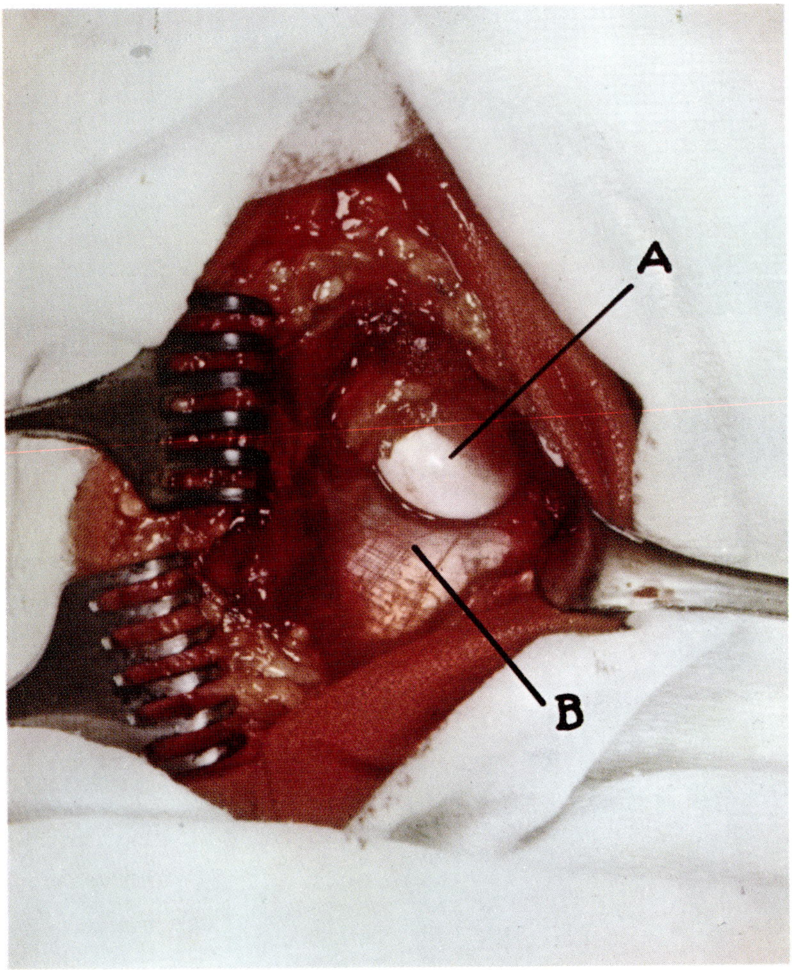

Surgery of the Elbow

Medial epicondyle of humerus displaced into the dislocated elbow joint. Photograph shows operative exposure of the medial aspect of the joint. (A) Trochlear process of humerus. (B) Flexor-pronator group of muscles curling into the joint just distal to trochlea. The medial epicondylar fragment comes into view only when the muscles attached to it are pulled upon and withdrawn from the joint. *(See Chapter X.)*

Second Edition

SURGERY of the ELBOW

By

FREDERICK M. SMITH, M.D.

Former Associate Attending Orthopedic Surgeon, Presbyterian Hospital, New York Orthopedic Hospital, and Vanderbilt Clinic

1972

W. B. SAUNDERS COMPANY

Philadelphia · London · Toronto

W. B. Saunders Company: West Washington Square
Philadelphia, Pa. 19105

12 Dyott Street
London, WC1A 1DB

833 Oxford Street
Toronto 18, Ontario

Surgery of the Elbow ISBN 0-7216-8382-7

 Press of W. B. Saunders Company. Library of Congress catalog card number 75-183457.

Print No: 9 8 7 6 5 4 3 2 1

To

MARY

Preface to Second Edition

The author has been gratified by the reception of the first edition of this book, especially by residents in traumatic and orthopedic surgery. The second edition has been revised not only to emphasize many of the principles brought out in the first, but to add some new illustrations of x-rays as well as to improve the quality of the sketches. Fortunately, not too much revision of the text has been necessary, but naturally new thoughts arise and these should be presented. Added also are comments on congenital synostosis, compound dislocations without accompanying fracture at the elbow, and on Monteggia fracture with radial neck fracture accompanying the radial head dislocation in children.

It is therefore hoped that residents and others not able to obtain the first edition may profit by the second.

FREDERICK M. SMITH

Preface to First Edition

THERE HAS long existed need for a book dealing with surgical conditions of the elbow. This region is subject to severe types of trauma (fractures, dislocations, lacerations, gunshot wounds, crushes, etc.) or to milder forms of trauma such as constant usage (occupation), sports (baseball pitching), or to irritation from mal-union after previous fractures or from post-traumatic arthritis. The joint may become the site of sepsis or tuberculosis and thus require operative surgery. Arthritis (gonorrheal or rheumatoid) does not require surgery in the early stage, but fibrous or bony ankylosis, the late result of either of these infections, may require surgery to increase joint motion. Other non-traumatic conditions of the elbow such as congenital deformities, neoplasms, osteomyelitis, paralyses, loose bodies, and bursitis often call for relief by operative surgery.

Although numerous monographs have been written upon such subjects as the shoulder, hand, hip and foot, the student must search through one or more of these or other text-books in order to cover the elbow region thoroughly. He must consult a text-book on fractures for traumatic lesions, many of which fail to warn against important associated soft part lesions, or fail to advise how to avoid incurring their complications. For late deformities or for tuberculosis of the joint, he must consult a text-book on operative orthopedics. In this is described one or more methods of treating such a lesion, usually stressing the particular method of the author, the latter well illustrated. Not only the medical student, but the resident or the younger surgeon may become utterly confused by the number of plausible methods of treatment suggested for a given condition. He is not in a position to decide for himself which method to choose from the information presented. He may recall the principles of treatment for fresh injuries; but for late deformities—this is something entirely different. It is just as important for the writer to inform his reader how a certain deformity might be avoided as it is to tell him how to correct it when present.

The purpose of this book is to deal with the various conditions in the region of the elbow that are amenable to surgical treatment or to a combination of surgical plus physiotherapeutic or radiotherapeutic measures. Inasmuch as trauma and the results of trauma make up a large part, the book will stress the principles of treatment, point out the danger spots, try to predict what can or may happen with good or bad treatment and thereby help the younger surgeon avoid the pitfalls that his predecessors have learned via "the hard way." For the purpose of impressing upon the reader the main principles of treatment and the importance of careful attention to details so necessary in the successful care not only of a particular patient, but of all patients coming under his attention, reiteration in the text is employed solely as a means of emphasis.

FREDERICK M. SMITH

Contents

Chapter I

Traumatic Lesions of the Elbow Region

GENERAL CONSIDERATIONS

THE ELBOW JOINT is an instrument of precision and one of complex mechanism. It is made up of three joints which, working together, give the function of one: the ulnar-humeral, the radio-humeral, and the (superior) radio-ulnar joints. The first two allow hinge-joint motion (flexion and extension); the latter two allow rotary motion of the forearm and hand (pronation and supination). It requires no intricate knowledge of anatomy and only a little common sense to realize that slight alterations in the joint structure may cause profound disturbances in its function. For example, a dicondylar fracture of the humerus with the condyles displaced in relation to the shaft and to each other may be compared to an ordinary door with its two hinges improperly aligned. Just as the door may be partially closed or opened, the elbow joint may be partially flexed and extended; but neither motion can be performed freely or completely. If one uses force to open or close this door beyond its free arc, the hinges may bind and squeak; if enough force is used one hinge may pull away from the door or wall or a portion of the hinge may break. If one uses force (passive motion or manipulation) to increase motion similarly following a fracture into an elbow joint, it also may bind, and if enough force is used, something must give way, i.e., a bone fragment, ligaments, or muscle.

Besides the importance per se of free flexion, extension and rotation in the elbow joint, it is important to remember that loss of one or more of these motions may seriously interfere with use of the hand. In many occupations complete pronation and supination are not absolutely essential and slight loss of either or both may not handicap the individual seriously since he can often compensate (sometimes imperceptably) for this loss by rotation of the humerus at the shoulder joint. Other individuals may be very greatly handicapped by the loss of only twenty or thirty degrees of one of these rotations. Consider the pianist who loses this amount of full pronation. For fifteen to twenty minutes he may compensate by abducting his humerus, but this becomes so tiring he has to stop playing, when formerly he was able to play the piano for two to three hours at a time. A violinist, should he lose thirty degrees of full supination in his left hand, may have his career come to a rather abrupt termination.

There are many reasons why pronation and supination may be interfered with following injury. Among these are development of irregularity or enlargement in the radial head, adhesions within the joint, loose bone fragments in the joint, and post-traumatic arthritis. These are but a few of the mechanical reasons for difficulty following injury. Pain and swelling are additional reasons for loss of function and use. (These disabilities, their etiology and treatment will be dealt with later in more detail in their proper chapters.)

So far nothing has been said of injuries to the surrounding soft tissues in the region of the elbow. Physicians with limited experience may forget that the soft tissues surrounding the bones and joints often exhibit more important pathology than the fracture or dislocation itself. The muscles, arteries, veins, lymphatics and nerves may be of much greater importance than the bone or the joint. For example, what good is an extremity which shows a well healed fracture, but also shows a Volkmann's ischemic contracture?

In general, injuries about the elbow give fairly successful results if treated with average consideration and intelligence. On the other hand there are many elbow fractures of a complicated nature which require some special knowledge and skill to be able to handle properly if the patient is to obtain a good functioning joint. Thirty or 40 years ago the treatment recommended for dicondylar fractures of the humerus in adults was reduction and immobilization for six to eight weeks in plaster casts or splints in such position as was considered optimum for the individual *should the joint become ankylosed.* The majority of them did ankylose after such prolonged immobilization. This is a peculiarity of elbow joints following severe injury when subjected to prolonged immobilization. The idea, however, was purely defeatist from the beginning. It is now encouraging that more and more surgeons who treat such injuries are beginning to be enlightened and are now getting these patients on early active motion in order to allow them to regain as much function as possible in this very important joint. It takes courage to sacrifice an excellent appearing elbow or a nice x-ray film of a perfect (?) reduction, if a sacrifice has to be made either in anatomy or function, and strive to restore joint function as fully as possible.

Furthermore, many of the commoner and less serious elbow injuries are often missed in respect to proper diagnosis and consequently are given improper treatment. The position of acute flexion is *not* the *routine* and *proper* position of immobilization in all elbow injuries. There should be no *routine* treatment of a particular type of fracture. Each patient should be examined and treated as an individual and the best method of treatment selected for him. It is better to vary or adjust the method to the individual than vice versa. Routine flexion, routine circular plaster and, what is worse, a routine surgical mind are probably responsible for more Volkmann's contractures than anything else. Too many times have we seen a child brought to the clinic or office months following injury and demonstrating little or no motion in the elbow joint, seeking help after his original doctor has mistaken a serious lateral condyle fracture for a "chip off the bone" and had resorted to forced stretching manipulations.

HIGH INCIDENCE OF ELBOW INJURIES

The elbow region is one of the common sites of injury both in the child and adult, being injured in the traumas of ordinary life (falls), sports, and in farm and automobile accidents. In large cities roller skating and traffic accidents become frequent causative agents of these injuries. At the Presbyterian Hospital, New York City, from 1929 to 1945 inclusive, fractures and dislocations of the elbow made up 9.9 percent and 18.8 percent of the total fractures and dislocations respectively treated on the Fracture Service. Omitting the dislocations, this amounts to more than twenty-one thousand fractures treated during this seventeen-year period.

WHAT ARE WE TRYING TO ACCOMPLISH?

The above question may best be answered in the words of Murray,[1] who said:

> In traumatic injuries what we as surgeons are trying to accomplish is the restoration, insofar as possible, of the individual to his former usefulness, in the shortest possible time, with as complete restoration of normal anatomy as can be accomplished under those circumstances.

From the Standpoint of the Patient. The writer has been taught in medical school and had impressed upon him thoroughly during his subsequent surgical training that the patient's welfare takes precedence over all else. This is a fundamental principle and as such deserves our immediate attention. All else, including teaching, research, etc., is of secondary importance. In other words, given an injured or ill patient, one must turn and devote all his attention, skill, and facilities within reason to relieve his suffering and to mend his injury.

This is an excellent principle and one that can and should be adhered to strictly in civilian practice. In the treatment of large numbers of war casualties it may be necessary and wise to forego the individual patient and to follow a method of treatment shown to be better for the entire group of injured, otherwise a few would be adequately treated at the expense of many. It is hoped that civilian surgery, however, will occupy the greater part of our future experience, and to this end is the majority of this book written.

We hope, therefore, to give the patient the best possible advantage anatomically, functionally, economically, and psychologically that can be furnished him.

From the Standpoint of the Insurance Company. Rarely is anyone sorry

---

1 Murray, Dr. Clay Ray.

because an insurance company has to reimburse a patient for damages or time lost. Actually this is beside the point. The honest surgeon with a conscience will treat and take care of the injured patient with the best of his skill and knowledge which means that he will not prolong the treatment unnecessarily. In the end the insurance companies should not be long in recognizing that good surgical care does not consist solely of keeping the "paper work" up to date. Good surgical care costs money, but if it is good, it will in the long run result in an actual saving of money.

From the Standpoint of Improving the Treatment of Trauma. Through being alert a constant search will be made for new methods of treatment and the management of traumatic injuries will be made clearer and less difficult. The surgeon, who is to be successful, must never hesitate to learn from others. He will do well to attend scientific meetings and enter into discussions. He must keep up with the current literature to be aware of the progress in his field. To think over the new methods of treatment and try to reason why these may or may not fit into the scheme of general principles of treatment is time well spent. It will stress the importance of these and will make him a better surgeon, because good surgical judgment improves from years of experience in following sound principles.

From the Standpoint of Teaching. There is no question but that medical students are molded by the type of teachers with whom they come in contact and the teaching which they receive. This cannot begin too early in their careers. They must be honest with themselves; they must seek the truth; they must face facts. They must be taught the importance of "giving the patient a break" first, and being purely scientific later. If this can be instilled into them, they in turn may be entrusted with the future of surgery.

The teaching of undergraduate students should be limited largely to the principles of treatment and should not take into consideration the various methods of treatment. Only those methods should be mentioned which help to illustrate a particular principle. Students are only human and look for short cuts, tending to classify a certain "cure" with a certain disease (or injury). They must be given enough ground work such as anatomy and physiology and be made to understand the pathology of injury as well as that of disease. They must be advised when, where and how to look for various types of complications and be taught their implications. None of this should be done solely with didactic lectures. These must be curtailed to a minimum merely to give a general survey of the particular subject at hand. The main part of his teaching in this type of clinical work should consist of demonstrations of actual clinical cases, roentgenologic examination, discussion of cases, observation over a period of time and actual participation in the care of the patient. This can be carried out with small groups of students studying cases in the out-patient clinic or on the surgical ward. In this way the student gets to see the actual management of a case and if he gets to discuss its possibilities, this form of teaching is infinitely more valuable to him than a dry lecture on the same subject.

The teaching of graduate students should augment this same teaching of sound principles by going into more detail as to various methods of treatment and the reasons for the choice of particular methods. It should also, if possible, permit them to participate in the actual treatment. In this fashion, they will learn refinements of diagnosis and technique that they had not previously acquired. Graduate students will benefit also if given an opportunity to carry out either a scientific or clinical research problem and in turn may help the professional staff or the institution under which they are working.

FRACTURES

Traumatic Etiology

Fractures in the region of the elbow are usually due to trauma, but they may have a spontaneous origin. Trauma may be divided into the direct and indirect types. Without identifying each and every variety it might be mentioned that of the slow-speed objects causing fractures by direct contact we have a pitched baseball, a club, a knife, pistol butt, falling glass, and other falling debris. High speed etiological agents consist of pistol or rifle bullets, shrapnel, shell, bomb or mine fragments. Then there are crushing injuries such as result from a window falling on the elbow, or a crush from a door, automobile or airplane accident. The elbow may be occasionally run over by a pneumatic tire of a car, or by the flanged wheel of a street car or train (in the latter case traumatic amputation usually resulting). Both the elbow and the object with which it comes in contact may be moving, and the combined speed of the two plus the mass result in a shattering, almost explosive injury to the elbow such as seen in the so-called "truck-swipe" or "side-swipe" injury sustained not infrequently by drivers of cars who insist on resting their forearm and elbow on the window sill while driving along the highway. Probably the commonest cause of elbow fractures comes from falls sustained by the patient in the home, at work, at play or on icy streets. Although many of these fractures come from hitting the elbow directly, many more come from a fall upon the hand, the force being transmitted indirectly to the elbow through the radius and ulna, but eventually knocking off the capitellum or radial head. Fractures resulting from pure indirect trauma are usually those caused by an avulsion mechanism as is sometimes seen in the olecranon after forcefully throwing a baseball; or in a dislocated elbow where the medial epicondyle epiphysis has been avulsed by the pull of the medial collateral ligament; or the bicipital tuberosity avulsed by a sudden violent pull of the biceps tendon.

Spontaneous

Spontaneous fractures in the elbow region are usually due to some localized bone pathology, the commonest of which is a metastasis from a malignant tumor. Giant cell tumors (benign) may also cause thinning of the bone sufficiently to allow it to become fractured without adequate trauma. The same may be said for bone cysts, although these are rare in the extremities of the bones making up the elbow joint.

Other Causes of Spontaneous Fractures. Osteoporosis due to senility, disease or paralysis; osteomalacia, coeliac disease, Paget's disease, primary bone neoplasms (sarcoma or myeloma), and osteogenesis imperfecta.

Epiphyseal Separations and Epiphyseal Trauma

In the growing child an injury to the extremity of a bone very frequently takes the form of a fracture passing along the epiphyseal line and separating the epiphysis and displacing it upon the diaphysis. These are true fractures even though the fracture line passes through cartilage. Usually when the epiphysis is displaced, it carries a small triangular shaped fragment of the diaphysis with it. All such cases, of course, should be treated by reduction and immobilization sufficiently long to permit healing to take place just as in a shaft fracture. Still more important is epiphyseal trauma without actual displacement demonstrable on the roentgenogram. The diagnosis must be made clinically on the finding of linear tenderness maximun along the epiphyseal line in the absence of roentgen findings. The importance of the diagnosis of epiphyseal trauma with or without displacement is the possibility of growth disturbance and later deformity. The chance of growth disturbance taking place is equally good whether or not there was displacement originally. In each case the extremity should be immobilized sufficiently long, i. e., until the linear tenderness limited to the epiphyseal line has disappeared.

Immediately after an injury it may be difficult to differentiate between a sprain of the elbow joint and an epiphyseal injury. In the child true sprains are *rare* at the elbow. Epiphyseal traumata are *very common.* If there is any doubt whatsoever, the injury should be treated as one of an epiphysis by immobilization, for this may prevent subsequent growth disturbance. Just as much and sometimes the worst growth disturbance may occur in those cases with the least amount of displacement or in those without any displacement of the epiphysis. Should the epiphyseal line tenderness disappear in four to seven days after injury we may assume that merely a sprain had occurred and discard the immobilizing splint. On the other hand if it should last for two or three weeks or more, one can be certain that the original trauma was of epiphyseal origin and should keep the joint splinted until the tenderness completely disappears. Only by treating these injuries conservatively will growth disturbances be minimized.

Whenever separation (fracture) of an epiphysis has been diagnosed or trauma to it suspected the surgeon who is wise will forewarn the child's parents or guardian of the possibility of growth disturbance. This can be done without alarming them unnecessarily, because the probability of disturbance in growth in non-weight bearing bones is relatively small (less than 20 percent).

It is also important in epiphyseal separations to perform reduction by closed methods, without undue force, and without frequent repetition. *Never* perform open reduction on a traumatically displaced epiphysis if it can be avoided, i. e., by obtaining reasonably good anatomical reposition through closed reduction. Open reductions and often repeated attempts at closed reduction definitely predispose to growth disturbance.

DISLOCATIONS

Dislocation means the displacement of one or more bones which ordinarily make up a joint so that the articular surfaces are no longer in contact. These may be pure dislocations, i. e., without associated fracture, or they may have associated fractures. Posterior or posterolateral dislocation of both forearm bones upon the humerus at the elbow joint not infrequently is accompanied by one of the following fractures: radial head, coronoid process of ulna, and avulsion of the epiphysis of the medial epicondyle of the humerus. Certain other dislocations almost invariably accompany certain specific fractures, such as an anterior dislocation of the radial head when there is a fracture of the upper third of the shaft of the ulna with volar angulation. This particular combination of fracture and dislocation is commonly known as a Monteggia fracture. Certain types of dislocation at the elbow *must* have an associated fracture in order to make possible the dislocation. The best example of this is the anterior dislocation of both forearm bones upon the lower articular surface of the humerus, which cannot possibly take place without a fracture of the olecranon process of the ulna.

Subluxations (or partial dislocations) can occur and these, as the name implies, connote only partial displacement of the bones at the joint. Fracture of the lateral condyle of the humerus often makes possible a lateral subluxation of the radius and ulna, and, if not corrected, may result in a considerable increase in the carrying angle as well as cause some loss of joint function.

The important fact to remember in a dislocation (especially in such a stable joint as the elbow) is that none can possibly take place without extensive damage to the ligaments and joint capsule. During the process of repair following an elbow joint dislocation calcium is frequently deposited in the collateral ligaments. This is so commonly seen in late follow-up roentgenograms that the presence of such deposits, even in a patient not previously seen, should lead the surgeon to question the patient concerning previous serious injury. It may also help to explain (on the basis of a previous injury) why function does not return fully as expected. Besides wide tearing of these structures which normally bind the bones to one another, there frequently is extensive damage to the soft tissues lying immediately superficial to the ligaments and capsule as does the brachialis anticus muscle, the ulnar nerve, and brachial vessels. (See Chapter XIX.)

COMBINED FRACTURES AND DISLOCATIONS

Mention has already been made about combinations of fractures and dislocations in the region of the elbow and these will be treated in detail. (See Chapters X, XI, XII.) Inasmuch as combined fractures and dislocations are extremely common at the elbow and often of a serious nature, it would be wise to be on a constant lookout for them. With a dislocation of both bones one should always search the roentgenogram for possible fractures and vice versa.

DEFINITIONS

Fractures

A fracture is a loss (or break) in the continuity of a bone or a portion of a bone or cartilage in a living individual. The fact that the fracture occurs in a *person* is stressed, because it is often more important to handle the individual with the fracture than the fracture itself. This means carrying out treatment with the patient's future well being in mind as well as his immediate needs.

There are in general two main groups of fractures—*Simple* and *Open* (compound). A *simple* fracture is any kind or variety of fracture not associated with a wound involving the skin or mucous membrane. These are *clean* (closed) fractures. An *open* (compound) fracture is any variety of fracture in which there is a wound of the soft parts extending from the fracture site to and *including* the skin or mucous membrane. These fractures are unclean, contaminated and may occur by an external object breaking or lacerating the skin (compounding from without) or by one or more sharp fragments of bone forcing their way through the skin (compounding from within). The differences between "compounding" from without or within need not be discussed here. The essential difference between a closed (simple) fracture and an open (compound) fracture is that the latter is an injury contaminated by unknown organisms, carries a potential serious threat to limb and life, and demands immediate treatment to prevent or minimize the possibility of infection.

Further definitions are in order for designating the types of fractures that are commonly met with in treating traumatic cases. Any of these may be closed (simple) fractures or open (compound) fractures.

Comminuted fractures are those with more than two main fragments, i. e., with actual fragmentation or with loose fragments. These can be either closed comminuted or open comminuted (the latter only when the skin is broken and the wound communicates with the fractured area of the bone).

Green-stick fractures are seen in children only, where, due to its greater springiness, the bone may bend and only one cortex shows a break in continuity.

Lead-pipe fractures are a form of *green-stick* fracture usually occurring in the cancellous portion of the bone and appear on roentgenograms as a wrinkling of the thin cortex.

Fissure fractures are usually short transverse fracture lines extending partially or wholly through one cortex of a bone. These occur commonly in Paget's disease of bone and often represent the first stage in a fatigue fracture before the fracture becomes complete.

Impacted fractures are those in which one fragment of a fractured bone is driven or jammed into the remaining bone or into another main fragment.

Pathological fractures are those occurring in a bone which is the site of pre-existing disease or other abnormal condition, and not due to adequate trauma.

Sprain-fractures are small surface chips pulled away from a bone by a ligament when it is sprained.

Articular fractures are those near the extremity of a long bone in which the fracture line passes across or through the articular surface into the joint proper.

Intra-articular fractures are those where the entire fracture line is within the joint cavity. The commonest of these at the elbow are fractures of the radial head, coronoid process of the ulna and the capitellum.

Avulsion fractures are those in which a portion of bone or epiphysis is pulled off the main bone by muscle, ligament, tendon, or a combination of these. Fracture and separation of the medial epicondyle epiphysis is an excellent example of this type.

Fracture-dislocation is a combination of a fracture of the extremity of a bone in which the fragment entering into the joint has been dislocated or displaced from its articulation with the remaining half of the joint.

Dislocations

The term *dislocation* applies to bones that form a joint and means complete displacement of one or more of these bones on the others so that their articular surfaces are no longer in contact.

Dislocations may be *incomplete* where there is a partial shift of the articular surfaces, but no complete displacement. These are also called *subluxations.*

As with fractures, dislocations may also be classified as closed or open, depending upon the absence or presence of a wound in the skin communicating with the affected joint.

Displacements

Deformities. In fractures as well as in dislocations the bone fragments or the bones themselves are often displaced. These displacements are sometimes called deformities, but it would seem more logical to use the term "deformity" in describing a clinical picture and to use the term "displacement" in describing the actual shift in the bones seen roentgenologically as well as clinically.

In designating any displacement it is usual to describe it in terms of displacement of the distal fragment upon the proximal. If everyone would do this, we should all be speaking a common language and it would be far simpler for physicians and surgeons as well as students to understand the terminology. The same should apply to dislocations, i.e., in describing a dislocation at the elbow as *posterior,* we mean that the radius and ulna have been displaced posteriorly upon the lower end of the humerus rather than implying that there is an anterior dislocation of the humerus upon the forearm bones.

The simplest type of displacement in a fracture is *lateral* or *antero-posterior.* If the amount of displacement equals the full diameter of the bone, it is usually accompanied by over-riding and shortening. In some oblique fractures there may be *shortening* without a complete lateral shift of the fragments. Another common displacement (or deformity) is *angulation* or *tilt* of one fragment upon the other. In describing this it is advisable to describe the direction in which the apex of the angle points in order to be consistent in the terminology. *Rotary displacement* is common and means a rotation of the distal fragment upon the proximal. This may be of any amount up to 180 degrees. Occasionally the fractured end of one fragment is found in direct contact with the side of the other fragment. This is known as an *end to side* position. It always requires correction if bone healing is to take place and if full return of joint function is to be made possible.

Dislocations may show similar displacements. The common ones at the elbow are posterior and lateral or a combination of the two. Medial dislocation at this joint is rare; anterior dislocations here cannot take place without a fracture of the olecranon. Dislocations may also be accompanied by a certain amount of rotation. Very rarely there is seen at the elbow a divergent dislocation. In this variety the forearm bones are not only dislocated from the humerus, but from each other as well, and their proximal ends are spread apart.

Other Traumatic Lesions

Many injuries in the region of the elbow do not involve the bones in a fracture or in a dislocation and are relatively minor in nature. By causing pain, deformity or partial loss of function these injuries bring the patient to the surgeon for relief. It would seem advisable to enumerate them here, but describe the pathology and treatment under a separate chapter reserved for that purpose. Such conditions are contusions, lacerations (especially over the olecranon bursa), sprains, hemarthrosis, acute and chronic olecranon bursitis, "tennis elbow" (radio-humeral bursitis), calcium deposit in the conjoined tendon of the flexor-pronator group of muscles, and rupture of tendons and muscles. (See Chapter XXII.)

Chapter II

Pathology of Fractures

ACUTE PATHOLOGY

WHENEVER fracture of any bone occurs the first pathological change to take place is immediate hemorrhage from the bone itself. This occurs around the bone ends and in the adjacent marrow cavity. Coincident with the original injury and displacement of the fragments and depending also upon additional secondary trauma from inadequate splinting and muscle spasm during transportation there is a variable amount of damage to the surrounding soft parts. With any degree of displacement periosteum is always torn. If displacement is marked or if the injured extremity is handled roughly or protected inadequately, there is in addition gross tearing of muscle tissue, ligaments, fascia, tendons and their sheaths, small caliber arteries and veins (occasionally vessels of major proportions), lymphatic vessels and nerves. Contusion of these same soft parts likewise occurs. Even with the lesser degrees of soft part trauma accompanying a fracture there are innumerable capillaries both venous and lymphatic that are ruptured and each of these is a potential source of hemorrhage and exudation of fluid.

Hemorrhage comes first, but is soon followed by exudation of inflammatory leucocytes and phagocytes and fluid into the injured area and immediately surrounding it. All the soft parts (whether damaged or merely adjacent normal tissue) become infiltrated, swollen, edematous and lose their elasticity. In addition to bleeding from countless small veins and capillaries, many of these become thrombosed as well. This leads to circulatory stasis and stagnation. A vicious cycle is created, due partly to the hemorrhage and partly to the chemical irritation of the free blood in the tissues as well as to the toxic products liberated by the death of bone cells and damaged soft parts. In addition to the acute local inflammatory reaction, a systemic reaction in the patient is manifested by malaise, fever, elevation of both the leucocyte count and sedimentation rate. Shock is often present and may be of a serious nature if much blood has been lost from injury to medium and large size vessels or if there has been extensive soft tissue damage. The treatment of shock, though helped very appreciably through replacement of blood loss by transfusion, may be very ineffective or slow to bring about recovery unless other measures are carried out to rid the traumatized area of its collection of toxic products (dead cells and tissue debris) which is a constant source for absorption of these products into the general system. Everything that can be done to assist the patient's minute circulation by physiological measures is justified. These would include active exercise of muscles, physiotherapy, gravity, and at times even operative evacuation.

During the early phase of exudation, death of tissue, and circulatory stasis the tissue fluids at the site of fracture can be shown to have an acid pH. Although bone repair begins certainly within the first two or three days after fracture, no great amount of calcium can be precipitated or deposited in the newly formed granulation tissue until the local tissue reaction has changed from an acid to an alkaline pH. This alkaline reaction can only be brought about early by removal of the products of tissue death and by overcoming the circulatory stasis. (For specific methods of dealing with the local acute pathology see Chapter XVIII.)

The clinical implications of the concomitant acute fracture pathology, circulatory stasis and early bone repair are that we must act early if we hope to reduce a fracture adequately and easily before tissue elasticity is completely lost and without causing additional damage in our attempt to do so. Immediately following a fracture there is a period of local tissue shock lasting from fifteen to thirty minutes. During this time there is little or no pain and no muscle spasm. When sufficient hemorrhage has occurred and local exudation of fluid and cells infiltrate the surrounding tissues (i. e., when the acute inflammatory reaction gets under way), the muscles go into spasm and the nerve ends regain their sensitivity. This spasm and increased tissue tension further increases circulatory stagnation and interferes with easy reduction. The acute reaction reaches its height between twelve to eighteen hours or even earlier. Much can be done in the first three or four hours following fracture that cannot possibly be accomplished at twenty-four hours by closed or open methods of reduction. Anyone who has operated upon a severe elbow fracture immediately after injury and has compared it to one operated upon after two to three days will testify to the advisability of the former procedure, because he can mobilize the fragments easily, he does not have to explore through highly edematous hemorrhagic tissue, or tissue that is completely rubbery and infiltrated, and, last but not least, he is able to close the wound with ease in the early case.

LATE PATHOLOGY

The late pathology at the site of a healed fracture (aside from the healed bone) will depend directly upon the extent of the original tissue trauma and upon the speed and ease with which the acute pathology was eradicated and function restored to the muscles and joints. Extensive early hemorrhage into muscle bellies and actual damage to these muscles will lead to fibrosis and connective tissue replacement, which in turn will render them less elastic and less strong, resulting in loss of joint function and early muscle fatigue and pain on use. Besides affecting muscles, increased amounts of fibrous tissue may by contraction cause pressure upon venous and lymphatic channels, resulting in prolonged or even permanent swelling. It may cause nerves to become adherent to bone or fascia with subsequent sensory or motor functional impairment. Again, increased fibrosis, the result of extensive hemorrhage and cellular infiltration, may cause definite thickening of ligaments and joint capsules with resulting loss of their pliability and limitation of full joint motion. This, when it occurs in the region of the anterior capsule of the elbow joint, may greatly handicap an individual either in his regular occupation or in his ordinary everyday activities. Should the original injury be an open (compound) fracture with infection necessitating prolonged healing by secondary intention, the resulting scar may cause adherence of skin and subcutaneous tissue to the bone with actual mechanical impairment of function.

REPAIR OF FRACTURES

Usual Repair of Bone

In the *adult* there is probably no specific osteogenetic cell. Whatever one's preference may be in describing the process of new bone formation following a fracture, it must be admitted that certain fundamental conditions exist. These may be enumerated as follows: Hemorrhage, death of tissue, local calcium concentration, granulation tissue formation and local adequate (minute) circulation.

Hemorrhage at and surrounding the fracture site if not excessive finally results in the blood forming a clot. The fluid portion is squeezed out and eventually absorbed by the circulation. The fibrin in the clot forms a network along which fibroblasts and new capillaries may grow, permeate, and replace with granulation tissue.

Hemorrhage and death of the damaged tissue as noted under the acute pathology, cause irritation and an acute inflammatory reaction, which changes the tissue reaction at the fracture site from one of alkalinity to one of mild acidity (acid pH). The fractured bone ends die for a slight but variable depth and the dead bone is bathed in this acid medium which in turn withdraws the calcium content from the dead bone and holds it *locally* in affinity with the fibrin in the blood clot. Comminuted fractures frequently heal with more callus than those without comminution, and an explanation for this is the greater area of fracture surface from which a greater amount of calcium may be obtained. After the fibrin has become replaced by new granulation tissue (undifferentiated connective tissue) and the products of tissue death have been carried away by the venous and lymphatic circulation, the tissue reaction returns to its normal alkaline state. At this time the calcium held locally by the fibrin is rapidly "precipitated" and laid down in this new undifferentiated connective tissue to form a bony callus. This at first is very soft, but as resorption continues, more calcium is laid down, and the new connective tissue becomes more mature and more firm, the bony trabeculae increase in density and eventually form new cortical bone, completely healing the original fracture.

The most important aspect of bone healing to remember is that in order to form good bony callus, the calcium that goes into its formation comes from the local fracture site and *must* be laid down in the new connective tissue while this is still in an undifferentiated state. Once this connective tissue becomes differentiated into definite adult, fibrous tissue, calcium cannot be deposited in it to form healthy callus. Instead there will be granular deposits of calcium completely surrounded by scar tissue, but not forming bone trabeculae. This delay, therefore, results in either a delayed or non-union. It is readily seen that there is an all important time element in the healing of bone. If for any reason circulatory stasis is permitted to persist by inadequate elevation of the injured part, by constricting dressings, or by failure to give *early* physiotherapy in the form of heat, massage, and active muscle contractions, the pH of the tissues will remain acid. Should such be the case, the optimum time for the deposition of calcium will have passed and the factors for delayed union will be brought into play, one of the important of which is the formation of dense scar tissue between the bone ends without adequate deposition of calcium within it.

There are of course other factors that influence the healing of bone. Those having an unfavorable influence are: (1) the site of injury—where the bone may have a poor blood supply owing to lack of highly vascular surrounding soft parts as in the lower third of the shaft of the tibia, or in a fracture of the radial head where the fragment by its intra-articular displacement has become completely deprived of its blood supply; (2) the extent of the injury may so disrupt the local circulation (as well as larger arteries and veins) and cause damage to the surrounding soft parts that bone healing will be slow at best; (3) extensive hemorrhage may, by virtue of the large amount of fluid present, cause a mechanical block to ingrowth of the new granulation tissue so necessary to the formation of early callus; (4) compounding of the fracture may give rise to infection at the fracture site, which, even if not of a virulent nature, may cause marked delay in bony healing; (5) interposition of muscle or other soft parts between the fracture fragments cannot do else but delay or prevent bone union.

Some of these factors are controllable by the surgeon (as well as by lay people) in rendering first aid treatment or by the former in carrying out definitive treatment of the injured individual. We cannot, of course, control the site of the fracture or the extent of the original injury, but much secondary trauma both to bone and soft parts can be minimized by careful handling, application of emergency splints and dressings, and by careful transportation. This will prevent increased hemorrhage and shock, may lessen comminution, nerve and vessel damage, and may avoid interposition of soft parts between bone ends and keep a simple fracture from being converted into an open (compound) one.

The type of bone in which the fracture occurs has a bearing on the healing process. Cancellous bone, being spongy and very vascular, always heals well and rapidly; cortical bone on the other hand is dense or hard, poorly vascular, and often heals with difficulty or not at all.

General or systemic factors have little or no influence at all in the healing of fractures. Fracture healing is the result of local factors as described above and not due to age, diabetes, generalized arteriosclerosis, or such metabolic or endocrine conditions as hyperparathyroidism or Paget's disease, or to skeletal conditions, such as osteogenesis imperfecta or senile osteoporosis. Actually, most non-unions after clean fractures of the shaft of a long bone occur in individuals below the age of thirty-five years rather than after middle age.

Delayed Union

Ordinarily any fracture becomes solidly healed in three to four months at most and is sufficiently strong to allow weight-bearing even in the lower extremity, except for some fractures of the femoral neck. With fractures in the region of the elbow bony healing becomes solid ordinarily in six weeks and unrestricted active motion may be freely permitted sooner than this.

The causes of delayed union are: inadequate reduction of the fracture fragments, inadequate immobilization of the reduced fragments either from splints that are too short or not applied for a sufficiently long time, from over-pull or distraction of the fragments (if treated in traction) which leads to formation of dense scar tissue between bone ends without actual callus formation, to interposed muscle or other soft parts, to an impaired local circulation and lack of nutrition or to circulatory stagnation, and to too early use. When may a fracture be said to show evidence of delayed union? Usually this has been considered to be anywhere up to six months following the injury. Perhaps it would be better to define delayed union as a period anywhere from four to six months following injury where monthly roentgenograms have shown slight but progressive diminution of the fracture line, but not complete union or evidence of increased absorption of the bone ends. Delayed union may be accompanied by subjective symptoms such as pain (especially on weight bearing in the lower extremity) or on use, or by such objective findings as persistent tenderness or a continued false point of motion at the fracture site.

The avoidance of the factors causing delayed union must be kept in mind from the beginning and none of these allowed to persist. Should delayed union occur, it will be advisable to eradicate any of the factors that may still be acting. If this cannot be done, the fracture will very likely go on to a non-union, and operative measures will be necessary.

Non-union

This is a stage beyond delayed union in which there is no further hope of union taking place across the fracture site without operative interference by drilling of the bone or by the implantation or laying on of bone grafts. The causes are identical to those of delayed union but carried on for a longer period of time. Just when delayed union ceases and non-union begins is difficult to define from the element of time. It varies with different bones and with the level of the fracture in these bones, but in general it occurs anywhere from the eighth to the twelfth month, following fracture.

There are altogether too many cases of non-union. The majority of these (excepting those following compound fractures or injuries with severe soft part damage) could be avoided if the surgeon treating the case was more aware of the pathology of acute fractures, the process of bone repair, and would follow the fundamental principles of fracture treatment instead of following a particular or routine method of treatment.

Avascular Necrosis

Aseptic or avascular necrosis of bone means death of a bone fragment due to loss of circulation to that fragment rather than the result of any infectious process. The commonest sites of avascular necrosis are the head of the femur and the proximal fragment in a high fracture of the carpal scaphoid bone. At the elbow intra-articular fractures of the radial head and capitellum may exhibit this same condition.

The condition of avascular necrosis becomes evident late after bone healing should have been completed and appears on roentgenograms as an increased density of bone. Actually this bone density is relative. During the process of bone healing and physical inactivity, the surrounding bones having a good circulation have become somewhat decalcified and less dense due to increased inflammatory hyperemia. The dead fragment having no circulation, has not become equally decalcified and therefore appears on the films as having greater density than the others. Later, even if the dead fragment becomes revascularized and unites, its blood supply may be greatly diminished as compared to normal and this portion of the bone may not be able to stand continued and prolonged function or weight-bearing. It undergoes a slow degeneration and its articular surface becomes irregular and rough and may later become the cause of a post-traumatic arthritis. Occasionally, late symptoms develop and become progressive and function may decrease. If so, operative measures of treatment may be necessary.

REPAIR OF SOFT PARTS

The repair of soft tissues anywhere in the body except for epithelium (epidermis and mucous membranes) and nerve axones is by scar tissue. Periosteum, muscle (striated or smooth), blood vessels, fascia, tendon, tendon sheaths and adipose tissue whenever they are incised or injured accidently, even if carefully approximated by sutures show healing by connective (scar) tissue. There may occasionally be a slight regeneration of muscle fibers, but this, if present, is minimal in amount.

In extensive injuries to soft parts due to displacement of bone fragments with stripping or tearing of these tissues, crushing, or severe interstitial hemorrhage, healing may result in excessive amounts of scar tissue formation which may interfere mechanically with function or the circulation. Contusion of a vessel may cause its thrombosis. Contusion of a nerve trunk with hemorrhage within its sheath may result in enough scar formation to interfere with or prevent the regeneration of axones into the distal portion of the nerve. Severed nerves, if not sutured relatively early, may have their ends caught in a mass of dense scar tissue and may give rise to traumatic neuromata.

It behooves the surgeon to do everything within his means *early* to prevent or minimize the formation of excess scar tissue if he wishes his patient to have a chance to recover full function.

Chapter III

Anatomy of the Elbow Region

ONE MUST KNOW the normal anatomy of the elbow region to understand the pathology and displacements incident to trauma found in patients of any age group. A thorough understanding is absolutely essential for the successful approach to the problem and in restoring the anatomy to as nearly normal as is possible without impairing the return of joint function.

BONY STRUCTURE

The elbow joint is formed by the articulations of three bones: the lower extremity of the humerus and the upper extremities of the radius and ulna. As the lower extremity of the humerus is approached from the shaft above its shape changes from a triangular cross-section to a flatter and broader expanded portion. As the bone widens out medially and laterally into the supracondylar ridges, it becomes thinner in its antero-posterior diameter. It finally forms the two condyles, medial and lateral which again are thicker but made up of less dense cancellous bone. The condyles contain at their most distal ends the articular surfaces of the capitellum and trochlea. The capitellum is dome-shaped for articulation with the shallow concave proxi-

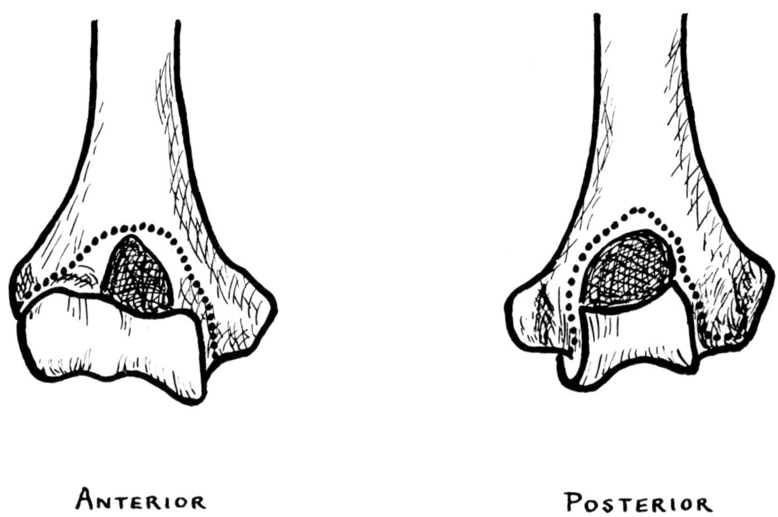

Fig. 1. Sketch of lower humerus showing capsular attachments in relation to articular surfaces of trochlear and capitellar processes.

mal surface of the radial head. Just proximal to the capitellum there is a shallow fossa on the anterior surface of the lateral condyle which receives the margin of the radial head on full flexion of the elbow. There is no articular cartilage on the posterior aspect of the capitellum, since in full extension of the elbow joint the head of the radius is in line with the long axis of the humerus and does not swing around behind as does the ulna. The trochlea is the articulating process on the medial condyle which receives the hook-shaped upper extremity of the ulna. It is somewhat spool-shaped and its medial margin extends distally from the condyle at least 1 to 1.5 centimeters. The articular surface of the trochlea extends completely around the distal end of the humerus and on to the posterior surface as far as the olecranon fossa for articulation with the olecranon process when the joint is fully extended. Just proximal to the trochlea the broad portion of the humerus becomes thinned out into deep hollows known as the coronoid and olecranon fossae for reception of the coronoid process of the ulna in full elbow flexion and for the tip of the olecranon process in full extension.

The supracondylar area curves slightly forward upon the axis of the humerus. The condyles and articular processes tilt forward upon this, so that the long axis of the articular surface slants forward approximately forty degrees upon the axis of the humeral shaft. Inasmuch as the transverse axis of the lower articular surface of the humerus is not perpendicular to the long axis of the shaft, but tilts downward slightly at its medial end (due to the distal extension of the trochlea), the forearm when fully extended at the elbow deviates away from the body or into abduction. This forms a definite angle with the arm of approximately fifteen degrees less than a

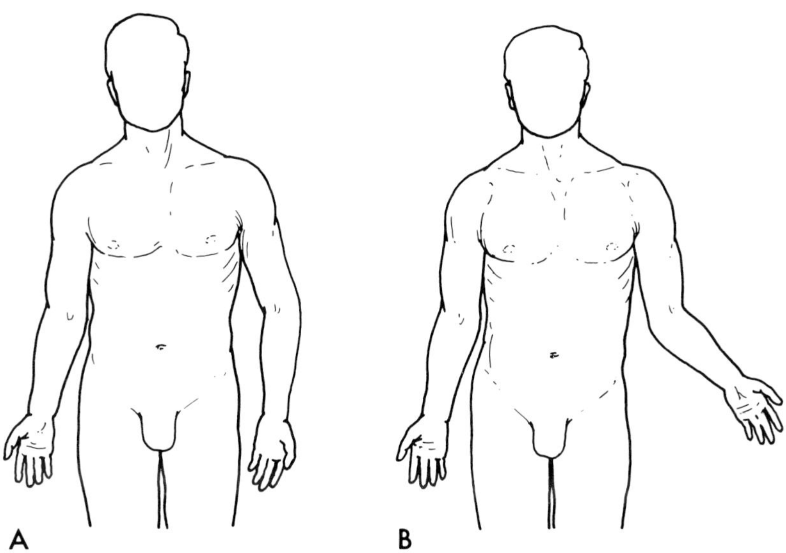

Fig. 2. The carrying angle at the elbow. (A) Right, normal; (A) left, reversed carrying angle (cubitus varus or gun-stock deformity). (B) Right, normal; (B) left, increased carrying angle (cubitus valgus deformity).

straight line, known as the *carrying angle* at the elbow. The carrying angle varies in different individuals, but in normals (without previous injury) it is rarely less than five or more than twenty degrees. Following injuries and due to either incomplete reduction of a fracture or due to growth disturbance from epiphyseal trauma, the transverse axis of the lower extremity of the humerus may eventually become increased or decreased in relation to the longitudinal axis. This will result in extreme carrying angle deformities known as cubitus valgus where the deviation of the forearm is away from the body, or cubitus varus where the deviation of the forearm is towards the body. In the latter type the carrying angle may become very markedly reversed, and if so, is often called a "gun-stock" deformity owing to the similarity of its shape to the wooden stock of a rifle or shot gun.

Surmounting the expanded condyles of the humerus there are two palpable prominences known as epicondyles. These are both readily palpable and represent muscle attachments. The medial epicondyle gives rise to the common tendon of origin of the flexor-pronator group of muscles and at its posterior-inferior aspect to a portion of the medial collateral ligament of the elbow joint. The lateral epicondyle gives attachment to the origin of the extensor muscles of the wrist and fingers. The medial epicondyle is much more prominent than the lateral. Both epicondyles lie in a portion of the bone outside the elbow joint proper.

The upper extremity of the ulna is the most expanded portion of this bone and is considered as the direct extension of the humerus. Its broad notch (or hook) is formed by the coronoid and olecranon processes. The

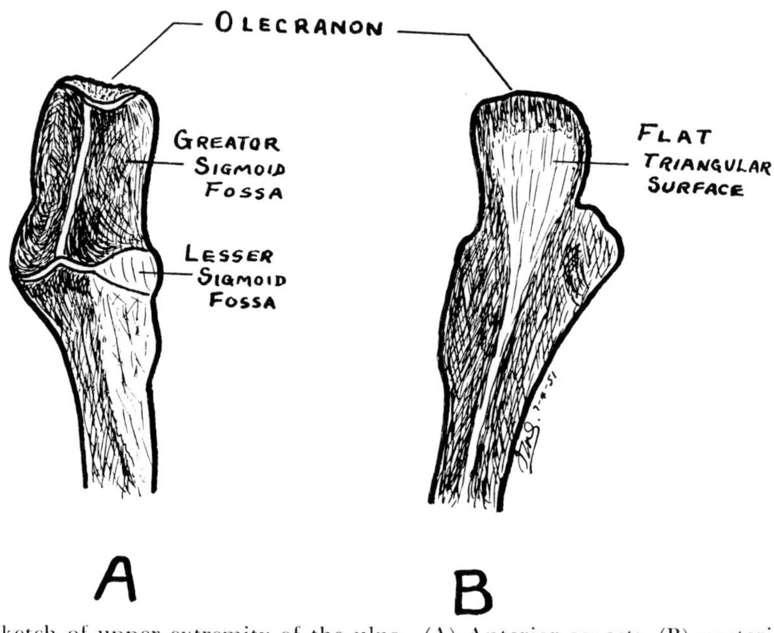

Fig. 3. Sketch of upper extremity of the ulna. (A) Anterior aspect; (B) posterior aspect.

former is distal to the latter and the two together form a deep semilunar notch called the greater sigmoid fossa (incisura semilunaris) covered with cartilage for articulation with the trochlea of the humerus. The proximal end of the olecranon is slightly rough for the insertion of the triceps tendon. The anterior surface of the coronoid process at its base is rough where the brachialis anticus tendon inserts. The posterior crest of the ulnar shaft flattens out into a triangular plateau slightly below the olecranon into which is inserted periosteum and the triceps expansion. Overlying this area is the olecranon bursa closely attached to the periosteum. Situated on the lateral side of the ulna just distal to the greater sigmoid notch there is a shallow groove concave laterally and running antero-posteriorly, known as the lesser sigmoid fossa (incisura radialis) covered with cartilage for articulation (pronation and supination) with the peripheral margin of the radial head.

In the upper extremity of the radius the neck is a continuation of the shaft. At the proximal extremity of this is the head which is a thick disc-shaped portion of the bone. The head of the radius is covered with articular cartilage on its proximal end which is concave and shallow for articulation with the capitellum and on its circular periphery for articulation with the lesser sigmoid fossa of the ulna. Approximately two and one-half to three centimeters distal to the lower margin of the radial head and located on the shaft of the bone is the bicipital tuberosity (tuberositas radii). This projects medially and anteriorly, and inserted into it is the inferior tendon of the biceps brachii muscle.

EPIPHYSES AT ELBOW

In view of the large majority of fractures and dislocations that occur in children's elbows as compared to adults it is important to appreciate the anatomical differences that occur in these age groups. The configuration of the bone ends of the humerus, radius and ulna are practically identical in the child and adult. The soft tissues are identical except for lesser muscular development in the younger child. The great difference between the two is that in the very young child the entire lower extremity of the humerus and the upper extremities of the radius and ulna are composed of cartilage and not merely covered with cartilage on the articular surfaces. This may to some extent explain the greater frequency of certain types of injury in the child, the epiphyseal cartilage being less strong and more readily subject to trauma than is fully developed bone.

For this reason it is essential that the physician or surgeon have a thorough knowledge of the roentgenologic appearance of the numerous epiphyses forming the elbow joint from birth to the time these epiphyses fuse with the diaphysis. The roentgenogram of a young child is often very confusing and frequently it fails to show a bony lesion, because the fracture line may pass through a portion of the articular surface which has not developed a visible ossification center. The various ossification centers appear at different ages,

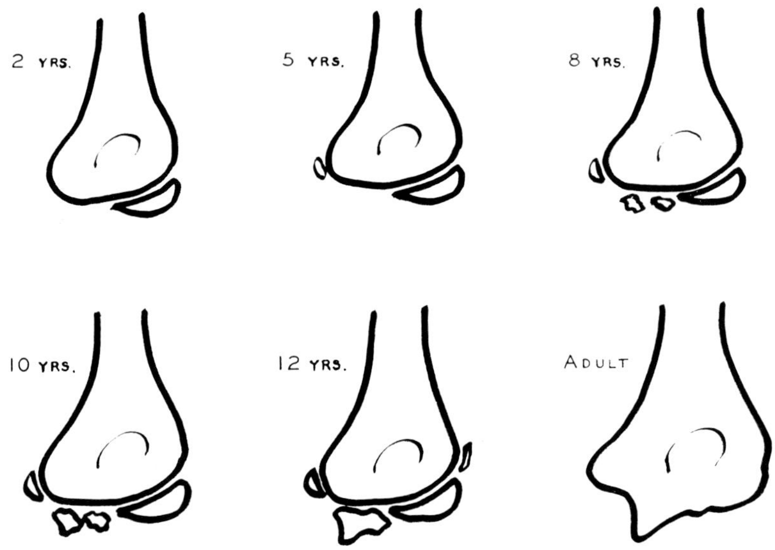

Fig. 4. Sketch showing development of ossification centers at lower end of humerus as seen on roentgenograms from age two years to the adult stage.

enlarge and eventually fuse. This development often leads to additional confusion because one center when displaced may be mistaken for another unless one knows what to suspect and keeps a sharp watch for it. Such an example may be seen in a separation of the medial epicondyle epiphysis which becomes displaced into the elbow joint and may be mistaken as one of the ossification centers of the trochlear epiphysis. The following table gives the time of appearance of the epiphyseal ossification centers and the times at which they eventually unite with the shaft in the bones forming the elbow joint. It is well to note that considerable variation occurs due to racial characteristics, etc., and that these figures are rough averages. It may therefore be necessary to make an allowance of one or sometimes two years in the extremes of this table.

EPIPHYSES IN REGION OF ELBOW

(As seen on roentgen examination)

	Appears at:	*Unites with shaft at:*
Humerus		
Capitellum (and outer part of trochlea)	2 yrs.	16 yrs. (both)
Trochlea (inner half)	10 yrs.	
Medial Epicondyle	5 yrs.	18 yrs.
Lateral Epicondyle	12 yrs.	16 yrs.
Ulna		
Olecranon	10 yrs.	16 yrs.
Radius		
Head of Radius	5-7 yrs.	18 yrs.

There is fortunately in most cases of elbow injury the opposite normal arm for comparison by roentgenograms as well as by clinical examination. In case of doubt films should be taken of the uninjured elbow to prevent such common errors as mistaking a displaced medial epicondyle for a part of the trochlear epiphysis. There are many other conditions that may also lead to errors in diagnosis unless the good arm is used for roentgenologic comparison.

BONY LANDMARKS

There are three easily palpable bony prominences that define what is known as the bony triangle of the elbow. These are the two epicondyles and the tip of the olecranon process. The base of the inverted triangle is a line drawn from one epicondyle to the other. With the elbow at 90° of flexion and examined from behind the apex of this triangle is the tip of the olecranon, which is practically equidistant from each epicondyle. With the elbow still at 90° of flexion and examined from the side all three of these points lie in the same vertical plane as the axis of the shaft of the humerus. Knowing this, it is not difficult to make a differential diagnosis clinically between a supracondylar fracture of the humerus and a posterior dislocation of the radius and ulna upon the humerus. When the elbow is examined in the fully extended position and from the posterior aspect the three bony points above

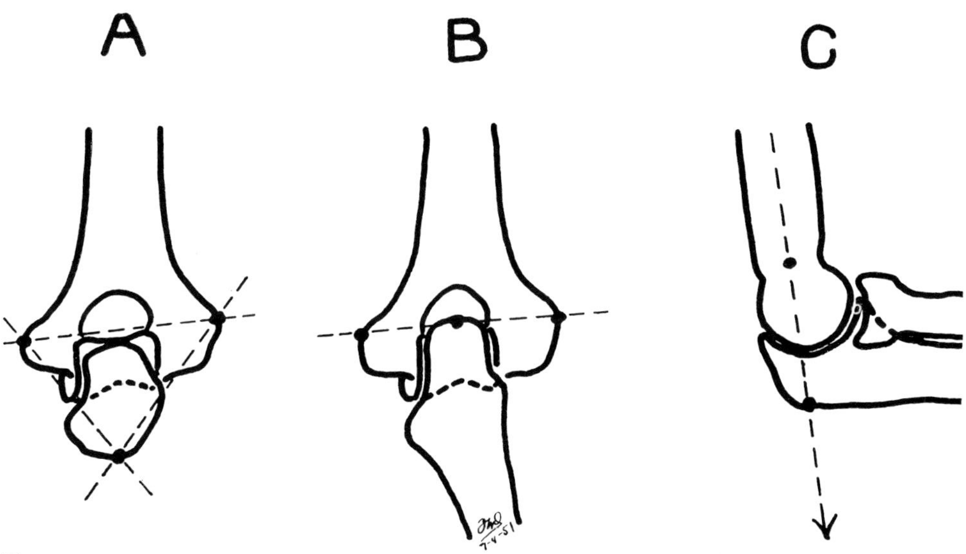

Fig. 5. Sketches of the normal bony landmarks at the elbow the relations of which may be altered clinically by displacements following fracture or dislocation. (A) posterior view with elbow in 90 degrees of flexion. There is seen an isosceles triangle with the base passing through the medial and lateral epicondyles of the humerus and the apex or third point of the triangle represented by the tip of the olecranon process. (B) All three points are on the same straight line when the elbow is in 180 degrees of extension. (C) Lateral view showing the three points in the same plane and lying in the axis of the shaft of the humerus.

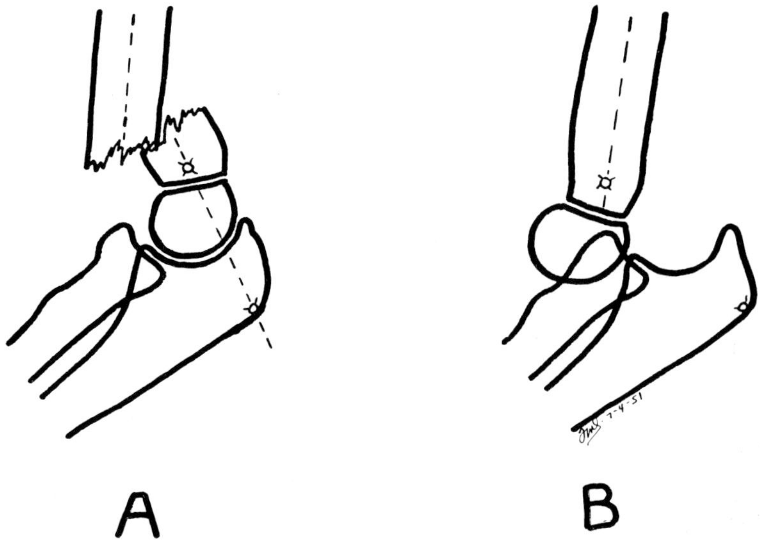

Fig. 6. Sketch showing the landmarks at the elbow. (A) Supracondylar fracture of the humerus. The three points of the bony triangle are in normal relation to each other, but are all displaced posterior to the axis of the humerus (compare with Fig. 5 C). (B) Posterior dislocation at the elbow joint in which the point of the olecranon is displaced behind the epicondyles which in turn remain in the normal axis of the humerus.

described will be found to lie along the same transverse line. If they do not on clinical examination, there is obviously a displacement of one or more of these points due to fracture or dislocation.

The radial head is readily palpable and can be felt to roll beneath the tip of the thumb when the forearm is either pronated or supinated. Along with the lateral epicondyle and tip of the olecranon the radial head forms another triangle which is frequently useful to know. Within this triangle lies the anconeus muscle and deep to it the postero-lateral capsule of the elbow joint. With an intra-articular fracture, such as a crack in the radial head, which leads to a tense hemarthrosis, the capsule of the elbow joint bulges most prominently in the center of this triangle. An aspirating needle inserted equidistant from these three bony landmarks and directed slightly forward and distally will easily enter the joint and permit evacuation of the entrapped blood. (See Chapter XII.)

JOINT STRUCTURE

The bony structures of the elbow joint have been described. It is time to review and describe the ligamentous connections holding these bones firmly together yet allowing a full range of motion; also to describe the capsule and the synovial lining of the joint. The main supporting structures of the joint aside from the configuration of the bones which give additional stability are the two collateral (medial and lateral) ligaments. Each of these takes its origin from the lower edge of its respective epicondyle on the humerus. It then fans out in a distal, anterior and posterior direction to become attached to the forearm bones. The medial (internal) collateral ligament becomes attached to the medial margin of the ulna along the edge of the greater sigmoid fossa, olecranon, and base of the coronoid process. The lateral (external) collateral ligament becomes attached to the lateral margin of the olecranon and greater sigmoid fossa and into the orbicular (annular) ligament surrounding the radial head with which it blends and with the capsule distal and medial to this. Both of these ligaments are thickenings in the joint capsule, are very tough and strong and normally prevent any abnormal lateral motion at the elbow joint. The orbicular (annular) ligament is a thickening in the capsule and is attached at either end to the anterior and posterior margins of the lesser sigmoid fossa of the ulna and surrounds the peripheral margin of the head of the radius except for the portion in contact with the notch itself.

The capsule envelops the entire joint and except for the thickening of the ligaments described above it is thin and pliable in order to allow for free motion in flexion and extension. It is reinforced anteriorly by the brachialis anticus muscle and tendon and posteriorly by the triceps muscle, tendon and its expansion, each of which lies in direct contact with it. The capsule is lined by a synovial membrane which is reflected on to the humerus above the coronoid and olecranon fossae and extends to the margin of the articular cartilage. It forms small cul-de-sacs where it is reflected on to the neck of the radius and lower humerus. The synovial lining secretes synovia (joint fluid) which in turn lubricates the joint surfaces. The radial head and a portion of its neck are by virtue of the capsular attachments and synovial reflections located entirely within the joint. The importance of this is seen when frac-

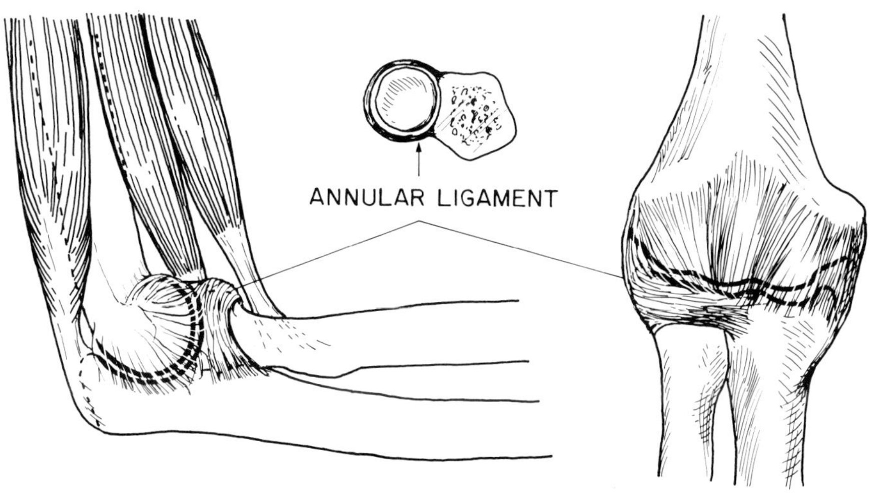

Fig. 7. Sketch showing the relations of capsule and ligamentous thickenings holding the humerus, radius and ulna together at the elbow joint.

ture occurs, because of the possibility of a loose fragment, because being intra-articular such a fragment is usually devoid of a blood supply, and finally because of the resultant hemarthrosis. The tip of the coronoid process is likewise intra-articular in location and may also give rise to hemarthrosis or loose body formation when fractured.

JOINT FUNCTION

The elbow is a diathrodial ginglymus or hinge joint. It is actually three joints in one. Hinge motion takes place between the lower extremity of the humerus and the upper extremities of the ulna and radius. The range of motion is best measured theoretically starting with the elbow in absolute flexion and considering this to be an angle of zero. Normal extension is therefore to an angle of 180° (or a straight line). It is of course impossible for an elbow to be flexed to an angle of less than 25° to 20°. The average adult has a range of motion in his elbow therefore from approximately 30° to 180°. This means he *actually* has hinge motion amounting to a total of one hundred fifty degrees. Some thin individuals can flex to less than a 30° angle and some young girls and women may be able to hyperextend the elbow as much as ten or twenty degrees, i. e., to an angle of 190° to 200°. When elbow motion is limited following trauma or disease, the limitation may be in any of the hinge or rotation movements or all of them. The neutral position as far as flexion and extension are concerned is with the elbow flexed at an angle of 90°. Any motion to decrease this angle is therefore known as flexion and any motion to increase it is known as extension. If the motion by actual measurement in the joint is from 60° to 120°, then the total motion range is sixty degrees. This range is often described as thirty degrees each of flexion and extension. If the arc of motion is from 80° to 140°, the total range of motion is likewise sixty degrees, but this represents flexion of ten and extension of fifty degrees. Consequently, it is not

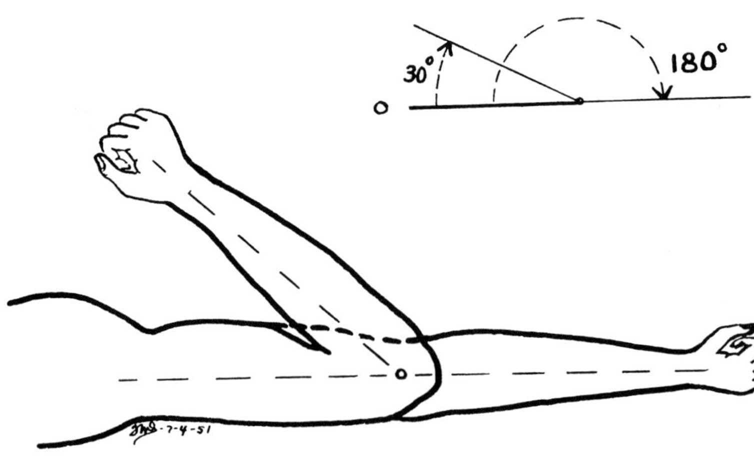

Fig. 8. Sketch demonstrating how to measure the arcs of motion at the elbow.

only simpler but more logical to train oneself to express elbow ranges by designating the extremes of motion. In this way the total range of motion can be readily understood and the arc in which this range is possible can be easily figured. The arc of motion may be of extreme importance to the patient if his range is limited. For example, one person may have a very useful arm when his arc of limited elbow motion is from 50° to 110°; but suppose his total range were the same (sixty degrees) and his arc is 100° to 160°, he would be unable to eat with this hand, tie his necktie or do anything else very useful around his face or head.

Rotary motion (pronation and supination) at the elbow occurs at the radio-humeral joint and at the proximal radio-ulnar joint. For rotation to be possible at the elbow it is also necessary that there be rotation at the distal radio-ulnar joint as well. The ulna does not rotate at all in pronation and supination. This seems to be a difficult fact for students to appreciate. The upper end of the radius turns on its long axis, the head rotating within the orbicular ligament in contact with the lesser sigmoid notch of the ulna and the capitellum of the humerus. The lower end of the radius swings around the head of the ulna as its proximal portion rotates at the elbow. The long axis of the radius if projected proximally on a lateral roentgenogram *always* passes through the center of the capitellum or capitellar epiphysis of the humerus. This is normally constant regardless of what degree of flexion or extension the joint may be in or what degree of rotation the radius may be in.

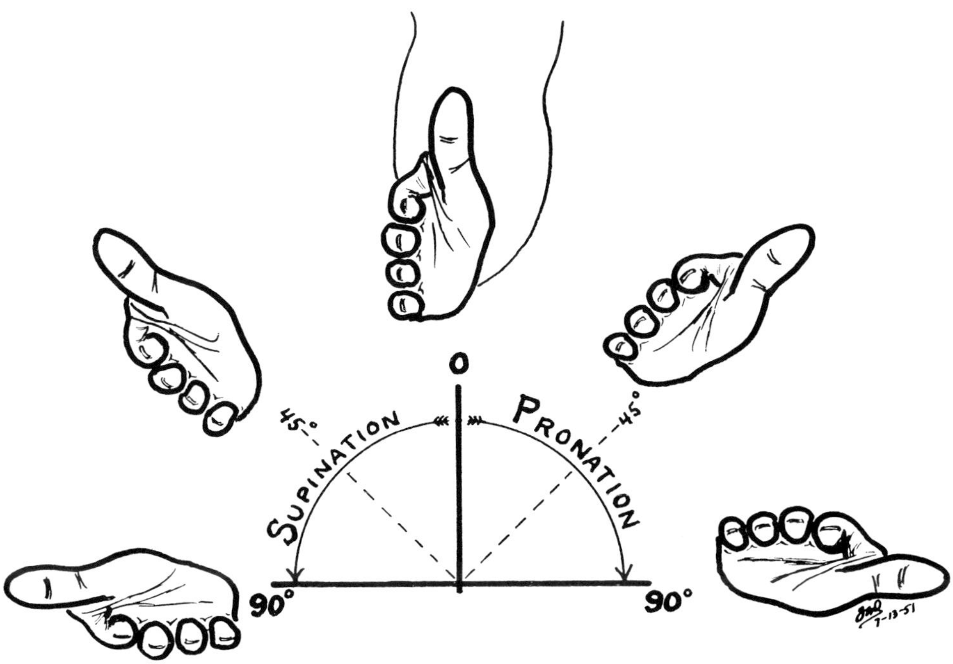

Fig. 9. Sketch showing method of measuring degree of pronation and supination from mid-point of rotation when the elbow is held against side of the chest.

Pronation and supination are difficult motions to measure accurately because of the tendency of the patient to compensate by abduction, adduction, or rotation of the humerus at the shoulder joint. A uniform method for this measurement should be used. In the first place, rotation and other motions of the humerus must be made impossible and therefore ruled out as a possible source of pronation and supination. In order to do this properly it is necessary to have the patient hold his upper arm (humerus) along the side of his thorax and hold the elbow flexed at approximately a right angle. Any rotary motion of the forearm with the arm and elbow thus held represents pure pronation or supination. Actual measurement of this motion is best determined by starting in the neutral position, i. e., in mid-rotation with the abducted thumbs pointing towards the ceiling. This point is considered as zero degrees. Any pronation or supination should then be estimated in degrees rather than in percentage figures or fractions of the normal. The reason for this is that the "normal" varies considerably in different individuals. The usual normal pronation range is ninety degrees, but some people can only pronate normally through an arc of 70°; some patients can supinate through an arc of 110°, but this is rather unusual.

The importance of getting an accurate comparison of the rotary range with the uninjured forearm is obvious when it comes to rate end-results of function and disability, especially in compensation cases. Pronation and supination is usually designated as 0/90°, (0/90°) or 0/50°, (0/80°). (Figures in parentheses represent the rotation range of the uninjured side for comparison.) If for any reason there is marked limitation of rotation so that the neutral position cannot be reached, but some further rotation to this same side is possible, this can be designated as follows: pronation 0°, (0/90°), supination 20/75°, (0/90°). From reading such a record it will easily be recognized just what arc of rotation is lost. In other words this patient has no true pronation and his supination begins at 20° and rotates to only 75°; his actual range of supination therefore is fifty-five degrees.

Loss of pronation or supination may interfere considerably with some patients' occupations or earning capacity or with their daily usage or avocation.

SOFT TISSUES OF THE ELBOW REGION

From a practical standpoint the soft tissues surrounding the elbow will be considered in the order of the superficial to the deep. The skin and subcutaneous tissue is freely movable upon the deep fascia. The skin is thin anteriorly and laterally, but thicker posteriorly especially overlying the olecranon. Situated anteriorly but superficial to the deep fascia are a number of rather large veins, the cephalic and the basilic with their communicating veins which form roughly a letter M. These are the veins most commonly used for venipuncture. Likewise situated at this same level there are found branches of the following sensory nerves—the lateral and medial antibrachial cutaneous nerves. The next layer consists of the deep fascia. This not only covers each muscle group, but binds these muscle groups together. Posteriorly the deep fascia blends with the periosteum of the upper ulna and the expansion of the triceps tendon. This fascia is composed of a tough inelastic membrane. Medial to the biceps tendon it received additional strength from the fibers of the lacertus fibrosus (bicipital fascia) which insert into and blend with it. The fascia is not only of importance from its anatomical function, but may be still more important from the standpoint of the pathology it creates in supracondylar fractures with marked displacement of the fragments and extensive hemorrhage into the underlying muscle. It is thus possible for dangerous tissue tension to be built up by confining the extravasated blood beneath this deep fascia, which in turn may compromise the circulation sufficiently to cause a Volkmann's ischaemia. The fascia and lacertus fibrosus may likewise be responsible for angulating the brachial artery and veins over the lower end of the humeral shaft fragment in these fractures. It is for these reasons that many surgeons advocate splitting the deep fascia in a threatened Volkmann's ischaemia in order to decompress the underlying muscular compartment by allowing the escape of blood, cellular exudate and edema fluid.

The main muscles acting upon the elbow joint are the triceps (extension)

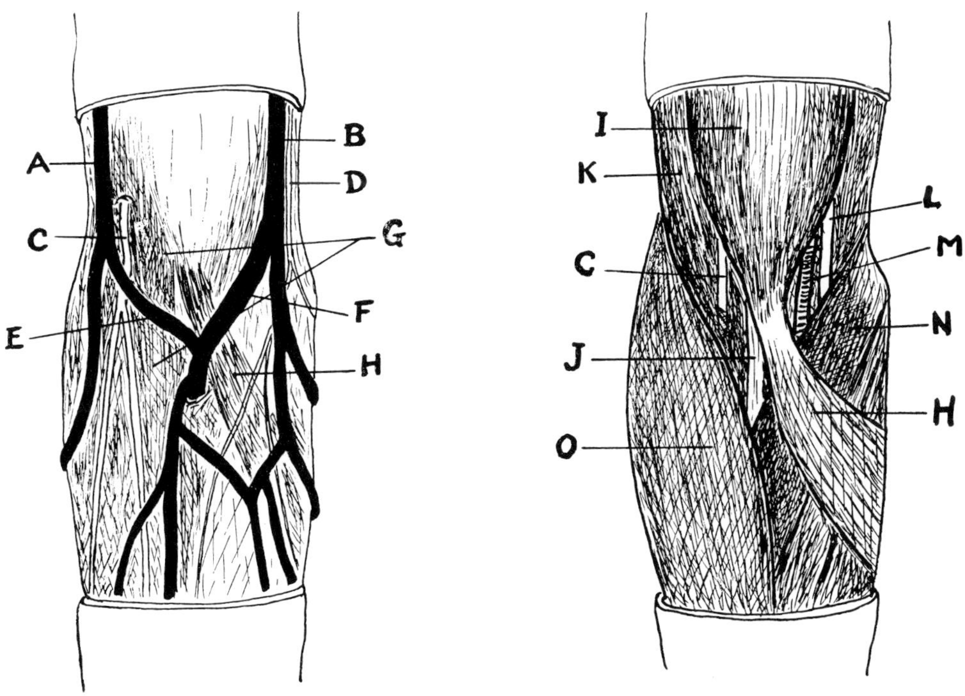

Fig. 10. Sketch of soft tissue structures on anterior surface of elbow: (A) Cephalic vein; (B) basilic vein; (C) lateral Antibrachial Cutaneous nerve; (D) median Antibrachial Cutaneous nerve; (E) median Cephalic vein; (F) median basilic vein; (G) deep fascia; (H) lacertus fibrosus; (I) biceps muscle; (J) biceps tendon; (K) brachialis anterior muscle; (L) median nerve; (M) brachial artery and veins; (N) pronator teres muscle; (O) brachio-radialis muscle.

and the brachialis anticus and biceps (flexion). The biceps in addition is a very powerful supinator of the forearm. The latter two muscles cross the anterior aspect of the joint to insert into the base of the coronoid process of the ulna and into the bicipital tuberosity of the radius (and deep fascia via lacertus fibrosus) respectively. As these muscles become narrowed down into tendons two other groups of muscles come into prominence from the medial and lateral aspects. These consist of: (1) the flexor-pronator group (pronator teres, flexor carpi radialis, palmaris longus, flexor digitorum sublimis, and flexor carpi ulnaris) taking its origin from a conjoined tendon attached to the medial epicondyle of the humerus; and (2) the brachio-radialis originating from the lateral supracondylar ridge of the humerus and the extensor group of the wrist and fingers (extensors carpi radialis longus and brevis, extensor digitorum communis, extensor indicis proprius, and extensor carpi ulnaris) which takes origin from the lateral epicondyle of the humerus. These two groups come together to form a V. When the deep fascia is divided between these groups and between them and each side of the biceps muscle, a clear-cut intermuscular plane is found to open-up medially and laterally. The neurovascular bundle consisting of the median nerve, brachial artery and veins is found which passes deeply into the antecubital space medial to the biceps tendon and deep to the lacertus fibrosus. Deep in this space the

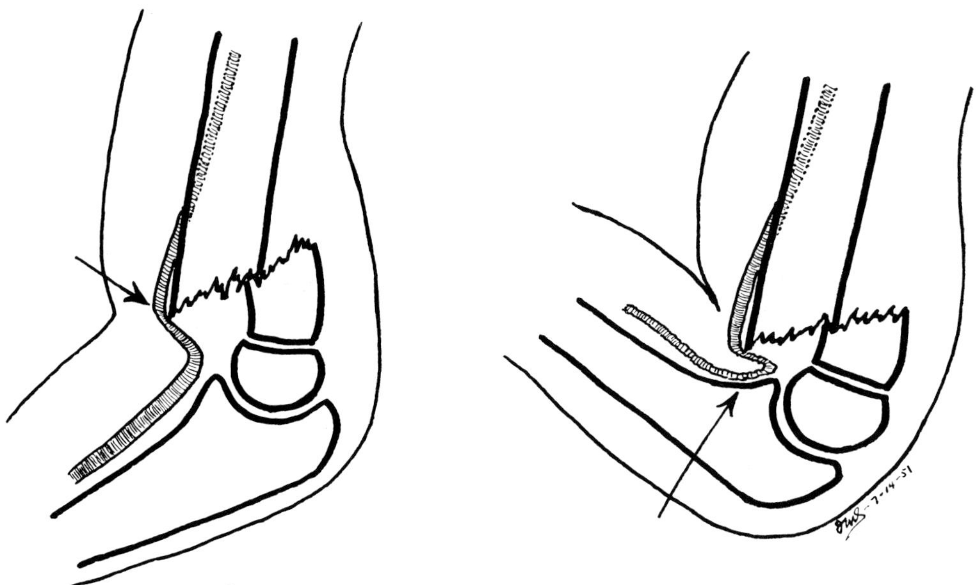

a b

Fig. 11. Sketch of brachial vessels (arrow) in relation to the proximal fragment in a supracondylar fracture of the humerus: (a) with posterior displacement; (b) compression of vessels is inevitable if the elbow is put in flexion *without* obtaining correction of the bony displacement. The fragments *must* be reduced before flexion of the elbow can be carried out.

brachial artery is found to divide into its radial and ulnar branches, the former coursing distally beneath the brachioradialis muscle and the latter passing medially and distally beneath the pronator teres, flexor carpi radialis, flexor sublimis, palmaris longus, and median nerve.

The median-nerve dips deeply into the antecubital fossa, beneath the pronator teres and then emerges more distally upon the surface of the flexor digitorum profundus muscle. Branches of the radial recurrent vessels are found extending laterally which must be divided and ligated before the intermuscular space on the lateral aspect and joint can be fully explored. Deep in the more proximal portion of this lateral intermuscular plane is found the radial nerve lying between the brachioradialis and the brachialis anticus muscles. Approximately three to four centimeters proximal to the radio-humeral articulation the radial nerve divides into: (1) a motor branch (posterior interosseus nerve) which courses distally and then laterally to wind around the lower portion of the neck of the radius between the superficial and deep bellies of the supinator muscle and finally reaches the posterior compartment of the forearm; and (2) a sensory branch which passes distally beneath the brachioradialis muscle and lateral to the radial artery and finally to the back of the hand and thumb. Before the radial nerve divides into these two main branches it gives off several small muscular branches from its *lateral* side which innervate the brachioradialis and extensor carpi radialis longus and brevis muscles. It is therefore perfectly safe in exploring the antero-lateral aspect of the elbow joint if the operator retracts the nerve laterally and incises the joint capsule medial to the nerve. In so doing none of these small or main branches can be harmed.

On the posterior aspect of the joint the triceps tendon covers the capsule before coming to insert into the olecranon. The fascia overlying the triceps muscle spreads out medially and laterally into expansions similar in nature and function to the expansions of the quadriceps muscle at the knee. These expansions insert into the deep fascia of the forearm and into the periosteum of the upper ulna. It is these expansions that prevent wide separation of an olecranon fragment when fractured. If the expansions remain intact the fragment can only separate a minimal amount and it is *possible* for the patient to extend the elbow against gravity. On the other hand if the expansions are widely torn when the olecranon is fractured, the fragment will become badly displaced and the patient will *be unable* to extend the arm against gravity. Operative repair is therefore necessary in this latter type of such fracture, and it is just as important to repair the expansion as it is to fasten the bone fragments together.

Medial to the triceps muscle can be found the ulnar nerve which passes just posterior to the medial epicondyle of the humerus. As it crosses the epicondyle it lies in a shallow groove in the bone which is covered by a rather tough roof of fibrous tissue. After leaving the epicondyle the nerve passes into the forearm deep to the humeral head of the flexor carpi ulnaris muscle. The close proximity of the nerve to the epicondyle and medial collateral ligament of the elbow joint predisposes it to direct injury in fracture or dislocation. Late disturbances (neuritis) in this nerve may develop as a result of an increased carrying angle following growth disturbance. Transference of the nerve anterior to the medial epicondyle when necessary shortens its course, removes the tension of stretching, and does away with its being crowded by the extended olecranon. (See Chapter XXI.)

Some mention should be made of the lymphatics in the elbow region. These consist of both superficial and deep vessels. Any serious injury not only causes laceration of many of these, but superimposed swelling compromises lymphatic drainage.

Chapter IV

Symptoms and Signs of Fractures and Dislocations

SYMPTOMS

THE OUTSTANDING symptom of a fracture is *pain*. This is subjective and is usually what brings the patient to the doctor or hospital for relief. It occurs in pathological fractures as well as in those following trauma. Pain may precede a pathological fracture and lead to the taking of a roentgenogram which may reveal the presence of metastasis from a distant malignant neoplasm. It may reveal the presence of other expanding lesions such as a giant-cell tumor of bone which has thinned the cortex sufficiently to make one wonder why a pathological fracture has not already occurred. Radiation (x-ray and radium) osteitis may cause persistent bone pain and very often does in the region of the hip following intensive radiotherapy for carcinoma of the cervix uteri. This pain frequently precedes a pathological fracture through the area affected by the radiation for a period of one to two months and should enable the surgeon to predict that a fracture may occur spontaneously at a later date.

Immediately following injury there may be very little pain due to local tissue shock. It is in this period lasting about fifteen to twenty minutes that some fractures and dislocations may be reduced easily without the necessity of an anesthetic. Hemorrhage, infiltration with fluid and cells into the surrounding tissues soon causes increased tissue tension and muscle spasm results. Pain then begins and may become severe. Intra-articular fractures such as those of the head of the radius without displacement gradually develop a hemarthrosis. When this increases to the point where tension is created within the intact joint capsule, pain, which was originally mild in character, then becomes severe.

Pain being a subjective symptom is difficult at times of evaluation when there are no other physical or roentgen findings associated with it. Patients vary in their sensitivity of pain. Those with a low threshold may describe a mild to moderate pain as very severe. Others may have very little pain or at least complain of very little when it would appear that they should have considerable.

Whenever active or passive motion is attempted in a joint adjacent to a fracture or dislocation muscular (protective) spasm will occur and pain will be increased. Motion at the fracture site whether involuntary or attempted by the examining physician will also give spasm and pain. In some fractures a small amount of active or passive motion may be obtained without increasing pain, but the moment the motion is increased beyond a certain amount, severe pain will be felt.

Stiffness, swelling, or inability to use an extremity are other symptoms that patients with fractures or dislocations complain of frequently. Less commonly do they complain of an actual deformity. When major nerves have been traumatized the patient may complain of numbness or inability to move the fingers as well as before, but this is rather rare. He usually does not offer this complaint until he has been questioned about it and the motor and sensory function of the nerves have been tested clinically. Occasionally, radiation of pain down the course of or in the skin distribution of a nerve will be offered as a symptom.

Physical signs on the other hand if carefully looked for and compared to the opposite uninjured extremity are far more reliable in making the diagnosis of a fracture or dislocation than are symptoms.

The first sign to look for in a suspected fracture or dislocation is *deformity*. If present, the diagnosis may be obvious or it may show characteristics that limit the actual bone injury to one of two or three types. Starting from here one should be careful in his examination in order not to hurt the patient or cause additional local trauma. On the other hand, there are a great many fractures in which there is no obvious bony deformity, so that it will be necessary to examine the extremity carefully and gently to elicit other positive signs and rule out false signs.

Swelling will almost certainly be noted unless the patient be very obese or unless the fracture be early and located purely within the joint (radial head). Swelling often gives the false impression of bony deformity and the latter can only be ruled out by very careful palpation.

Redness and **localized heat** may be noted in the region of the swelling, but represent inflammatory reaction in the soft tissues and not necessarily a bone or joint injury.

Ecchymosis may or may not be present in a fracture or dislocation. It is often stated that this is one of the cardinal signs of a fracture, but actually it is not usually an early sign to appear. Whenever ecchymosis appears early, i. e., within the first hour or two following a fracture, it means that there has been severe injury to the soft parts as a result of one of the bone fragments having ruptured through the overlying muscle and its over-lying deep fascia, thus allowing the escape of free blood into the immediate subcutaneous area. Early ecchymosis may also imply that one will have difficulty in reducing the fracture because of interposed muscle between the bone fragments. It is a sign that warrants great respect when noted early. Ecchymosis appearing four to five days after a fracture is of no practical assistance as a physical sign.

Tenderness is one of the most valuable of physical signs in helping to make a diagnosis of a bone injury. This may be of two types—direct or indirect. Direct tenderness is that which is elicited when pressure is applied directly over the fracture site. There may be mild tenderness on either side of this, but it is maximal at the line of fracture. One may occasionally be fooled by direct bony tenderness when the only injury is a severe contusion. Indirect tenderness in such cases is often a more reliable sign. This is elicited by pushing proximally upon the shaft of the bone suspected of being fractured or by tapping or percussing this bone at some distance, but along its axis. If on doing this the patient complains of pain at the suspected fracture site, the diagnosis is almost certain.

Crepitus is a sign which is pathognomonic of a fracture. It may be felt as a definite grating of two bone ends together and in such case is known as bony crepitus. It may be felt to give the sensation of rubbery surfaces slipping or skidding on each other. This is called soft tissue crepitus and usually implies the presence of interposed muscle between the bone fragments. Crepitus is a most valuable sign when elicited, *BUT* the examiner should not repeatedly attempt to elicit it because, by so doing, he may cause additional injury to the bone ends, muscle or any vessels or nerves that may be caught between the fragments.

False motion is motion elicited in the region of a bone where there normally is no joint and is pathognomonic of a fracture. Continued attempts to elicit this sign should be avoided in order to lessen trauma and additional pain.

Limitation of joint motion does not necessarily imply the presence of a fracture, but frequently is associated with one. Motion of the extremity against gravity often is limited and causes pain whereas supported motion may not. Immediately following an injury joint motion may not be limited appreciably according to the patient, but within an hour there is very noticeable limitation and after two hours joint motion is markedly impaired and pain becomes extreme. This suggests the development of a hemarthrosis. With other injuries joint motion may be markedly limited from the beginning even before pain becomes severe. This suggests an intra-articular fracture with displacement of a fragment that is causing an actual mechanical block. This may be seen in cases of fracture of the radial head or of the capitellum with displacement. Instead of there being simply limitation of motion, the complaint and finding is weakness of certain motions or inability to move the joint in certain directions against the pull of gravity. A fracture of the olecranon with displacement and separation of the fragment is a good example of this type. Motion limited or absent due to nerve injury is usually found not at the joint affected by the fracture, but at a more distal joint.

Hemarthrosis as a physical sign has already been mentioned as being a cause for delayed loss of motion in a joint after injury. The actual presence of the hemarthrosis can be detected clinically by noting a bulging, tense joint capsule which is tender to pressure. This is often seen on the outer side of the elbow in the triangle bounded by the three following bony landmarks; lateral epicondyle, radial head and tip of olecranon. The importance of looking for this is because, if present, aspiration of the blood from the distended joint will not only relieve pain instantly, but will allow freer motion and make it unnecessary for it to be absorbed (which is a slow process normally), and lessens the chances of formation of intra-articular adhesions.

Circulatory disturbances may be arterial or venous in nature or both. Diminution in the volume of the radial pulse as compared to that in the normal wrist usually means that there is pressure on the brachial artery from the lower end of the humerus or from the pressure of swelling in the antecubital fossa plus perhaps too much flexion at the elbow. If no radial pulse can be felt even when the elbow is extended and traction applied, it means either contusion of the brachial artery with subsequent spasm or thrombosis or perhaps even laceration. Any lessening of the palpable pulse calls for emergency measures such as Kirschner wire-traction, removal of all splints, discontinuance of the flexed position, or at times even operative exploration. To permit a feeble or absent pulse to continue will very likely be disastrous. The great majority of Volkmann's ischaemias and contractures are avoidable.

Nerve disturbances can be motor or sensory or both. Motor impairment may be found to be merely weakness (palsy) or it may be complete paralysis. Sensory disturbances are more often a diminution in skin sensation to pin prick, but may be complete loss of sensation. Occasionally a hyperesthesia is noted. (For complete details of nerve involvement associated with elbow injuries see Chapter XIV.)

A wound of the skin situated anywhere near the site of a fracture and from which there oozes old blood should be considered a communicating wound. The fracture should be considered as an open (compound) fracture and treated as such until operation proves that contamination of the fracture site does not exist. (See Chapter XV.)

Numerous symptoms and signs of fractures and dislocations have been described, many of which are found in other surgical lesions of an inflammatory nature as well as following trauma. The *cardinal signs* of a fracture are: bony deformity, indirect bony tenderness, false point of motion and bony crepitus. When these signs are all present it does not take a physician or surgeon to make the diagnosis. It is self-evident even to the average layman. Where trained surgical experience does count, however, is in making the diagnosis or at least suspecting the likelihood of a fracture when none of these signs are present and in splinting the injured part for transportation and roentgen examination in order to prevent the four cardinal signs from becoming evident.

Chapter V

Physical Examination of the Elbow

(AND ITS RELATION TO THE ARM AND HAND)

EXAMINATION of the elbow region, forearm and hand should be carried out just as systematically and thoroughly as physical examination elsewhere in the body for the purpose of eliciting abnormal physical signs which with the history of the case will assist in making a clinical diagnosis. Even though a completely accurate diagnosis cannot be made clinically, due to excess swelling which may obsure all the bony landmarks, a careful examination will give very definite clues as to the probable diagnosis which should subsequently be verified by roentgen examination. Simply because roentgen examination is usually made as a short-cut to diagnosis and visualization of bony displacements, it should not be used as a substitute for careful physical examination and thorough clinical evaluation of the injured extremity. Roentgen examination though helpful in disclosing accurately many displacements (though not infallible in very young children) is of no assistance whatsoever in aiding the surgeon or practitioner to decide whether or not urgency in treatment or even if special treatment is indicated from the standpoint of the circulation or of a nerve injury. It should be most embarrassing to reduce a fracture or dislocation and to later discover a paralysis without knowing whether this paralysis existed prior to manipulation. Still more important, a different form of treatment might have been indicated in the presence of a definite nerve lesion.

As in physical examination of the heart and lungs a definite system should be followed in examining an extremity. The four main methods of examination should be adhered to religiously and in this order: inspection, palpation, percussion, and auscultation.

1. By **inspection** can be determined the presence of bone or soft part deformity, swelling, ecchymosis, redness, bleb formation, the general attitude of the patient and whether or not he guards the elbow to prevent pain or discomfort. The general contours of the limb may indicate a particular injury. The color (pallor or cyanosis) of the hand and fingers can be noted. It is also possible to note the attitude of the fingers and their function or lack of function which may give direct evidence of nerve or vessel damage at the elbow. Atrophy of muscle and of the pulp of the finger tips may indicate nerve injury of long standing. Scars should also be looked for, and if

found, the patient questioned as to previous injury or operation. Very often loss of function may be due to a previous nerve or tendon injury and not to the injury of the moment.

2. **Palpation** will elicit deformities and displacements often missed on inspection as a result of swelling. It will also give one some idea of the amount of swelling and tissue tension surrounding the injury or the degree of tension in a joint capsule, the result of a hemarthrosis. Tenderness, both direct and indirect may be found and if carefully sought for will give a strong clue as to whether or not a fracture exists and in what region of the bone it lies. Crepitus and false motion may be discovered on palpation. The presence of and the quality of the radial pulse can be evaluated by comparing it to that in the uninjured arm. The temperature of the hand and fingers should be tested by palpation to determine the presence or absence of vascular impairment. Muscle action, strength and muscle tone may be determined by palpation often better than on inspection alone. Muscle spasm may be similarly appreciated.

3. **Percussion** though not resorted to routinely in examination of traumatic injuries is sometimes of aid in determining the presence of indirect tenderness. It may also be useful in detecting deep bony tenderness in the presence of a lesion such as a Brodie's abscess.

4. **Auscultation** is most commonly used at the elbow in determining the patient's blood pressure with a sphygmomanometer and stethescope. Occasionally it is useful in determining the presence of intra-articular crepitation. Where it may be of extreme importance is in detecting the presence of an arterio-venous fistula formation following a stab wound or gun-shot wound.

DIAGNOSIS

A. Clinical Diagnosis

Clinical diagnosis must be based upon a careful history of the case, whether it be traumatic in origin or of an insidious onset, and upon careful physical examination. Very often the history alone may give a clue as to the diagnosis or actually make the diagnosis. As an example of this we may consider the so-called "pulled-elbow" (subluxed radial head) in very young children who have had their arm jerked by the nurse or parent when being hurried or in an attempt to check their falling when they stumble. Another example might be a fall on the hand followed by pain in the outer aspect of the elbow which did not seem serious at the moment, but which after several hours became much more painful and less easily moved by the patient as is often the story with fractures of the head of the radius with gradual development of a hemarthrosis. Again, the patient may give a story that following a fall his arm or elbow was "out of shape" and that a friend pulled on it, causing reduction. This history very probably indicates that the patient has had a dislocation. In view of such a history and being unable to detect any definite bony deformities on physical examination, one should keep in mind what lesions are commonly associated with dislocations and check further for these clinically as well as making a special search for them on roentgenograms.

It should be remembered that the three bony points forming the triangle at the elbow can be of great assistance in helping the surgeon or practitioner to make a clinical diagnosis. The three points (medial and lateral epicondyles and olecranon process) form an inverted isosceles triangle with its base lying on the trans-epicondylar line and its apex at the olecranon when the elbow is held at 90°. On viewing the elbow from the lateral aspect these three points should be in line and in the same axis as the shaft of the humerus. If all three points maintain their proper relationship to each other, but all three are behind the shaft of the humerus, a supracondylar fracture with displacement must be present. If the triangle is distorted, yet the epicondyles remain in the axis of the humerus and the olecranon is situated posteriorly, there must obviously be a dislocation of both forearm bones upon the humerus. (See Fig. 6b.) At least this is the main diagnosis, and other fractures must be sought for and ruled out.

So complicated may many elbow injuries be that a complete diagnosis is frequently impossible from a clinical standpoint. This may be due to excessive swelling that prevents accurate determination of the bony relations or it may be due to inability to perform a thorough examination in a child on account of pain or fear. In such cases it is justified at times to do only what is necessary to convince oneself that a fracture or dislocation exists and to determine its general nature and resort to roentgen examination for the actual diagnosis of the bone or joint lesions. Again, after examination of roentgenograms, one may wish to re-examine the hand and fingers for the possible presence of a specific nerve injury. It is always wise to check ulnar nerve function if the film discloses a displacement of the epiphysis of the medial epicondyle of the humerus.

Likewise with obvious compound fractures in the region of the elbow clinical examination of the local lesion may be curtailed, the wound and fracture protected with a sterile dressing and splint and the patient sent for roentgenograms without delay. The reason this is permissible here is because inspection and debridement of the wound is to be carried out in the operating room as soon as possible and can be more safely done there than in an office or hospital emergency room.

B. Roentgenologic Diagnosis

Roentgenologic diagnosis is not always as satisfactory or as easily made as one might suspect. In the first place, in acute traumatic injuries it is often extremely difficult to obtain perfectly satisfactory views in two planes i. e. anteroposterior and lateral. This is because of pain, because of rotation of the extremity or a major fragment, because of inability to hold the extremity quiet during the examination and because of the size, shape and opacity of the emergency splints. With many elbow lesions, chronic as well as acute, it is impossible for the elbow to be extended beyond 120° to 130°. In such cases it is therefore impossible to obtain a satisfactory anteroposterior roentgenogram by the usual technique. If the tip of the olecranon is balanced on a film holder with the shafts of the humerus and forearm bones slanting away from the plate, all of the bones at the region of the elbow will show great distortion when projected upon the film. The only method by which a good anteroposterior roentgen examination can be made under such conditions is to take two separate views—one with the humerus resting flat on the plate and the second with the forearm bones resting flat on the plate.

Roentgen examination in the very young patient may be difficult owing to the lack of ossification of the numerous epiphyseal centers. A thorough knowledge of the time of appearance of these, their development, and final fusion with the diaphyseal portion of the bone is essential in the treatment of elbow injuries and diseases. (See Fig. 4.) All that the film may show is a small crack in the lower end of the diaphysis which may appear rather minor in nature. Some lateral condyle fractures of the humerus are of this type and unfortunately the only diagnosis made is a "chip fracture." If one understands the films and, what is more, realizes that there may be and likely is an extension of the fracture line down into the joint, existing in the epiphyseal cartilage not visible on the films, he will not miss the most important aspect of this and other types of fractures.

Certain roentgenologic diagnoses can be made only by taking comparative films of the uninjured extremity. Owing to the large number of epiphyseal ossification centers in children's elbows, internes, residents and younger surgeons in practice should always get these comparative films to keep them from missing minor fractures and displacements and also to familiarize themselves with epiphyseal development at various ages.

Most surgeons who treat traumatic cases read their own films and this is

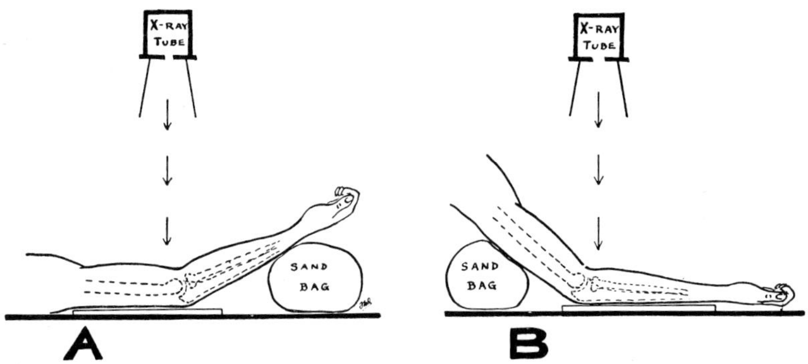

Fig. 12. Sketch showing method of taking roentgenogram of elbow when it is impossible to fully extend the joint. This technique gives a good view of the lower humerus in (A) and of the upper radius and ulna in (B). (Smith, F. M.: Displacement of medial epicondyle of humerus into the elbow joint. *Ann. Surg.*, *124*:410, 1946.)

as it should be. The roentgenologist should not be expected to describe all the smaller details shown on the film which are of no interest to anybody but the clinician who is caring for the patient. The roentgenologist can be aided very materially if the clinician ordering the films will be specific in designating exactly what region and views he wishes taken in the examination and also if he will state on his requisition what his tentative diagnosis is. Requests for post-reduction or post-operative films should also have these details stated if the roentgenologist is not expected to guess at them. The clinician will receive not only a more complete report, but also one more to the point if he takes the time to cooperate thus with the roentgenologist.

Chapter VI

General Principles of Fracture Treatment

WITHOUT a thorough knowledge and understanding of the accepted principles of fracture treatment it is hopeless to attempt to furnish intelligent and completely adequate care to fracture cases beyond the immediate period of emergency. New methods of treatment are being constantly devised and new instruments or gadgets are being just as constantly placed on the market with the idea that they help in the treatment of this or that fracture, either by facilitating reduction, maintaining reduction, or by helping to get better and quicker bony union. No doubt many of these are extremely helpful in particular fractures, but if they are used without regard to following the general principles of treatment they may very well do the patient more harm than good.

To be specific, consider a fracture of a long bone treated by pins through each fragment and fixed by external bars of one sort or another. If the pins are not put in at the correct angle, the fragments may slide back and forth upon them, the pin tracts become contaminated and eventually infection gets into the bone at the site of the pin hole. This leads to a low grade osteomyelitis and the formation of a ring sequestrum; a sinus tract persists and will often not clear up until removal of the dead and infected bone is resorted to by operation. This may be more annoying than serious, but may prolong the patient's convalescence until long after the fracture site has solidly healed. On the other hand, suppose the same method has been used in a fracture where there has been extensive stripping of the soft tissues surrounding the bone and suppose one pin passes through this area and the adjacent hematoma and in its tract there develops infection; the result may be extensive osteomyelitis at the fracture site with loss of bone fragments and possible non-union. One or more operative procedures may be necessary to combat the infection and assist in the sequestration of dead bone fragments. Late bone grafting may be required. All this may take years to accomplish with very dubious possibilities as to the ultimate results.

Similarly, these pins have been known to lead to suppurative arthritis when they have been applied close to the joint and pass through the joint capsule. The principle violated in the above examples is lack of adequate fixation due to either improperly applied apparatus or to the apparatus itself which was inadequate in being able to maintain the reduction. These types of apparatus if not readjusted two or three weeks following application may tend to hold the ends of transverse bone fragments apart and thereby act as a distracting force which may result either in delayed or non-union of the fracture.

Although methods of treatment may undergo a constant change and be in a state of flux, the general principles remain the same over a period of many decades. It is not the intention of the author to condemn any particular method of treatment so long as its advisors have worked it out on sound surgical principles and as long as its users keep these principles in mind when using it and apply the method properly instead of attempting various modifications according to their own whims.

Another extremely important factor in the treatment of a fracture is to know when a particular method of treatment is working and accomplishing what it was intended to do. Blind use of any method even though it was indicated at the beginning does not mean that it should be continued for two months without adjustments being made or without change to another method once the first has accomplished its prime purpose. In other words the average surgeon or general practitioner will be able to do very much better with his fracture patients and his ultimate results will be vastly improved if he rigidly follows the accepted principles and plans his methods of treatments for the specific injury based on these principles. Treatment otherwise may be good or it may be poor, but it is far from intelligent.

In medical schools and hospitals students and internes are not only taught how to take a complete history and perform a proper physical examination, but they are given ample practice and constant repetition in doing these things. The reason for this is that by so doing they train themselves in a logical, well-planned method of obtaining clinical data which establishes a basis from which to determine what laboratory studies are necessary to complete the diagnosis and also to begin a plan of treatment. In other words they are not taught merely the short cuts to diagnosis and treatment. Why? Because, first, the diagnosis is not always clear cut; second, a particular treatment does not always work; and third, the complications of the disease are often more serious than the disease itself. Just so with fractures which have tremendous variability, numerous associated lesions, frequent complications, and take a long time to heal, unless one follows a well organized plan based on sound and accepted principles which have stood the test of time, he will have a hard and rocky road to hoe. These principles are not difficult to learn and understand. They represent merely an orderly, logical, common sense list of principles which everyone should know, but which are frequently not followed. It makes little difference where one is working. Whether it be in a large well equipped hospital or in a small hospital less well equipped the treatment rendered will be no better than is the surgeon's ability to follow and stick to principles of treatment in deciding upon what methods or apparatus he should use.

Below is a list of principles to be followed in carrying out the treatment of fractures (and dislocations). Each of these will be amplified in some detail in the paragraphs to follow.

PRINCIPLES OF TREATMENT

1. Protection
   a. For the injured part.
   b. For the patient.
2. Early (and adequate) reduction of the fracture.
3. Adequate immobilization for the fracture.
   a. Types
   b. Length of time.
4. Employment of means to lessen local pathology and to promote bone and soft part healing.
5. Restoration or maintenance of function.
6. Restoration of the individual to his pre-injury status in so far as possible.

The purpose of treatment of any fracture or dislocation may be stated briefly as follows: *to restore the injured person to as nearly a perfect condition anatomically, functionally, and economically as is possible.* It is also common practice in evaluating the results of treatment to judge these on the same basis.

1. Protection

(a) Protection to the injured part means "splint 'em where they lie." It also means careful handling during transportation. The purpose is obvious: (1) to prevent additional injury to the fractured bone; (2) to prevent laceration of adjacent blood vessels and nerves; (3) to prevent the interposition of soft parts between the bone fragments; (4) to prevent a simple fracture from being converted into a compound fracture with its possible threat of infection; (5) to lessen pain and bleeding and thereby diminish the tendency to surgical shock, and (6) to make the ultimate treatment much easier for the surgeon as well as the patient.

Various methods of emergency immobilization may be used, the best of which is the Thomas splint for the lower extremity and the Murray-Jones splint for the upper extremity with or without fixed traction. Numerous other splints may be improvised from basswood or other boards padded with cotton, pillow splints, cardboard splints (padded), etc. In some elbow cases a sling alone is sufficient for emergency splinting. A padded wood or folded newspaper splint may be applied medially across the angle formed by the humeral shaft and forearm bones. This along with a sling gives protection and comfort. Figure-of-8 adhesive dressings are not good for emergency splinting, because they constrict the circulation and are extremely difficult and painful to remove since they are usually applied on the unshaven skin. They also interfere with the taking of the roentgenograms.

(b) Protection of the patient implies the use of methods to prevent hemorrhage (tourniquet, pressure dressings, morphine); to prevent pain (morphine, demerol, codeine and protective splinting); to prevent shock. The prevention of pain and hemorrhage will both help to prevent shock or lessen the degree of it. Whole blood, plasma, or other blood substitutes should also be given as a protective measure where shock is either imminent or already present. Early operation by its evacuation of the hemorrhage removes many toxic products from the injured extremity that would otherwise have to be absorbed systemically and which tend to prolong the condition of shock.

Above all, it must constantly be kept in mind that for the protection of the patient with an obvious serious injury a complete physical examination must be made. Injuries are *frequently* multiple. Very often a serious compound fracture may "steal the show" and everyone's attention and all treatments are directed towards this, while at the same time the patient may have a ruptured liver or bladder which requires more immediate attention if his life is to be saved.

2. Early and Adequate Reduction of the Fracture

The reasons for performing *early* reduction are obvious from a study of the acute pathology that occurs at and surrounding the fracture site. These are mainly swelling and infiltration of the surrounding soft tissues, especially muscle tissue which thereby loses its elasticity. This infiltration plus spasm makes it very difficult to stretch the muscle by manual and other forms of traction. Since the soft part pathology reaches its maximum approximately twelve to sixteen hours after injury, it will be seen that any delay in treatment will increase the difficulty of reduction with each hour that passes. Also, if reduction is attempted after twelve hours, it may necessitate more force being used which in turn may cause additional tearing of inelastic muscles further.

There are instances when patients come for treatment after the ideal time for reduction has passed. Suppose the first time a patient is seen is two days after injury; swelling is tremendous and immediate reduction is out of the question. The principle holds, however, that reduction should be done just as soon as it is possible. The injured extremity should be highly elevated or suspended and heat applied in order to hasten disappearance of the excess swelling and extensive infiltration so that the deformity may be reduced as soon as the soft parts permit.

Early reduction has been stressed. *Adequate* reduction must also be stressed. The term adequate is emphasized because it is not always possible to obtain a completely perfect anatomical reposition of the bone fragments by any means, closed or operative. Adequate reduction also means that what is adequate for over-coming the deformity (angular or shortening) of the particular fracture and region of the bone affected is at the same time adequate to permit maximum function later of the adjacent joints. It also means what is adequate for the particular individual according to his age and needs. In other words a fracture of the olecranon without displacement or with minimal displacement requires no reduction. Its position *is* adequate. One with marked displacement should be reduced in a young to middle aged individual, but in an elderly arthritic person it would be better to ignore the displacement, not reduce it and not immobilize the joint, which would very likely stiffen if kept splinted for four to six weeks. Minor deformities in children frequently require no reduction and will correct themselves by subsequent growth. Consequently the position of these may be considered adequate and merely splinted for protection against further injury and for the relief of pain.

3. Adequate Immobilization for the Fracture.

(a) **Types.** If fracture fragments must be held in position following reduction it usually means that the adjacent joints must be immobilized. Sometimes it is necessary to apply molded splints or circular plaster casings to accomplish this. In the elbow region it is preferable not to apply circular plaster owing to the danger of swelling, etc. and it is difficult to immobilize the shoulder joint even by placing the patient in a plaster spica. In supracondylar fractures of the humerus, the elbow is placed in flexion *after* reduction is obtained, and a posterior molded plaster splint is applied from the axilla to the metacarpophalangeal joints. It might be asked how this type of plaster can give adequate immobilization without including the shoulder joint. The answer is that the plaster per se does not, but the plaster and dressing keep the elbow in flexion while the triceps muscle and tendon act as a direct splint upon the posterior surface of the lower humerus and the flexed position keeps this muscle taut. Suspension of the flexed elbow by a cuff at the wrist with a halter around the neck accomplishes the same purpose even without the splint.

Traction (skin and skeletal) may be used to carry out immobilization and at the same time allow active exercises in the adjacent joints. Some fractures require no immobilization and frequently do better if given none or only minimal immobilization. A radial head fracture without displacement is a good example of this type. Internal fixation often gives more adequate immobilization as well as maintenance of anatomical reposition and at the same time replaces external apparatus and permits immediate active function of the adjacent joints.

(b) Time of Immobilization. The duration of immobilization cannot be stated in general terms. Different fractures vary so greatly in their healing time that it is best to judge the time necessary for immobilization by the study of specific fractures and by experience. At the elbow we have a highly specialized joint with both hinge and rotary motions. Function is far more important in this joint than perfect anatomy. It is a joint that is prone to become partially or entirely stiff if completely immobilized for long periods of time after injury. Probably the longest that an elbow should be immobilized is six weeks. The majority of elbow injuries (including severe supracondylar fractures in children) need not be immobilized beyond four weeks. Other injuries, certain radial head fractures and mild displacements of the medial epicondyle epiphysis in children, take an unusually long time to recover full function if they are immobilized for as long as two weeks. Most radial head fractures with little or no displacement do best if the joint is aspirated (for relief of pain) and started on immediate active motion, thereby preventing the formation of intra-articular adhesions.

4. Removal of Local Pathology

The local pathology surrounding the fracture site has already been described in detail. Any measures that can be used to diminish swelling, tension and rid the area of its cellular infiltration and products of tissue death, which are toxic to the system and interfere with the treatment of shock, are justifiable. This is because the tissue reaction will the sooner be converted to an alkaline pH which will enhance the deposition of calcium in the new granulation tissue to form early bone callus. Ridding the tissues of its local pathology also acts mechanically in making it possible for muscles and joints to be actively exercised and hastens rather than delays the return of their function. Needless to say any healing of the soft parts is improved as well as healing of the bone.

Means of promoting improvement of the local pathology are by the avoidance of any more extensive immobilization than is necessary to maintain the fragments in position, by avoidance of any constricting dressings, splints or other apparatus, by the elevation of the injured part to assist in gravity drainage of the veins and lymphatics, by the use of low intensity heat, and active contraction of the muscles in the extremity even though joint motion is not possible. All of the above measures if carried out from the beginning as they should be will improve the entire circulatory status of the extremity, improve the chances of early bone healing, will lessen the functional recovery time, and do away with prolonged measures of late rehabilitation.

Open reductions with rigid internal fixation of the bone fragments by plates and screws where feasible and possible will do away with the necessity of external splints for more than a few days following operation. Active motion may thus be begun almost immediately with comfort, and these patients really never lose their function or require more than a minimal amount of physiotherapy. What little is needed may be carried out in the home by soaks in hot water and by frequent active exercises. Under this same regime muscle atrophy remains at a minimum and joint stiffness as a result of prolonged immobilization does not have a chance to occur.

Chapter VII

Anesthesia

(A) PURPOSE

THE PRIME purpose of an anesthetic in order to reduce or otherwise care for a fracture or dislocation is to make the procedure painless. If the patient does not experience pain during the manipulation, there is no muscle spasm to overcome and the whole procedure may be done with greater ease as well as with greater thoroughness. Much less force is necessary and therefore the risk of causing additional damage to bone and soft parts is lessened.

Some patients may feel that they can stand the procedure without anesthesia, but if a real reduction is necessary and not merely a single quick push to straighten a simple angulation, it is unfair to the patient and to the surgeon as well not to administer an anesthetic. During the period of after-care cooperation of the patient is very necessary. This is very likely to be lacking in a child who has been made to stand severe or prolonged pain.

(B) CHOICE OF ANESTHETIC AGENT

Anesthetic agents may be grouped into three classifications; those that act by local application, those that give regional anesthesia by nerve and plexus block, and general anesthetics.

Local anesthesia obtained by the injection of a one percent solution of procaine hydrochloride or proper concentration of some other safe local anesthetic into the region of the hematoma surrounding the fracture site is advocated by many surgeons, especially Böhler. Its advantages are: (1) It does not require the services of an assistant (or anesthetist) to administer; it may be given by the surgeon himself and in his office if necessary; (2) if properly administered and sufficient time (15 to 20 minutes) is allowed for the procaine or other agent to diffuse thoroughly throughout the hematoma, excellent anesthesia and relaxation may be obtained; (3) it is valuable where a general anesthetic is contra-indicated due to the presence of an upper respiratory infection, cardiac decompensation or when the patient has eaten a meal too recently to expect its digestion to have been completed.

There are several disadvantages in the use of local anesthesia in the treatment of fractures and dislocations which should be carefully balanced against the advantages before the surgeon should decide upon its use. The disadvantages are: (1) frequently too little time is allowed to elapse between injection of the procaine and starting the manipulative reduction; the patient experiences pain and is unable to relax; (2) it is a poor type of anesthesia in young children who in general are apprehensive and hate needles; (3) though it may be useful in the region of the wrist or ankle, the author believes it to be a poor agent for elbow fractures owing to the presence of excessive swelling and the risk of increasing this by the addition of fifteen to twenty cubic centimeters of anesthetic solution; (4) occasionally the solution when injected gets into a vein and into the general circulation and, if this happens, the patient may expire.

Nerve or brachial plexus block anesthesia has very little use in the treatment of elbow injuries. Its chief advantage is where it is either impossible or inadvisable to administer a general anesthetic for the reasons stated above under local anesthesia. The disadvantages are numerous: (1) it requires considerable practice and skill to administer properly; (2) it should *not* be used as an office procedure, because it is too complicated; (3) it is of no use in children and frequently of no use in over-apprehensive adults; (4) there is also considerable risk in getting the anesthetic solution into a large vein or in creating a pneumothorax by inadvertently puncturing the pleura over the apex of the lung.

General anesthesia when it is possible to give without undue risk, is in the opinion of the author the very best type of anesthesia for use in reduction of elbow injuries. Its advantages are many: (1) the patient is unconscious and not worrying about possible pain; (2) he cannot over-hear bits of conversation or discussion about difficulties during reduction or other remarks by the surgeon or assistants that he as a layman is in no position to understand and will very likely misconstrue if he tries to do so; (3) he is completely relaxed which makes easier the procedure of reduction; (4) he is not frightened by the array of surgical instruments or apparatus visible in the room; (5) it may be prolonged for any necessary length of procedure. The disadvantages of general anesthesia administered by inhalation are: (1) its risk in upper respiratory infection and cardiac decompensation; (2) possible prolonged anoxemia if nitrous oxide is used without sufficient oxygen, and (3) the hazard of explosive mixtures, however small, in the presence of static electrical sparks or those from the control switch of the fluoroscopic machine. General anesthesia is not as well tolerated as is local, regional or nerve block anesthesia in patients in shock or in incipient shock.

Pentothal sodium given intravenously as a general anesthetic is excellent except in young children. Its chief advantages are the ease of induction and the complete relaxation obtained. It is excellent in long or short procedures, and the patient usually recovers consciousness fairly quickly and has less frequent after effects of nausea or vomiting than following some other general anesthetics. Its chief disadvantage is that it occasionally causes laryngospasm. Patients who have just recovered from such an anesthetic and are ambulatory should not be permitted to go home alone. They frequently lose all sense of direction and may be almost completely oblivious to external surroundings, thus either wandering off and getting lost or injured in a traffic accident. If a friend or member of the family can accompany the patient, it is perfectly safe to let him go home. The effect of the drug wears off completely after two or three hours as a rule. It is contra-indicated in patients with extensive renal damage.

(C) SAFETY OF ANESTHETIC AGENT

The use of local anesthetic agents such as procaine, metycaine, nupercaine, or monocaine, or the use of any of these for nerve or plexus block is relatively safe provided it is not injected directly into a vein or a pneumothorax does not result from the procedure, and provided the safe dose of the drug is not exceeded.

Most of the agents used for inhalation anesthesia are explosive in nature when mixed with oxygen, whether the latter be from the room air or from a tank. Ethylene or cyclopropane with oxygen, though two of the very best, are so highly explosive that special precautions must be taken to ground the patient, anesthetist, and anesthesia apparatus against the possibility of static electrical sparks. Ether and oxygen or nitrous oxide and oxygen are much less explosive mixtures and therefore far safer from this standpoint. It may be very difficult to anesthetize a chronic alcoholic with either one of these without giving him so much of the agent that it tends to asphyxiate him. In working with colored people this may be a real hazard owing to the difficulty of being able to detect cyanosis. It is therefore far safer for the patient to have either one of these agents administered by means of a machine such as the Connell or McKesson type which measures accurately the percentage mixture of agent and oxygen. It should be kept in mind, however, that since any mechanical device may lose its accuracy, the mechanical regulator cannot be considered a substitute for careful observation of the patient. In children under the age of seven years it is usually considered not particularly safe to use nitrous oxide and oxygen.

Young children needing a reduction or operation do best and are more safely handled with open-drop ether. The initial induction can be obtained in a few seconds with ethyl chloride inhalation and then changed to ether. This gets away from much of the fear and struggle so often present with ether induction alone. Open-drop ether except for its definite contra-indications is probably the best and safest anesthetic agent for use in all age groups including the aged and hypertensive cardiovascular risks. Nitrous oxide and oxygen alone is not a good agent in this latter group because of its tendency to increase the blood pressure and possibly cause a cerebral vascular accident. Nitrous oxide with oxygen inhalation along with intravenous sodium pentothal is an excellent combination in adults, even in the aged. The use of pentothal makes it unnecessary to have to administer more than a very weak mixture of nitrous oxide and oxygen.

Owing to the fact that a patient coming in for an emergency procedure may have recently eaten or because gastric emptying is frequently slowed following injury, it is not only beneficial but extremely desirable to induce vomiting before induction of a general anesthetic. This can be accomplished by tickling the patient's posterior pharynx with a finger. This method of emptying the stomach is far better than attempting to do it through a stomach tube, owing to the large quantity and large pieces of undigested food often obtained that could not possibly pass through even a large tube. Such a procedure may save the patient the risk of aspiration pneumonia, atelectasis, or even aspiration asphyxia since such food would almost unquestionably be vomited during the anesthesia.

A new drug, Ketamin-HCL, can be administered intravenously for general anaesthesia even in patients who have eaten shortly before sustaining their injury. Its chief advantage is that it does *not* knock out the cough and gag reflexes and therefore gives little or no chance of aspiration of stomach contents should the patient vomit. Most people recover quickly enough so they can be discharged in a reasonable time. One disadvantage of the drug is its tendency to cause disturbing dreams or hallucinations in certain individuals.

When it comes to the choice of anesthesia for a particular patient, this should be made by the surgeon responsible for the care of the patient and his injury. The surgeon should consider the patient's age and general physical and mental condition, he should know how much shock or strain the reduction or operation will cause the patient, how long it should take (including application of and "setting" of plaster-of-Paris splints), and how much relaxation is going to be required to accomplish the procedure satisfactorily. After weighing all of these factors, experience and sound surgical judgment should cause the surgeon to choose whatever type of anesthesia and form of anesthetic agent he believes is best (not necessarily ideal) for the particular patient with his particular injury and his particular general condition.

Chapter VIII

General Considerations of the Patient

(A) THE INDIVIDUAL AS A WHOLE

WHENEVER WE are called upon to treat a patient with an injury we must consider him as a whole. It is therefore necessary to consider his age, sex, his interests in life aside from his regular occupation, his possible fear of doctors, needles or anesthetics as well as hospitals, his tendency to blame his condition on someone else if he feels he has a just complaint and can sue for damages. There is also the patient who has been under the treatment of another physician and who comes in on the advice of a friend. This patient comes somewhat reluctantly and often with a preconceived idea in his own mind as to just what his condition is. He names the diagnosis and relates just what Dr. So-and-so said about it. After taking a history and examining the patient it is sometimes obvious that the patient's condition is something other than his version of it. Considerable tact may be required to handle the situation, especially if a radical change in treatment is to be advised and the patient is to be sent back to his original physician.

Age is very important. There are times when complete and accurate reduction of the fracture fragments is inadvisable. This, of course, depends to some extent upon the particular fracture, but very often considerable displacement may be allowed to remain in young children because growth can be counted upon to correct certain deformities. As long as the general axis of the fragments is good, even though there be lateral displacement, the chances of correction by growth are excellent. Angular deformities on the other hand do not correct so readily by growth and often take four or five years to become corrected. Fractures along the epiphyseal line or across the cartilagenous plate of the epiphysis may result in actual growth disturbance (retardation). For this reason it is often wiser to accept an incomplete reduction of the fragments (as seen on roentgen examination) after one or two attempts to manipulate them than to keep repeating the manipulations in the hope of obtaining perfect position and at the same time subjecting the injured part to additional trauma, which almost certainly will predispose to growth disturbance. Similarly, it is in general unwise to perform open reductions upon epiphyseal displacements if a reasonably satisfactory closed reduction can be obtained. These if opened are very prone to show growth disturbances of a severe nature. An occasional exception, however, must be made and this must depend upon the individual case and the judgment of an experienced fracture surgeon.

In healthy, active adults who must use their arms and hands, it is important to restore the maximum amount of function in their elbows that the particular injury will allow to be recovered. In elderly individuals who no longer need to work for a living, strength and maximum function are not so important. It is important, however, to restore enough function so that the patient may be able to dress and feed himself and for a woman to be able to fix her own hair without being completely dependent upon someone else for these everyday necessities of life. In young and middle-aged adults it might be imperative to operate on certain elbow fractures such as one of the olecranon, but in a patient older than 65 years this would perhaps be foolhardy. Decision as to the actual treatment of the case requires judgment and depends upon how active the particular patient is and how anxious he is to regain full use of the elbow. Some elderly individuals look upon an injury as an excellent excuse to "slough" off household duties upon a younger generation. Others cannot get back to work soon enough.

The sex of the patient may have a bearing upon the treatment advised and upon the rapidity and completeness of his functional recovery. Boys and men in general go in for rougher sports and more strenuous occupations. Treatment designed to restore full strength as well as maximum function in order to allow them to continue with heavy work is imperative. Formerly, the man was the bread winner in the family and therefore it was important to restore him to this full capacity. Women are more and more entering occupations which make them important in the family economic circle, so their injuries now also demand treatment offering restored function and strength rather than just a good cosmetic result.

We must not neglect the fact that almost every individual has some interest outside his occupation. He may like to play golf, shoot, paint, knit, or play a musical instrument and if it becomes necessary to give up his avocation he may become exceedingly unhappy. Some persons with several hobbies are in luck. Others who have but one hobby and are so mentally inflexible as to be unable to take up another are in a very sad position if they have to give their's up.

There are also patients who have a real fear of a doctor or a hospital. This is sometimes a very real problem in a child who fears the doctor is going to stick him with a hypodermic needle or who has had a previous anesthetic of ether and becomes terrified at the thought of another. Sometimes these may be reasoned with, but oftentimes not. Sometimes the parent is the one who is worrying for the child and fusses over him. The child mainly wants to know if it is going to hurt "when the bone is set." If it is possible not to hurt him (and for this reason general anesthetics are advisable in children) we should do what we can to avoid pain. If it is going to hurt and this cannot be avoided, *always* tell the child beforehand that it will hurt for a moment, but try to make the moment a brief one. Never tell a child that it will not hurt him and then do something that does; you will never regain his confidence and cooperation. His subsequent care will be difficult and the result very likely unsatisfactory.

There are patients who look upon an injury as an opportunity to collect for damages. Many of these have justification and should collect. Others injured while working are protected by law and should be taken care of and paid compensation while definitely unable to return to their former or other gainful occupation. Nobody will argue about either of these types of patients. There are, however, those who feel sorry for themselves even though their slight injury was not the fault of another or of their occupation. These individuals unfortunately and frequently get into the hands of unscrupulous doctors and lawyers who see an opportunity of making a good case out of it and financial gain to themselves. This is bad practice and should be frowned upon by all reputable professional men and medical societies. Such a patient should be discouraged in forcing his suit. The surgeon in charge should keep accurate and complete records of the case from start to completion of his treatment. If the case later comes to court, actual factual evidence may save an innocent defendent from a large claim.

(B) AN INDIVIDUAL WITH AN INJURY

We must not overlook the fact that when a patient is presented with an injury, he is not just a case. True, it may be an interesting case from a surgical point of view, and the patient may also be pleased to know that his is an interesting case. But John Doe is mostly interested in John Doe, the pain he is suffering and what are the prospects of his relief and ultimate recovery. He may be interested in knowing what was done for the last twenty similar cases and their results, but only in so far as these may help him to get well. Long academic discussions and explanations of treatment techniques cannot be understood by the patient. It is best to size up the whole situation and then to explain to the patient in brief but understandable terms what must be accomplished and how this should be done. With a child this should be discussed with the parents. With patients of low intelligence or in which there is a language barrier, a relative, friend or interpreter should be used. If there is some doubt in the surgeon's own mind as to what is the best form of treatment, he will do well to carry out what he thinks ought to be done for himself or on a member of his own family with a similar injury. He should not be influenced by any personal prejudices to methods of treatment if he feels that the method chosen offers the patient the best possible chance of recovery in the shortest possible time.

It is extremely important in treating an injured patient not to allow him or his family to talk or argue the surgeon out of what he feels is the correct treatment and persuade him to substitute a compromise method. This in the end will only lead to increased trouble both to the patients thus treated and to the surgeon.

(C) OCCUPATION

Consideration of the individual patient's occupation is most important in selecting proper treatment for him. What is ideal treatment for one person may be improper for another. A violinist with an injured left elbow must recover full supination of this hand and practically full elbow extension. Any form of treatment or position of immobilization that results in much limitation of either of these functions will put an end to his professional career. Also, any form of treatment that prolongs his recovery unnecessarily or the application of physiotherapy (such as diathermy alone) to help him regain motion is useless and causes a hardship to him financially and mentally and may be hard on his employer or the insurance carrier as well if he happens to be a compensation case.

Not infrequently certain types of injury preclude the patient ever returning to his original occupation. Severe, comminuted compound fractures at the elbow or injuries with severe nerve damage may so affect the forearm and hand that a skilled workman will become totally disabled for his particular kind of work. Individuals whose work does not require skilled use of their hands and those whose work is in an office or other sedentary work may very well be able to carry on their usual occupation and continue with the same earning capacity even with one arm useless or amputated. It is far more important in general to save an arm than a leg. If the question of amputation arises as a result of tissue damage and inability to reconstruct the injured extremity, one should try to save the hand or as many fingers and thumb as possible, provided there is adequate circulation to sustain nutrition. If gangrene occurs or serious infection develops, it may be imperative to amputate to save the patient's life. No artificial arm or hand can ever substitute for the patient's own even if he retains but a thumb and two functioning fingers. Many such patients become expert though seriously handicapped and are able to return to their regular occupation. It is therefore extremely important to try to return a man to his former occupation and earning capacity because above the age of 45, it may be difficult or impossible for him to adapt himself to a new job and new surroundings particularly if he has to work at the same tempo as his unhandicapped fellow workers.

(D) PATIENT'S ECONOMIC STATUS

This brings up the question of the patient's economic status. Any serious injury requiring a prolonged period of treatment, convalescence and rehabilitation is an economic catastrophe to the average individual. Even if he be a compensation case, the amount he is paid while away from work can never equal what his earnings would have been had he been working. His and his family's living expenses probably do not change during this period except by absolute necessity when his savings have been used up or until he has to sell his house or car to furnish enough money to feed his children. If his injury has been received at sports and is not compensable, he then has to stand the entire expense of treatment himself and may at the same time receive no wages or salary. This patient if not covered by accident insurance may have to borrow money, sell property, or use up his savings. If he cannot do any of these, he may have to submit to treatment at a city or other charitable institution against his wishes. It is therefore important from the standpoint of any of these reasons noted above to give this man a planned course of treatment that will get him back to work as soon as possible and return him to his former economic status. If this is not possible, it may take much work on the part of physiotherapists, occupational therapists, physicians, social service workers, etc., to get him a job that he can do or to get him trained for another type of occupation.

(E) MORALE OF THE PATIENT

The morale of the patient is based on so many factors and is so complex that it is only possible here to discuss a few of these. The morale of an injured child recovers almost as soon as the pain disappears. He has no family worries or occupation to think about; his next meal will come automatically; he has no mortgages to pay off, or life insurance premiums to keep up or any of the multitude of other responsibilities that an adult would have. The morale of the adult is subject to all these and other factors plus the acquisition of an incapacitating injury even though not hopeless of recovery. The longer he is hospitalized and the longer he sits around the home convalescing (and not working), the longer it will take to rehabilitate him and return him to his regular work. This is especially true in compensation cases. Whether the case comes under compensation status or not, many fractures become completely healed and function may be fully restored in three months. The patient may lack full muscle power and may fatigue easily at this time; he may have a little residual swelling and possibly some mild ache and pain. Should he stay away from work until "perfectly" well and strong? The answer is "no." To do so will keep his morale low. He gets used to taking it easy and is in no hurry to get to work. He sits around feeling sorry for himself and finds plenty of reasons in his aches and lack of full strength to justify (or alibi) his waiting another few weeks before going back to work. The only trouble with this attitude is that it tends to repeat itself at the end of those few weeks just when he said he would go back to work. Very often this may lead not only to financial but also to family difficulties and these again react unfavorably upon the patient's morale.

Compensation cases may act the same way. Countless numbers of patients with minor injuries aside from serious injuries continue to "sit around" waiting for the treatments to make them better and in the meantime receiving their compensation checks at regular intervals. This is why many of these patients come to be called cases of "compensationitis." It is not always the patient's fault, though an occasional true malingerer is found. The responsibility is the fault of the labor laws, the employer, the insurance carriers, the referees and the doctors.

To cite but two of these—the employer and the insurance carrier—much could be accomplished to the benefit of themselves as well as to the patient and his morale if they would get together and allow him to return either to light work or half-time work when he is able to do this, rather than insist that he return to his regular, full schedule of heavy work. This would get a lot of patients back to work at three or four months, boost their morale, get their minds off their troubles, give them an earning capacity, and, last but not least, allow them to be doing something useful.

Chapter IX

Classification of Elbow Fractures

THE TYPES OF injury encountered in the region of the elbow are extremely varied. Fractures are by far the most frequent especially in children. Dislocations are also common, but not quite so varied (Chapter XIX). There is a group of combined fractures and dislocations which though not so common is a very important group because of the possible poor prognosis and the difficulty of handling properly.

Owing to the variability of the lesions occurring at different age groups it would seem best to classify the injuries accordingly. Below is a classification which is felt to be useful especially for medical students, internes, and hospital residents. It is a general classification and cannot of course embrace every individual variant of injury. This classification is also not intended to differentiate between fractures with displacement as against those without displacement. It would also seem advisable to list the different types of fractures according to the nature and region of the bone affected rather

SPECIFIC FRACTURES AT THE ELBOW

(In order of their frequency in each bone)

Children	*Adults*
Lower Extremity of HUMERUS (Chapter X)	
Supracondylar (Transcondylar)	Dicondylar Y or T
Medial Epicondyle (Epiphyseal separation)	Lateral Condyle
Lateral Condyle	Capitellum
Capitellum	Supracondylar
Epiphyseal Separation (entire)	Medial Condyle
Medial Condyle	Trochlea
	"Side Swipe" Fractures
	(usually involve radius and ulna also)
	Medial Epicondyle
	Door-Handle Injury
	Gun-Shot Wound of the Elbow
Upper Extremity of ULNA (Chapter XI)	
Shaft, upper 1/3	Olecranon
Olecranon or epiphysis	Coronoid
Coronoid	Shaft, upper 1/3
Upper Extremity of RADIUS (Chapter XII)	
Head (epiphyseal separation)	Head
Neck (with or without impaction)	Neck
	Bicipital Tuberosity

than list them according to etiology or type of displacement. In doing this, it is made easier for anyone looking up a particular type of injury, to refer to the chapter and section dealing with its treatment and locate any variations which he wishes to study or adopt.

COMMON COMBINED TYPES OF FRACTURE AND DISLOCATION AT THE ELBOW

a. Fracture of Coronoid with Posterior Dislocation of Radius and Ulna.
b. Separation of Epiphysis of Medial Epicondyle with Postero-Lateral Dislocation of Radius and Ulna. (Epicondyle may be displaced into the elbow joint cavity.)
c. Fracture of Head of Radius with Posterior Dislocation of Radius and Ulna.
d. Anterior Dislocation of Head of Radius with Fracture of Upper 1/3 of Shaft of Ulna (Monteggia Fracture).
e. Lateral Subluxation of Radius and Ulna with Fracture of Lateral Condyle of Humerus.
f. Anterior Subluxation of Ulna (and Radius) with Fracture of Olecranon.

The majority of the fractures listed above are simple rather than open (compound) fractures. The one type of fracture in this region that is almost always compounded is the "side-swipe" or "truck-swipe" variety. Other types that not infrequently become compounded are fractures of the olecranon, supracondylar or dicondylar Y or T fractures, and Monteggia (upper 1/3 of ulna shaft) fractures. In the case of a gun-shot or blast injury most anything can happen to the bones as far as fragmentation, compounding and extensive soft tissue damage is concerned.

Chapter X

Fractures of Lower Extremity of Humerus

DICONDYLAR (INTERCONDYLAR) "Y" AND "T" FRACTURES

General Considerations

THE DICONDYLAR "Y-" or "T-" shaped fracture (also called intercondylar, diacondylar, or bicondylar) of the lower extremity of the humerus is a relatively common injury in adults. It may occur in young adults, but is more frequent in those of middle age or older. It is caused by a fall directly upon the elbow, the patient landing on its posterior aspect or upon the flexed elbow causing the upper ulna to act as a wedge, thus splitting the humeral condyles. There is usually considerable separation of the fragments as a result of the original force and these are spread apart and tilted upon each other in one or more planes by the constant pull of the muscles attached to each epicondyle. Thus the articular surface of the humerus is disorganized and offers irregular contours and axes for articulation with the ulna and radius unless the fragments can be reduced and held in reasonably good position. There is also the likelihood of adhesion formation in addition to possible bony block that may cause subsequent pain as well as limited joint motion. Unfortunately many of these fractures exhibit extensive comminution of the lower humerus with as many as six or eight separate bone fragments, thus presenting an impossible situation for reconstruction of the joint by open operation. If the fracture should consist of two or three main fragments only, and these are relatively large, it may be a wise procedure to perform open reduction and apply internal fixation, provided the surgeon has had adequate experience in this type of work and can perform the operation in a hospital properly equipped and staffed for taking care of open operations in acute bone and joint trauma. More will be said about treatment further on in this chapter.

The soft part injury accompanying dicondylar fractures is often extensive and it in itself may lead to permanent disability. Associated with the fracture, especially if marked comminution and displacement of the fragments exists, is laceration of the joint capsule, periosteum, muscle, and not infrequently injury to one or more of the major nerves. A fair number of these fractures are accompanied by a compounding wound in the skin. The circulation may be considerably disturbed owing to the displacement of the fragments, resultant hemorrhage and swelling. There may be accompanying fracture of the olecranon process or of the radial head.

The lesion is serious because it involves joint surfaces. It is extremely difficult to reduce by closed means with any assurance of regaining perfect function. Any closed reduction followed by prolonged plaster immobilization is very likely to result in fibrosis or bony ankylosis of the joint. So serious is the threat of permanent stiffening in the joint if the fracture be fixed in plaster that it was not unusual to find the older text-books advocating fixation in a position "optimum for ankylosis." This suggestion of treatment seemed to assume that the recovery of reasonable joint motion was never to be expected. Such an attitude would now be regarded as purely

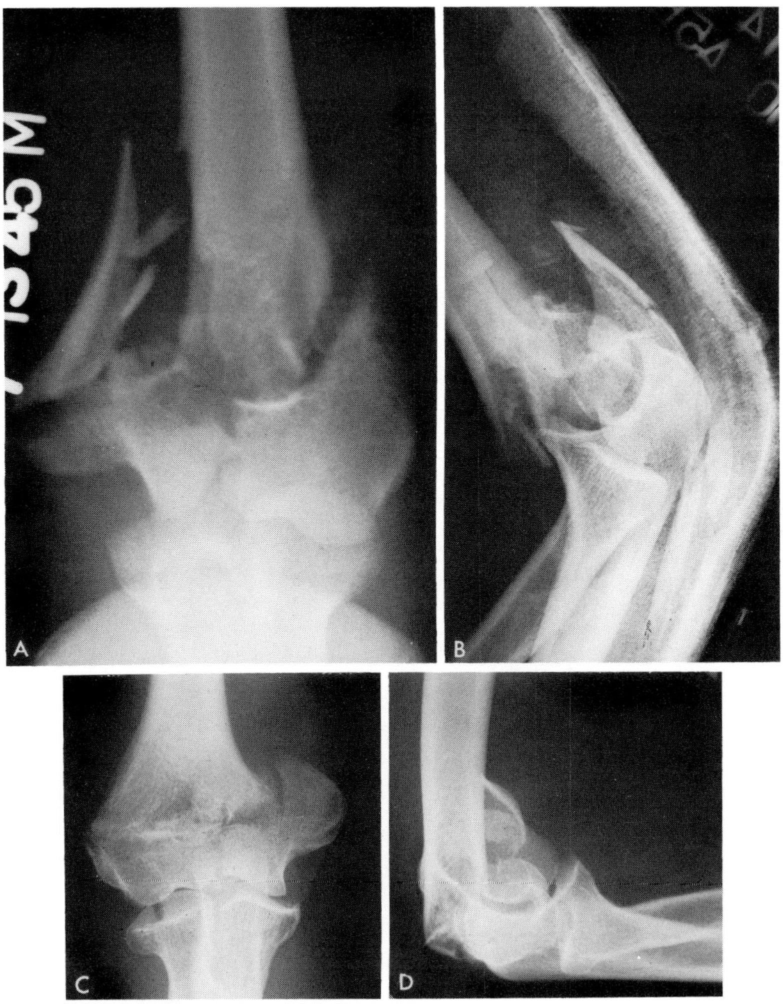

Fig. 13. Roentgenograms of dicondylar fractures of lower humerus. A and B, anteroposterior and lateral views, respectively, of 27 year old woman. This patient also had accompanying radial and ulnar nerve palsies. C and D, similar views of a 50 year old woman. Note the marked comminution and displacement of the distal fragments.

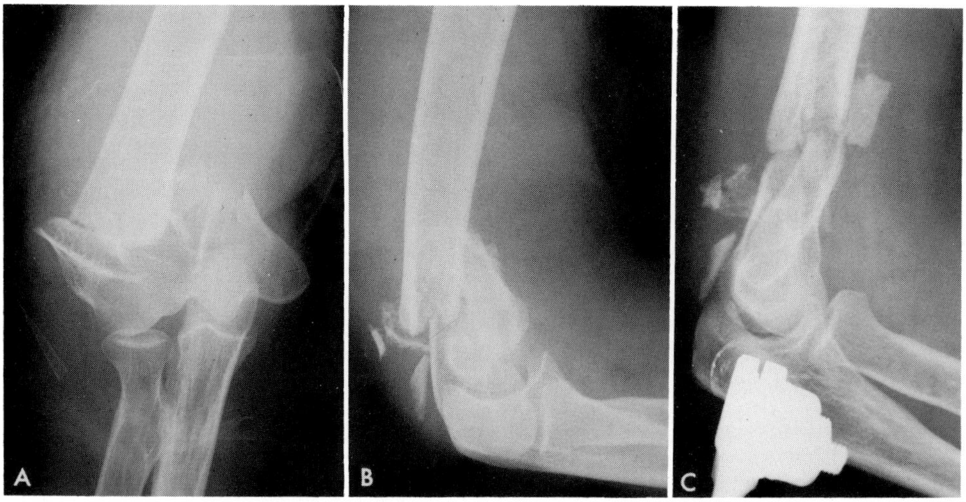

Fig. 14. Dicondylar fracture of lower humerus with comminution. (A) Antero-posterior, and (B) lateral views of original bony injury. Owing to the comminution the fracture in this 55 year old woman was treated with skeletal traction by means of a Kirschner wire passed through the olecranon. (C) shows lateral view in traction.

defeatist. The present trend and the only logical form of treatment strives to regain joint function and not to worry so much about the cosmetic appearance of the elbow or necessarily try to obtain excellent reposition of the fragments as seen on roentgen films. In other words with this type of fracture it is frequently impossible to give the patient a good looking elbow and a good functioning elbow at the same time. Consequently, it is often necessary to compromise, and, if such a compromise must be made, it should be made early in the treatment and usually for the more important return of function.

Treatment

Closed Reduction. Several methods have been advocated, but none is completely satisfactory. Wilson and Cochrane have advised closed manipulation, molding of the fragments and fixation in a neck halter. If reduction is obtained by this method (which is frequently impossible), immobilization in the halter must be continued for at least four weeks to allow sufficient bone healing to take place to prevent slipping of the fragments. Such prolonged fixation even though active flexion is permitted is very likely to lead to intra-articular adhesions, periarticular fibrosis, and marked loss of joint extension regardless of the quality and persistence of after-treatment.

Since the advent of the "hanging cast" in the treatment of shaft fractures of the humerus as introduced by Caldwell, some surgeons have tried the method in the treatment of dicondylar fractures with good results in the milder forms of displacement. The method cannot be expected to give satisfactory results with such a fracture where separation of the fragments has been extreme. The author believes this method of treatment should be reserved for what it was originally intended, i. e., fractures of the shaft of the humerus.

There is often great difficulty in applying a plaster cast, splint, or other dressing for fixation that is competent to maintain reduction of the dicondylar fragments unless it be employed in conjunction with some form of traction or traction and suspension. A good form of traction for these injuries has been described by Magnuson which employs the use of a felt cuff applied to the upper anterior surface of the forearm (flexed to 90 degrees) and with ten to fifteen pounds of weight furnishing the traction force. The patient lies supine in bed with the forearm suspended vertically by skin traction with just enough weight to keep it in this position. The elbow is at a right angle. The weight attached to the felt cuff applies traction to the upper forearm in a dorsal direction and through the muscles and ligaments to the condyles of the humerus in a distal direction. It may be advisable to manipulate and mold the condylar fragments under anesthesia after a day or two of this traction to overcome angulation and spreading. If the tendency to spread persists, it may be wise to apply a well-molded plaster compression splint of the sugar-tong type. The elbow is usually kept in this traction for two to three weeks, followed by a posterior molded splint and sling. Active elbow exercises are carried out at frequent intervals thereafter, the splint being removed to permit these. As a matter of fact some active motion may be permitted as early as four or five days while the elbow is suspended in the traction apparatus. It would seem advisable to begin the motion as early as this, for the movement of the ulna and radius upon the humerus may help to mold the condylar fragments into a somewhat better position, thus improving the opportunity to regain more complete flexion

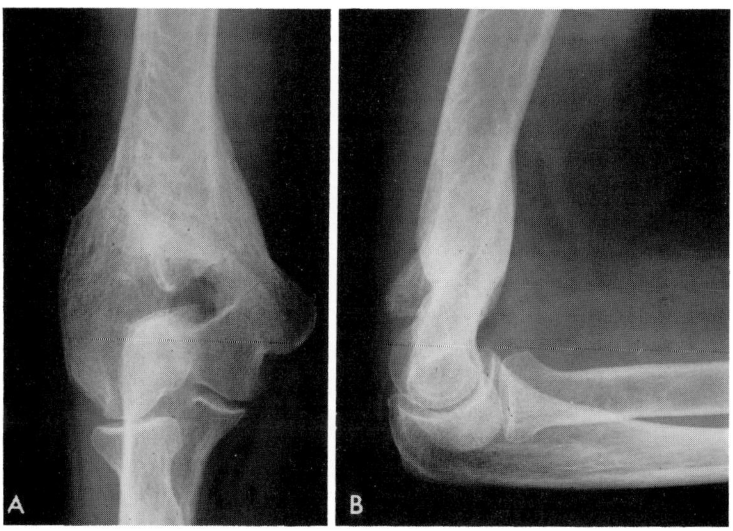

Fig. 15. Dicondylar fracture of lower humerus with comminution. (A) and (B) represent antero-posterior and lateral views, respectively, taken eight months after injury. (Same patient as in Fig. 14.)

and extension. Early motion also minimizes the formation of adhesions between the joint surfaces.

Skeletal traction is much more effective in assisting reduction of a fracture of this type and its use is therefore to be preferred over skin or felt-cuff traction. It may be employed by means of a Kirschner wire inserted through the olecranon as described under its use in some serious supracondylar fractures. (See Fig. 28.) In dicondylar fractures the surgeon, if he does not wish to suspend the elbow in over-head traction, may employ the Kirschner wire traction with the arm in the same position as is used for the Magnuson felt-cuff traction. Over-head position is often preferable, since it maintains the injured elbow at a much higher level than the shoulder and consequently permits swelling to recede more rapidly. Further manipulation may be performed in the traction if necessary and a posterior molded splint may be applied prior to removal of the wire if desired. Wire traction should be kept on for at least three weeks and in some instances it may be advisable to prolong it to six weeks to allow firmer bone healing. Active elbow motion is encouraged within the first week after injury while in traction and these exercises should be performed for five minutes every hour while the patient is awake in order to help mold the fragments into a more optimum position for flexion and extension and also to minimize the risk of adhesions. Heat and gentle massage may likewise be given to decrease swelling and improve the circulation around the injured elbow. (See After-treatment.)

The Jones traction splint has been advocated for the treatment of this fracture, but this has two very definite disadvantages: (1) it is heavy and cumbersome; and (2) it does not permit active motion in the elbow joint. If traction and early active motion are to be used, it is much more efficacious to employ the Magnuson cuff or the Kirschner wire skeletal traction.

Occasionally a patient may be encountered who, owing to senility, alcoholism or some form of mental agitation, makes the use of any ideal type of treatment inadvisable and dangerous. In such a case it may be imperative to discontinue traction and active motion if already instituted and to avoid all operative measures. In order to protect the patient from causing himself additional harm, it may be necessary to immobilize his arm, elbow and forearm in a well-padded circular plaster casing and allow him to be ambulatory. This type of treatment should be resorted to only when no better method can be employed.

Operative Treatment. As stated previously there are some dicondylar fractures which lend themselves to open reduction and internal fixation and are probably best treated by such a method if all the qualifications for the use of open reduction are met. There are many advocates of open reduction and likewise many critics. Open reduction should not be employed without experience in this form of surgery and without the proper equipment and materials for internal fixation. One reason the method is criticized is that the extensive comminution of the lower humerus in many cases makes it difficult if not impossible to re-assemble the fragments in an anatomical position without interfering with the blood supply to these and because it frequently turns out that the many fragments cannot be adequately and rigidly fixed by means of screws, plates, nails, etc. If such circumstance occurs, more harm may result than good and the elbow may have to be immobilized in plaster anyhow, which really defeats the prime purpose of the operation, i. e., to obtain reposition and fixation of the fragments, and to institute early motion in order to regain function.

Certain types of dicondylar fractures, where comminution is at a minimum and the roentgenograms reveal only two or three reasonably large condylar fragments that definitely appear amenable to internal fixation, may be and probably should be operated upon. This should not be performed in elderly individuals, in persons whose physical condition is poor, or where there is a dirty abrasion in the vicinity of the elbow. There are many cases, however, where operation can improve the bony anatomy of the elbow and also offer the patient the probability of recovering far better function than can be expected from any form of treatment.

If operation is to be performed in dicondylar fractures, it is best employed as a *primary* form of treatment and not after one or more other methods have failed to give a reduction. Also, if performed, it is best to do so within the first eight to twelve hours after the injury before soft part swelling has become too great and before extensive induration has made these soft parts non-elastic. This procedure is easier if performed early; and a better job may also be done.

Operative Method. Several different incisions may be employed for exposure of the posterior aspect of the condyles of the humerus. Some surgeons prefer the use of two lateral incisions in order that a bolt may be passed transversely through the two condyles. A U-shaped incision may also be used to advantage by turning the skin and subcutaneous tissue flap upwards and approaching and exposing the posterior aspect of the lower humerus on either one or both sides of the triceps tendon. The Van Gorder incision also gives an excellent exposure for this region (Chapter XVII). The ulnar nerve must be identified and protected from harm in any of these exposures. The skin margins must be well protected with towels before the fracture site and joint is exposed, since infection would be very serious and probably result in ankylosis. When the fracture site is exposed, blood clots should be removed and the main fragments handled as gently as possible in order not to strip more muscle and periosteum than is necessary to fit them together and fasten them securely. If any completely loose small fragments of bone or cartilage are found in the joint, these should be removed, since they will otherwise act as loose bodies and cause irritation. The main condylar fragments should next be re-assembled and also aligned with the lower end of the humeral shaft. At this point the operator will have to study the situation and decide upon the best and most rigid type of fixation that can be used.

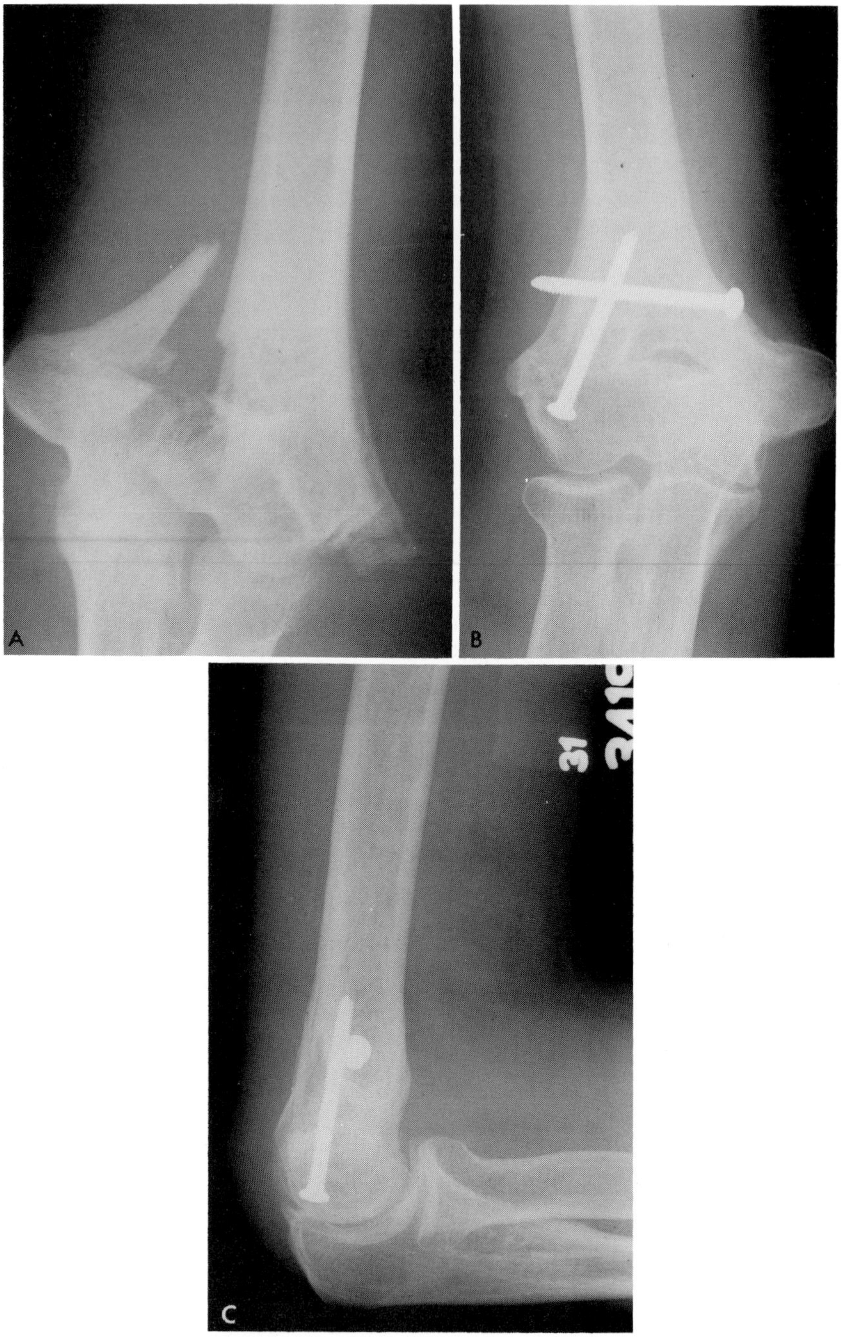

Fig. 16. Roentgenograms of lower humerus showing a dicondylar fracture in a 40 year old man with minimal comminution. (A) Original injury; (B) and (C) antero-posterior and lateral views of same elbow eight months after open reduction and internal fixation with two screws. Excellent functional and anatomical result obtained.

Some cases will require the use of a transverse bolt to fasten the condyles to each other; possibly one or two screws or nails may accomplish the same fixation. In any case neither the bolt, screws, or nails must pass through the olecranon fossa or they will interfere with joint motion. The most difficult part of the procedure may be in fastening the reduced condyles to the lower shaft. If, fortunately, a bony spike is found on one condylar fragment, this may be transfixed to the shaft by means of a screw. At other times one or more small or narrow (forearm) plates may be used to bridge the posterior or lateral surface of the condyles or shaft. These plates should be bent to conform to the surfaces upon which they are to lie. If a transfixion screw can be used in addition to the plate without causing unnecessary damage by further exposure, so much the better, for it will increase the firmness of the internal fixation and permit freer and earlier active motion which is desirable to regain full function. The author recommends the use of screws rather than nails for fixation since these obtain a better grip upon the bone and are less likely to loosen. Many surgeons prefer nails, however, and seem to have less difficulty in inserting them. Loops of wire, if used for fastening the condyles to the shaft, rarely give satisfactory fixation and plaster immobilization is usually required in the post-operative period. If for some reason it is found possible to lock the two condyles together by a bolt or screws, but impossible to fasten them to the lower end of the shaft, the elbow should be put up in over-head Kirschner wire traction following operation.

The metal used in the plates, screws, nails or bolts should be of a non-irritating type, such as stainless steel or Vitallium.

After-treatment. Following any of the methods of original treatment employed (closed or open) the elbow should be elevated and kept at rest for the first few days to assist in decreasing the swelling and to make the patient more comfortable. Low intensity heat may be applied continuously and gentle massage twice a day will help to improve the circulation to the injured part. Active exercises *within pain limits* should be started early in the treatment (five to seven days) and carried out for periods of five minutes each hour. This regime can be followed if the patient has been treated by traction or by open reduction with adequate internal fixation. No splint is necessary in the latter except for the first day or two following operation and at night thereafter for protection only for three weeks. A sling for support and rest is advisable after coming out of traction, but may be removed for exercise periods and discarded altogether after the end of five or six weeks. Soaks in warm water several times a day combined with active exercises are beneficial and may be started as soon as any wire holes or operative wounds have healed. Whirlpool baths may be substituted for the regular soaks. Occupational therapy may be employed to great advantage in these cases to assist in regaining function and muscular strength through active use. These patients should be started on light work and this gradually increased as their condition improves.

Again, it hardly seems necessary to caution against the use of passive motion, forceful manipulation, weight-carrying, etc. in the treatment of these injuries, but it is too often found to be employed frequently and to the detriment of the patient's recovery. Present day surgery respects tissues and calls for the gentle handling of these at operation. The same principle should and *must* apply in the after-treatment of traumatic injuries.

Complications

Nerve injuries may occur as complications of these fractures. These should be treated conservatively at first and only operated upon later if no improvement is noted in their function after four to six months.

Limitation of elbow motion in flexion or extension or both, particularly if the arc of motion is such as to greatly handicap the patient in his work or daily life, may have to be corrected by operative means. Some cases may develop this as a result of bony block; if so an ostectomy may have to be performed. Others may show limited extension because of fibrosis of the anterior capsule of the elbow joint; this may necessitate a capsular releasing operation (capsulotomy) after the manner described by Wilson in which the entire attachment of the anterior joint capsule is freed from the front of the humerus (Chapter XXI).

Should fibrous or bony ankylosis occur and constitute a grave handicap to the patient, some form of arthroplasty may later be performed in order to give him a movable and more useful elbow. (See Arthroplasty.)

Disability Time

If the injury has been treated by one of the closed methods described, the disability time is likely to be as long as four to six months. If it falls into the type that can be adequately treated by open reduction and internal fixation, the disability time will be shorter and in the neighborhood of three to four months.

Prognosis

In general the prognosis is far from excellent in dicondylar (intercondylar) fractures owing to the frequent occurrence of comminution and to the age of the patient. A reasonably good functioning and useful elbow, however, may be obtained in a high percentage of cases if traction and early motion are employed as treatment or if operation can be done with good fixation of the fragments. If closed reduction and complete immobilization in plaster is employed as treatment, the functional result is very likely to be poor.

The prognosis is better now that it is known that we must strive to recover function and not try so hard to obtain and maintain anatomical reduction by closed methods.

SUPRACONDYLAR (TRANSCONDYLAR) FRACTURE IN CHILDREN

The most frequent fracture sustained in the region of the elbow in children is the supracondylar (transcondylar) fracture of the lower extremity of the humerus. Some writers attempt to differentiate between what is considered to be a supracondylar or a transcondylar fracture of this bone. From a purely academic viewpoint there is a very slight difference, as the names imply. For all practical purposes when one considers the pathology accompanying the trauma, the type of treatment to be given, the complications, and prognosis, the two types are identical. For the purposes of description and clarity the author prefers to use the term "supracondylar" fracture, since he believes it will lead to less confusion in the following paragraphs.

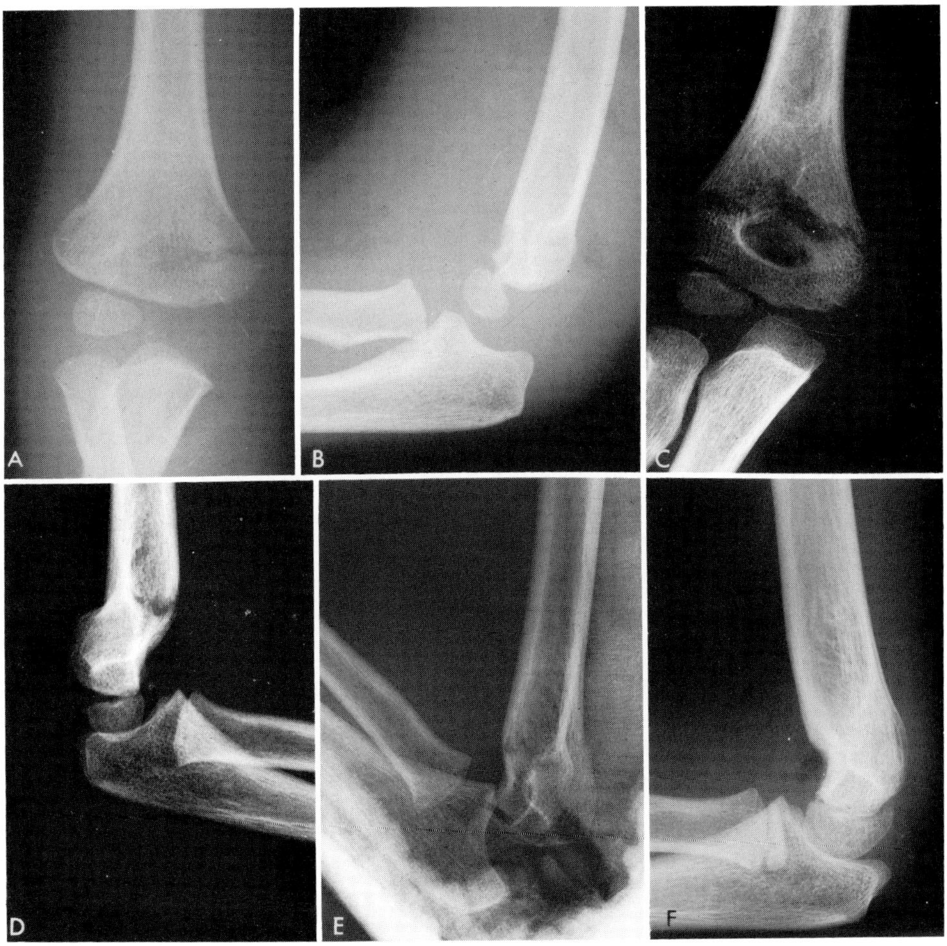

Fig. 17. Roentgenograms of supracondylar fracture of humerus. (A) and (B) Anteroposterior and lateral views barely showing fracture line and minimal displacement requiring no reduction. (C) and (D) Show similar views in another child with moderate displacement. (E) Lateral view after partial reduction, and (F) later view of same elbow two and one-half years later.

General Considerations

Supracondylar fractures are common injuries and may be serious. They usually occur from a fall upon the hand while the elbow is partially flexed. The force imparted travels upwards along the radius and ulna, and is transmitted to the lower extremity of the humerus which becomes fractured through or just above the broadest portion of the condyles. The most common deformity is thus a posterior angulation or displacement of the distal fragment of varying degree. In addition to the usual posterior displacement of the lower fragment, there is often a lateral or medial displacement and even rotation of this upon the shaft fragment.

(Very rarely there is an anterior displacement of the distal fragment, but

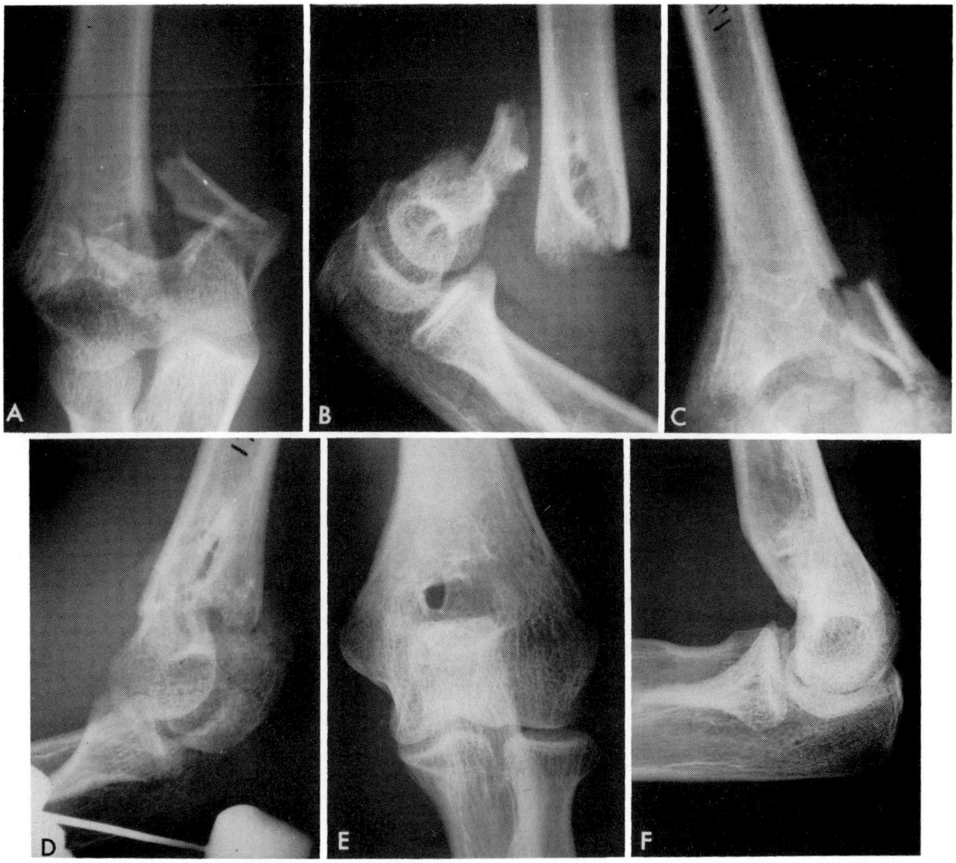

Fig. 18. Supracondylar fracture of humerus with marked displacement in a 12 year old girl with associated paralysis of posterior interosseus nerve. Patient was treated by Kirschner wire skeletal traction through olecranon and manipulation. (A) and (B) Antero-posterior and lateral views of original injury and displacement. (C) and (D) Similar views in skeletal traction six days after injury. (E) and (F) Similar views of the same elbow eight years after injury. The nerve recovered full function in two and one-half months. Except for five degrees limitation of flexion this patient regained full range of motion, including rotation.

this occurs in less than five percent of the cases. The latter type of displacement is usually due to a fall in which the patient lands upon the back of his flexed elbow.)

As mentioned above the bony deformity may vary considerably· there may be no deformity or it may be extreme. Besides the main types and degrees of displacement shown in Figures 17-21 the reader must keep in mind that there may be any degree of angulation or deformity between those pictured. He also must remember that these fractures may occur at practically any age from one and one-half to 14 years. The associated soft part pathology, swelling, hemorrhage, circulatory impairment, and possible nerve damage is in *direct* proportion to the amount of bony displacement. If the displacement has been sufficiently extensive, the distal end of the shaft fragment may puncture the skin on the anterior aspect just above the

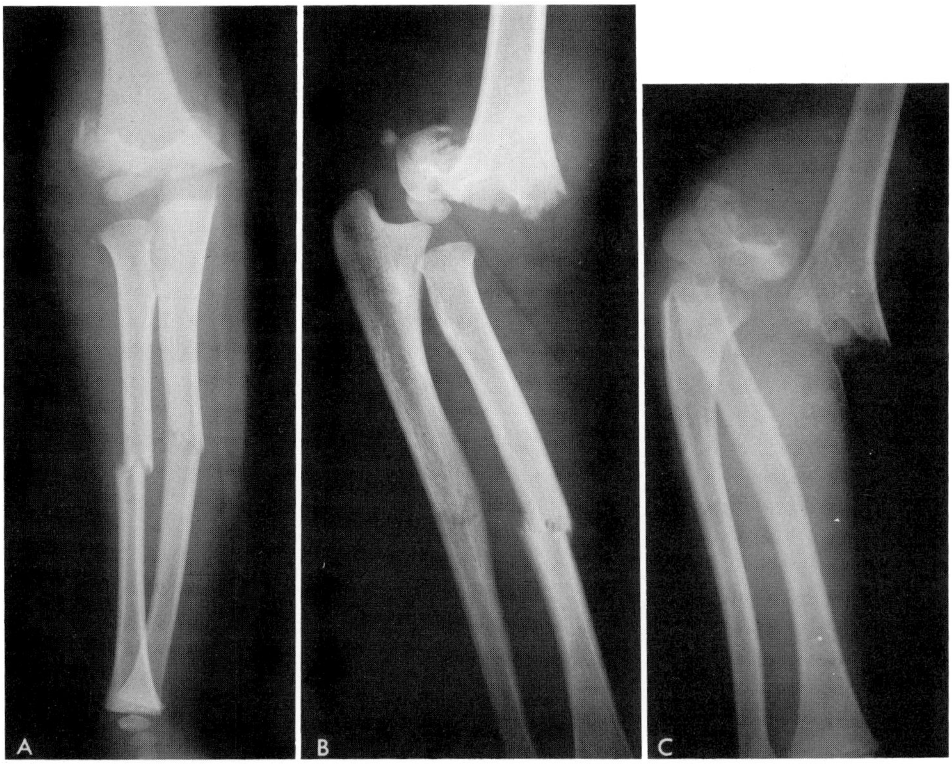

Fig. 19. Supracondylar fractures of humerus with marked displacement of distal fragment and associated injuries. (A) and (B) Antero-posterior and lateral roentgenograms of a six year old boy showing associated fractures in middle third of shafts of radius and ulna. This patient's elbow was treated by Kirschner wire skeletal traction and the forearm fractures by molded plaster splints. (C) View of elbow in another boy eight years of age in which the distal fragment of the humerus is displaced so far posteriorly that the lower end of the shaft perforated the skin, creating an open (compound) fracture. Kirschner wire skeletal traction and suspension were also used in this patient to maintain reduction of the fragments after thorough surgical debridement and cleansing of the contaminated wound.

elbow flexion crease, causing the fracture to be "compounded," e. g. (open fracture). Likewise with marked displacement the brachial vessels are compromised by pressure from the shaft fragment and the circulation below the elbow may be greatly impaired. If not treated judiciously and immediately, this may result in Volkmann's ischaemia and paralysis. Before discoursing further upon this whole subject, the author would like to empha-

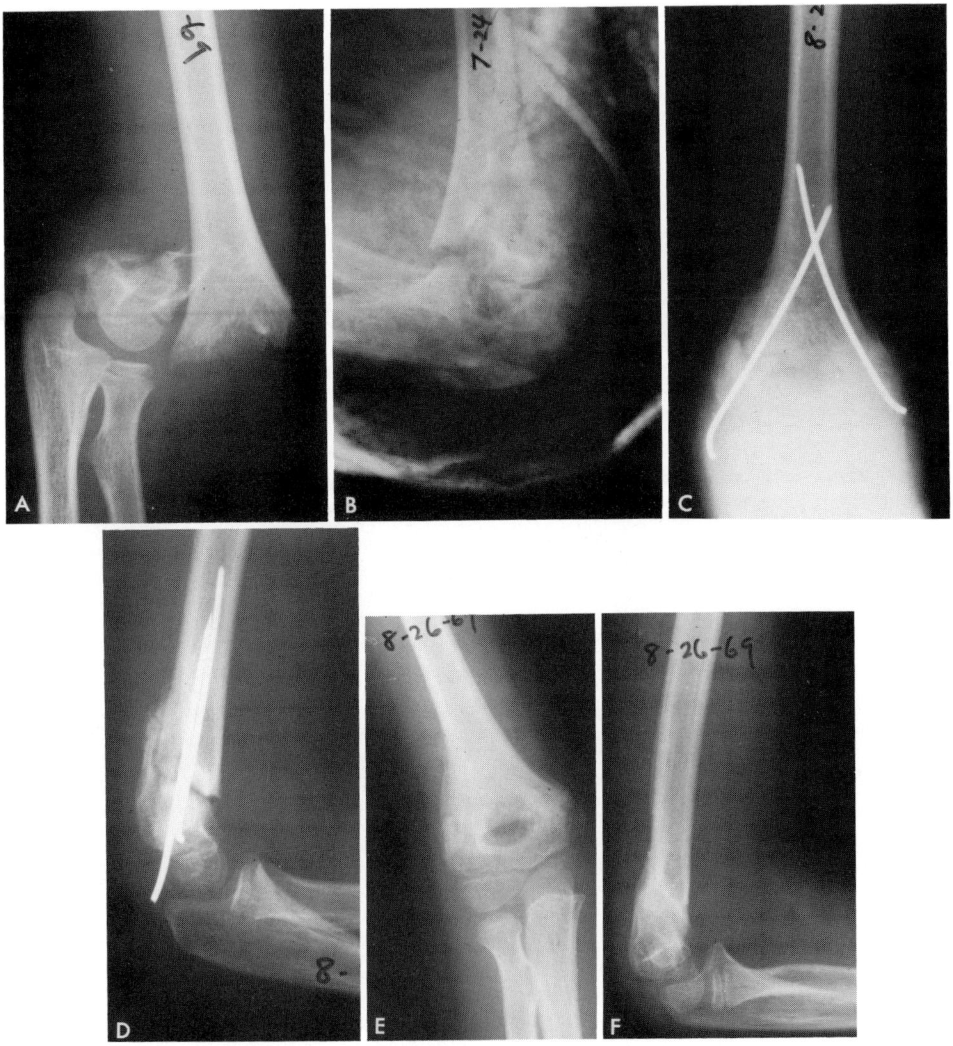

Fig. 19-A. Supracondylar fracture in a 9 year old boy with marked posterior displacement. (A) original view; (B) after closed reduction showed marked rotary displacement. Three days later posterior displacement recurred in plaster. Swelling was excessive. The patient was transferred from the original hospital on fourth day after injury. Pulse and nerves were functioning well. Instead of using over-head Kirschner wire suspension it was decided to perform an open reduction, and views (C) and (D) show the position of the fragments to be anatomical as held by Kirschner wire pins. At the end of 4½ weeks after operation under general anaesthesia the wires were removed and the fracture healed as in (E) and (F). The patient regained full return of elbow motion in 2½ months.

size the fact that **the best way to overcome an impaired circulation in a badly displaced supracondylar fracture of the humerus is to bring about immediate reduction of the fragments.**

Associated Lesions

Hemorrhage from the lacerated brachialis anticus muscle and small blood vessels may be extensive and cause marked swelling and difficulty in maintaining reduction in the flexed position thus further compromising the circulation.

Nerve injury is not infrequent, the radial or its motor branch (posterior interosseus) being the most commonly injured. The ulnar is next in order and the median nerve is the least frequently injured in this type of fracture. Impairment of nerve function is the result of contusion or stretching in most cases rather than from direct laceration. (See Chapter XIV.)

Circulatory impairment is present in all cases with displacement of the fragments. This is of two types: (1) the minute circulation, and (2) the gross circulation. The former is due to laceration of small veins, arterioles, and capillaries in the torn muscle tissue. This causes local hemorrhage and inflammatory swelling, stasis and tension beneath the deep fascia, which, if permitted to increase by lack of reduction, elevation, or by the application of too tight splints or bandages, may secondarily compress the larger veins, brachial artery and lead to Volkmann's ischaemia. The gross circulation (brachial artery and veins) may be compromised by the bony deformity per se, e. g., these vessels may be drawn tightly over the forward projection

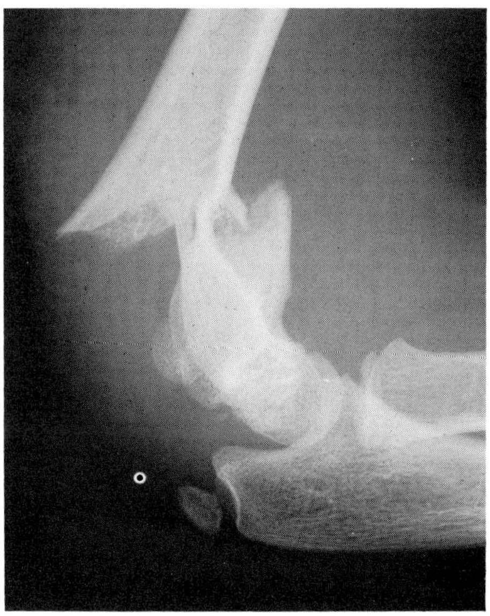

Fig. 20. Supracondylar fracture of humerus of the flexion type, i. e., with anterior displacement of the lower fragment. This is an extremely rare type of displacement and results from a fall with the patient landing on the posterior aspect of the elbow. The accompanying lateral view is of the elbow of a nine year old girl.

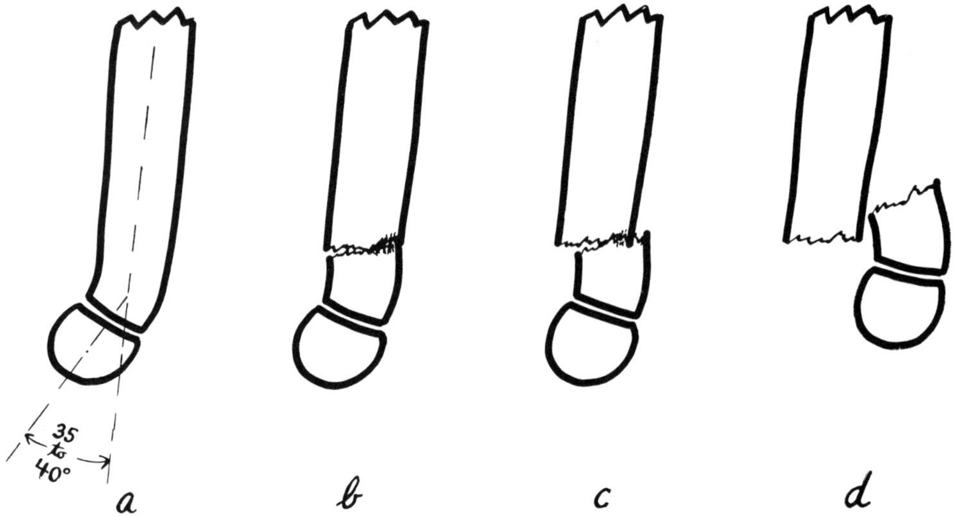

Fig. 21-A. Sketch of lateral view of lower humerus to show normal forward tilt of articular process (capitellum). (a) Varying degrees of displacement of distal fragment in supracondylar fracture. (b) Loss of forward tilt. (c) Same plus partial posterior displacement. (d) Complete posterior displacement with over-riding.

of the proximal fragment. The artery may be scratched or otherwise irritated by the sharp edge of this fragment and respond by going into extreme spasm, thus shutting off the circulation to the lower forearm and hand. Spasm may last until the irritation is relieved, hence the importance of performing immediate reduction of the fracture and of removing the irritating factor. This is the reason why "waiting for the swelling to go down"

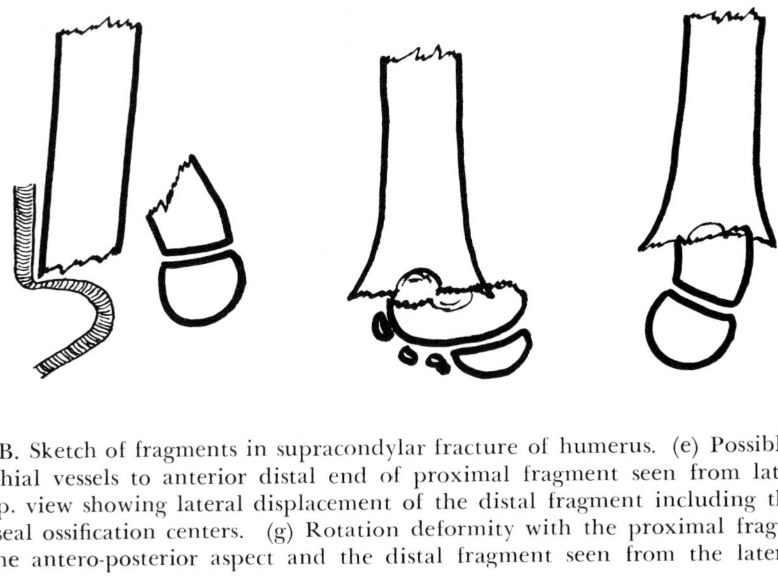

Fig. 21-B. Sketch of fragments in supracondylar fracture of humerus. (e) Possible relation of brachial vessels to anterior distal end of proximal fragment seen from lateral view. (f) A. p. view showing lateral displacement of the distal fragment including the various epiphyseal ossification centers. (g) Rotation deformity with the proximal fragment seen from the antero-posterior aspect and the distal fragment seen from the lateral aspect.

in badly displaced supracondylar fractures before performing a reduction is an inexcusable mistake and has accounted for many cases of Volkmann's paralysis. The artery is very rarely lacerated. The radial pulse will not return after reduction and the hand will remain blanched and cold if laceration of the artery is present.

Injury to the cartilagenous plate of the lower humeral epiphysis may occur at the same time that a supracondylar fracture is sustained. It is usually impossible to make an additional diagnosis of this injury unless roentgenograms reveal true displacement of the ossification center of the capitellum upon the lateral condyle. That epiphyseal injury may occur in this region we know from the fact that some of these patients develop growth disturbance after several years, leading to an alteration of the carrying angle that was not thus altered six months or one year after the original injury.

Hemarthrosis may also accompany the fracture and account for the extreme pain that some patients have when minimal displacement of the fragments exists.

Diagnosis

Supracondylar fractures must be differentiated clinically from posterior dislocation at the elbow joint. In fresh cases before swelling has completely obliterated the bony anatomy the differentiation should be easy. In supracondylar fracture the three landmarks (medial and lateral epicondyles of the humerus and the tip of the olecranon) forming the bony triangle of the elbow will all be found posterior to the axis of the humeral shaft when displacement is marked. If no displacement is present, the bony anatomy may be normal and the diagnosis will have to be made upon the finding of localized bony tenderness over both humeral condyles. In posterior dislocation

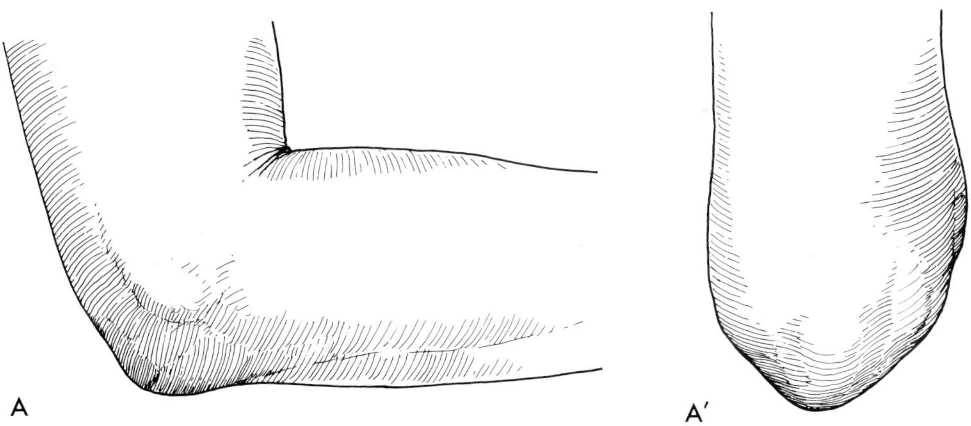

A A′

Fig. 22. Sketch showing outlines of normal elbow from (A) lateral and (A'), posterior aspects: note that the dorsal surface of the elbow in either projection shows *convex* contours from above downwards and from side to side.

the two epicondyle landmarks will remain in the same axis as the shaft of the humerus, but the tip of the olecranon will be displaced posterior to all of these. The posterior aspect of the elbow is normally convex from above downwards and also in a transverse direction. In this fracture the convexity is increased by swelling and the change from convexity to concavity (on lateral inspection) takes place three or four inches proximal to the elbow joint. In dislocation the triceps tendon is bow-strung, taut, and concave from above downwards and the subcutaneous tissues and skin are drawn inwards to make concave hollows on either side of the tendon behind the lower humerus.

The student may ask the reasons for performing detailed clinical differential diagnosis when roentgenograms are to be taken. One reason for the importance of the clinical examination is that the surgeon must perfect his diagnostic acumen and use the roentgen examination only to verify and augment his clinical findings. Too much reliance upon roentgenograms may lead to "sloppy" judgment in selecting treatment or in overlooking soft part lesions, such as nerve palsies. Another reason for careful clinical diagnosis is that some of these injuries occur where it is impossible to get the patient to a hospital for many hours or even longer. An elbow dislocation if seen within fifteen to twenty minutes after injury may be reduced readily by traction alone without the necessity of an anesthetic. This may save the patient many hours of pain and subsequent difficulty from attempts to reduce forcibly the dislocation after swelling and muscle spasm have set in. Reduction of a dislocation on the athletic field may be performed immediately by the team surgeon should he be certain that no

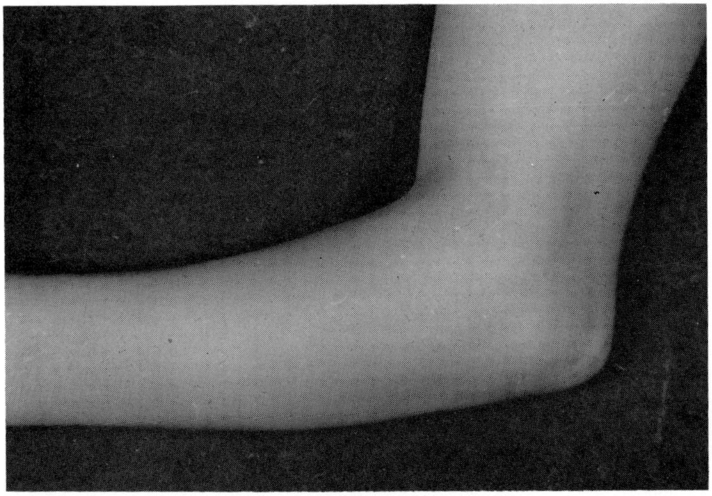

Fig. 23. Photograph of dislocated elbow deformity in a 12 year old boy. Note how the normal convex contours on the posterior aspect of the lower arm and elbow region have been changed to concavities from above downwards and from side to side.

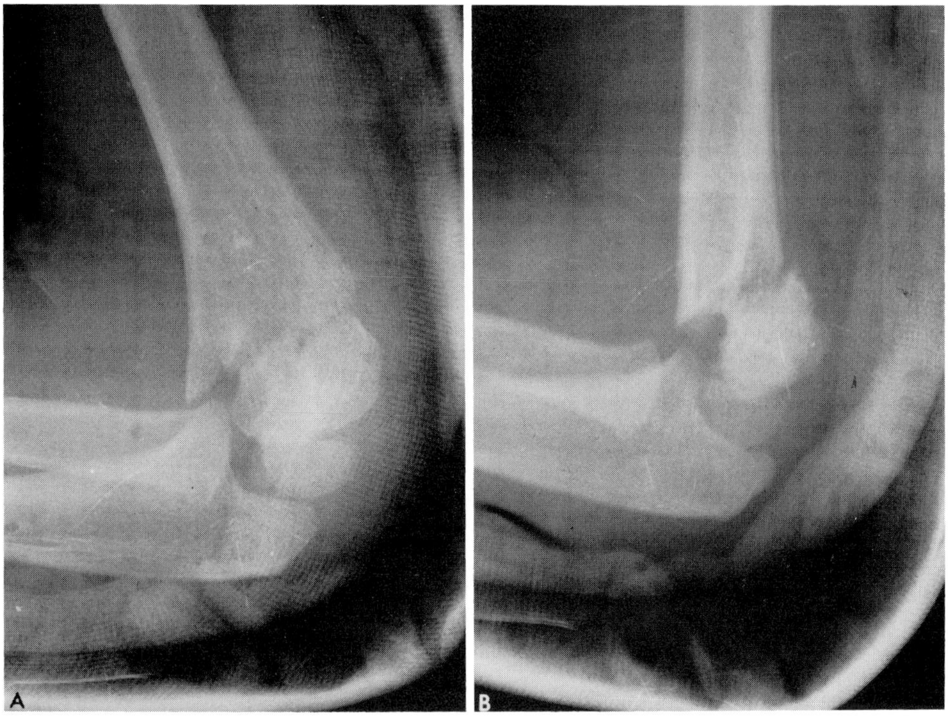

Fig. 24. Roentgenograms of supracondylar fracture of humerus in a six year old girl. (A) Lateral view two days after closed reduction showing rotation deformity. Note "fish-tail" appearance of lower end of humerus which means that it is not in a true lateral projection compared to the distal fragment. If such rotation deformity is allowed to persist, there will result a loss of or reversal of the carrying angle of the elbow. (B) Shows correction of the rotary deformity. A moderate posterior displacement of the distal fragment as noted in this view rarely gives more than a few degrees limitation of flexion as long as the general alignment and rotation are correct. Children do not correct angular or rotary deformities readily by growth.

serious fracture with displacement were present to complicate it. Any dislocation thus performed should be followed by roentgenographic examination to check on possible additional fractures of the radial head or of the medial epicondyle epiphysis with possible displacement into the elbow joint requiring further operative therapy.

Treatment

To simplify the description of treatment of supracondylar fractures it seems advisable to divide these into four main groups for those with minimal or the usual posterior displacement. Those with anterior displacement and those with associated compound wounds will be considered separately.

Posterior Displacement. The four types to be considered are:

A. Fracture with minimal displacement.

B. Fracture with mild displacement.

C. Fracture with moderate displacement.

D. Fracture with complete posterior displacement, angulation, rotation, and over-riding.

The student will do well to study and familiarize himself with the lateral sketches illustrating these four degrees of deformity. (See Figs. 17, 18, 19.) Again, he must realize that intermediate deformities may occur and he should try to formulate an opinion as to the proper treatment for each according to the nearest type into which it falls. Lateral displacement or rotation of the distal fragment of the humerus may occur in any of the types where considerable posterior displacement has occurred.

Rotation deformity in supracondylar fracture is not difficult to recognize if one will remember that on lateral roentgenograms of the elbow the thickness of the distal and shaft fragments should be identical. However, if on such a view the lower end of the shaft fragment appears to broaden out (flare of the supracondylar ridges) giving it the so-called "fish-tail" appear-

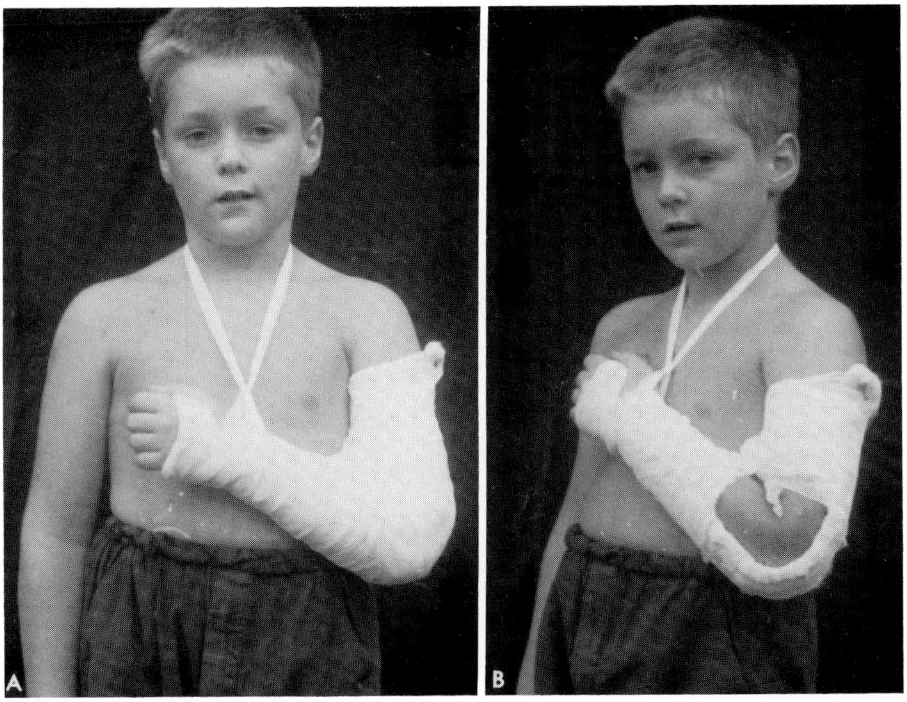

Fig. 25. Photographs showing the posterior moulded plaster splint bandaged in place. The splint should extend from the axillary fold to the metacarpophalangeal joints. If the lower end extends only to the wrist joint, its edge causes pressure and pain over the ulnar head or styloid process. (A) Splint bandaged snugly in position and suspended from neck by a halter or sling. (B) Cut-away view showing how the splint is held securely in place by figure-of-8 bandage which avoids passing through the antecubital fossa, thereby causing no circular constriction to impede the circulation. The gauze projecting from the antecubital fossa keeps the skin surfaces apart and also acts as a wick to assist in evaporation of perspiration. This prevents skin maceration by moisture that would otherwise collect in this area.

ance, while the thickness of the distal fragment remains normal, it is quite obvious that the shaft is being viewed in more of an antero-posterior projection than a lateral one. This means rotation of one fragment upon the other. This same discrepancy of "fish-tail" appearance noted on postreduction lateral films indicates the rotary deformity has not been corrected.

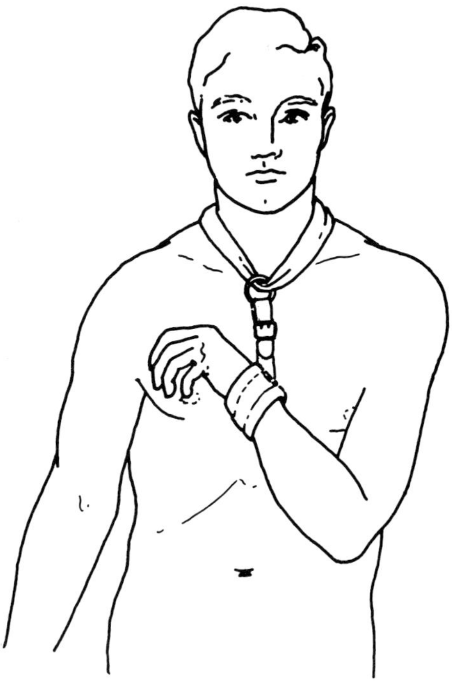

Fig. 26. Sketch showing neck halter and cuff employed to maintain flexion of the elbow.

A. Fracture with Minimal Displacement. Supracondylar fractures with merely a visible crack in the lower humerus, but with less than twenty degrees loss of the normal forward angulation of this portion of bone actually do *not* require reduction of the fragments. At most these need protective immobilization in a posterior molded plaster splint extending from the axilla to the base of the fingers. The elbow should be flexed to an angle of approximately seventy degrees in this splint, and, owing to the lack of excessive swelling in such cases, there is no real risk of compromising the circulation by this amount of flexion. A sling should also be worn to support the weight of the arm and splint. Instead of a splint some surgeons prefer to employ the halter type of sling, suspending the flexed elbow from the wrist (well-padded). Circular plaster casts are unnecessary and dangerous. They do not provide allowance for subsequent swelling, they mask increased swelling, and prohibit active elbow motion. Figure-of-8 adhesive dressings also present the same disadvantages and are difficult to remove later without hurting the child.

Healing is rapid in children, and in fractures of this type immobilization by more than a simple sling is unnecessary after ten days to two weeks. It is best to allow early active motion, for this will permit early return of function without harm. One may be sure that most children will not exercise or use the elbow to the extent of causing pain. Unnecessarily prolonged splinting may greatly delay recovery of function by falsely stressing the importance of the injury. (See After-treatment.)

B. Fracture with Mild Displacement. When the distal fragment of the humerus is angulated to the extent that more than 20 degrees of the normal forward angulation has been lost, it is usually advisable to attempt reduction. Certainly, if there is complete loss of normal forward angulation, reduction *must* be performed, otherwise the patient will be unable to

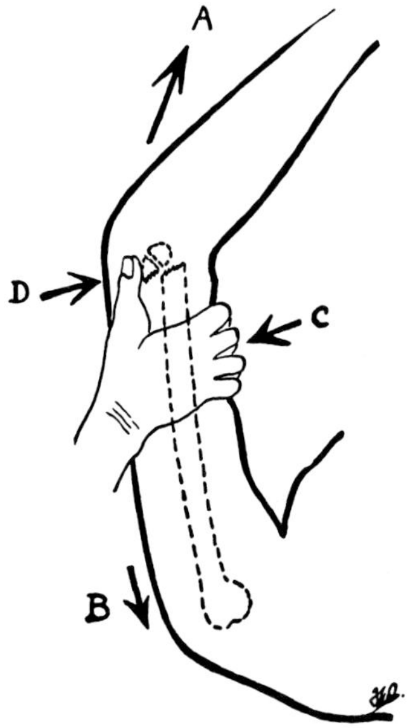

Fig. 27. Sketch showing technique of manual reduction for a supracondylar fracture of the humerus with posterior displacement of the distal fragment. (A) Traction on forearm; (B) counter-traction; (C) posterior push with *flat* of hand (not with finger tips) on proximal fragment; and (D) forward push on distal fragment with one or both thumbs. (Bancroft and Marble: *Surgery of the Motor Skeletal System*. Chap. 32, 2nd Ed., Lippincott, Philadelphia, 1951.)

accommodate for the loss by growth and will have a permanent impairment of elbow flexion of possibly 20 to 30 degrees. At the same time he will gain hyperextension at the elbow, which will serve no useful purpose and may predispose to his sustaining a posterior dislocation from a fall at a later date. If very little flexion needs to be regained, it is occasionally possible to reduce the loss of angulation by slow and steady flexion of the joint to an angle of 60° or 70°. In order to accomplish this the child must be cooperative and the procedure painless. If the manipulation (in flexion) is painful and the elbow cannot be flexed sufficiently, there is no advantage in leaving it thus, since the angulation will not have been corrected. In such case or where there would seem to be considerable pain, it will be best to give the child a short general anesthetic for the reduction manoeuvre. Under anesthesia and with the patient's muscles relaxed the operator may apply direct pressure with his two thumbs to the posterior aspect of the distal fragment and angulate this forward to its proper position. Following such reduction the elbow should be flexed to an angle of 60° or 70°. (See Immobilization and After-treatment.)

In case the greater part of the patient's pain seems due to hemarthrosis of the elbow joint rather than from the fracture, marked relief may be obtained by aspiration of the joint. (See Chapter XIII.)

C. Fractures with Moderate Displacement. In cases with moderate angulation, displacement in one or more directions and rotation of the distal humeral fragment a reduction should always be performed and under a general anesthetic if possible. This avoids all pain, gives complete muscular relaxation and permits the surgeon to perform reduction more easily, more completely and with less force and risk to the patient.

Reduction should be performed by first applying slow, steady traction to the forearm while an assistant gives counter-traction to the upper arm in order to gain relaxation and length. Any medial or lateral displacement of the distal fragment should next be corrected by pushing this in the direction necessary to overcome its displacement and using the other hand to give a "counter-push" upon the shaft in the opposite direction. Posterior displacement and angulation may now be corrected by having the assistant maintain the forearm traction while the operator uses his thumbs on the posterior aspect of the distal fragment and pushes this forward upon the proximal (shaft) fragment. The operator may use the flat surface of his fingers to furnish counter-pressure on the lower shaft in a posterior direction. While doing this he must be careful not to allow his finger tips to concentrate pressure upon the brachial vessels and median nerve, thus traumatizing them against the sharp, ragged lower edge of the shaft fragment.

Under no circumstances should flexion of the elbow be employed to *reduce* a supracondylar fracture when there exists moderate to marked displacement. The use of acute flexion (i. e., the Jones' position) *is for the maintenance of reduction only* and not for the purpose of securing reduction. To flex an elbow before the posteriorly displaced distal fragment in a supracondylar fracture has been brought forward and engaged in its axis with the shaft fragment is definitely harmful and will almost certainly obliterate the circulation, thus bringing on a Volkmann's ischaemia. Flexion of the elbow *following reduction* of this fracture is employed to maintain the reduced fragments in position. Flexion tightens the triceps tendon and muscle which acts as a direct splint on the fragments thus helping to stabilize and jam them together. The posterior molded splint used for immobilization is primarily for the purpose of keeping the elbow in flexion while the triceps furnishes the actual immobilization of the fragments. When the elbow is flexed after reduction this should be to a point at least ten to fifteen degrees short of weakening the radial pulse, which point will vary in different individuals depending upon the amount and tenseness of the soft part swelling accompanying the fracture. It may be possible to flex the elbow to an angle of 50° or 60°, but if much swelling is present it may not be possible to flex it to an angle of less than 75° or 80°. A safe rule to follow is to flex the elbow slowly (while keeping a finger on the radial artery at the wrist to palpate the pulse) until the pulse begins to weaken, then to extend the elbow ten or fifteen degrees until the full volume of the pulse returns. The elbow should therefore not be immobilized in any more acute flexion than at a point thus determined. The reason for leaving such a margin of safety is that swelling has probably not reached a maximum following the injury and because manipulative reduction may add additional trauma and cause added swelling.

Following reduction of the lateral and posterior displacement, the operator should next undertake to correct any rotary deformity. This is performed by manipulation with the thumbs and is best controlled by fluoroscopic check. In order to maintain correct rotary alignment of the two fragments the hand should be directed towards the shoulder joint when flexion of the elbow is performed to maintain reduction. By doing this the fragments are locked and the distal fragment will not be internally rotated upon the proximal. If the hand is brought across the chest as flexion is increased, internal rotation will result which, if left, will give a permanent loss of or a reversed carrying angle. If flexion of the elbow with the hand directed towards the shoulder is completed and the posterior molded splint applied in this position, then the entire splinted arm may be rotated medially to lie along the chest in a sling without the risk of then rotating one fragment separately upon the other. (See Immobilization and After-treatment.)

D. Fracture with Complete Posterior Displacement, Angulation, Rotation, and Over-riding. In supracondylar fractures with marked and complete displacement, angulation and over-riding of the fragments it is often possible to reduce these by closed reduction as described under the less severe type (C). A general anesthetic and firm, steady traction and counter-traction must be employed. The reduction procedure is identical except for correction of the over-riding of the fragments where it may be necessary to hyper-extend the distal fragment (while applying traction) in order to push it forward sufficiently to engage it with the lower end of the shaft fragment. (See Immobilization and After-treatment.)

So far only those supracondylar fractures have been described in which it has been possible to reduce and maintain reduction by ordinary means and which have not been accompanied by difficult procedures or soft part lesions of a serious nature.

Complicated Supracondylar Fractures
(Treatment by Kirschner Wire Skeletal Traction)

Approximately ten percent of supracondylar fractures are of such serious nature that some form of treatment other than the usual attempt at reduction and immobilization must be resorted to in order to secure and maintain reduction without running the risk of Volkmann's ischaemia and paralysis, or other serious complications. The method of treatment to be described employs over-head skeletal traction and suspension to reduce and maintain reduction of the fracture and has practically eliminated the necessity for performing open reduction. In general there are four varieties of serious supracondylar fractures where Kirschner wire traction is indicated.

1. Where it is impossible to reduce the fracture by other closed methods.

2. Where it is possible to reduce the fracture, but impossible to maintain the reduction by flexion without compromising the circulation.

3. Where swelling is excessive, circulatory impairment is present, or Volkmann's ischaemia already threatens.

4. Where associated lesions are present such as compounding of the fracture, additional fractures in the same extremity, or paralysis of a nerve.

The advantages of the Kirschner wire traction method are:

1. Skeletal traction is more effective than skin traction in reducing or maintaining reduction.

2. It does not require acute flexion of the elbow to maintain reduction, thus offering no impediment to the circulation.

3. No constrictive bandages or dressings are needed.
4. The injured extremity is kept highly elevated, thus permitting gravity to assist both the venous and lymphatic circulation in reduction of the swelling.
5. The patient remains under direct observation in the hospital and cannot fall and re-injure himself.
6. Early active elbow joint motion can be permitted in traction and suspension without risk of loss of reduction of the fragments.
7. Roentgenographic or fluoroscopic check-up for position of the fragments may be made as frequently as is necessary or desired.
8. Heat may be applied in the early stages to assist the circulation.
9. The method of treatment is comfortable which is especially important in children.
10. It allows access for change of dressings or inspection of an open (compound) wound without the risk of losing position of the fragments.
11. It does not interfere with the use of splints for other fractures or a cock-up splint for radial nerve palsy if desired.

Method of Application. With strict aseptic technique and under general anesthesia a small incision (three millimeters long) is made on the medial aspect of the ulna three centimeters below the tip of the olecranon in order to avoid its epiphyseal plate. A No. 13 needle is then introduced until its point reaches the posterior crest of the ulna. An assistant holds the point of this needle on the bone, but moves the whole needle anteriorly, thus crowding the soft tissues (muscles and ulnar nerve) away from the posterior crest. While the needle is thus held transversely with its point against the side of the ulna, it is used as a cannula and the Kirschner wire is inserted into its barrel, drilled through the bone, and brought out on the lateral side. Sterile dressings are applied to the skin at the sites of entry and emergence of the wire. A traction yoke is fastened to the wire and the latter tightened.

The arm should then be placed in traction and suspension according to Figure 28. It will be noted that the traction weight applied to the Kirschner wire (A) causes a pull in a distal and forward direction upon the lower fragment, while that applied to the swathe around the upper arm (B) forces the shaft fragment posteriorly. Body weight furnishes counter-traction. The swathe under the forearm furnishes support and counter-balances it. The operator may wish to manipulate the fragments once the traction and suspension have been set up in order to facilitate reduction. If it is impossible to accomplish satisfactory reduction at this time, another attempt may be made at the end of twenty-four or 48 hours of traction. Frequently it is thus possible to accomplish reduction under anesthesia (if the traction itself has not secured it) by simply giving a forward push to the lower fragment. Rotary displacement may be corrected by changing the transverse axis of the forearm and this may be checked by the fluoroscope. The amount of traction weight needed on the wire varies with the size of the child, but is

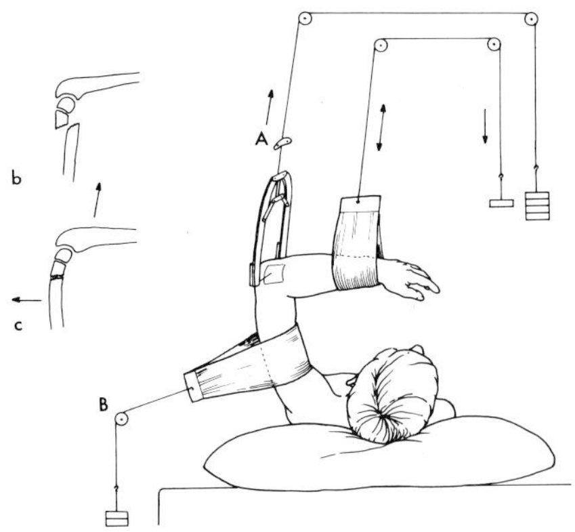

Fig. 28. Overhead skeletal traction and suspension by means of Kirschner wire through olecranon. This method plus manipulation helps to bring about reduction of the fragments and the traction maintains the fragments in the reduced position. (A) Traction on wire in olecranon; (B) pull to keep shaft of humerus in a posterior position if necessary. High elevation assists gravity drainage of veins and lymphatics and gets rid of excessive swelling rapidly. Note that the position of acute flexion is not necessary to maintain reduction achieved by this method; also note absence of constricting bandages around elbow. Insets (b, c) show position of fragments before and after reduction by this method. (SMITH, F. M.: Traction and suspension in the treatment of fractures. *Surg. Clin. North America*, Saunders, Philadelphia, April, 1951.)

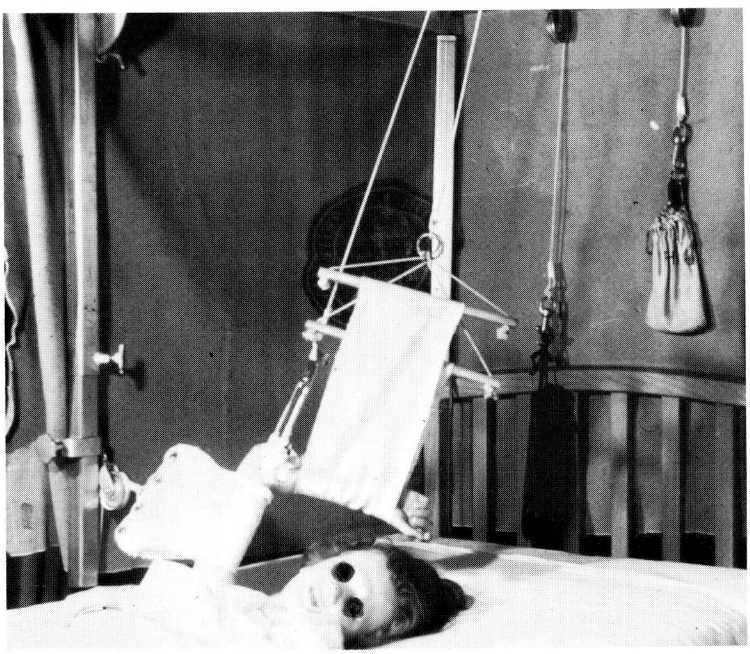

Fig. 28-A. An 8 year old girl with arm suspended over-head by means of a Kirschner wire through the olecranon and with a swathe affecting a posterior pull on the shaft of the humerus. Note how the swelling and congestion of the injured part is assisted by the high elevation.

usually about four to six pounds. Over-pull (distraction) of the fragments can best be detected by roentgenograms and guarded against by decreasing the traction weight.

The patients should be kept in this form of traction and suspension until good evidence of callus formation along the posterior margin of the humerus can be seen on lateral roentgenograms. This takes about two weeks on the average. At this point the Kirschner wire may be removed and the elbow immobilized in a posterior molded splint without fear of compromising the pulse.

In a series of thirty-nine cases thus treated, reviewed and published by the author in 1947 not a single case of Volkmann's paralysis developed. (See Immobilization and After-treatment.)

Dunlop Traction for Supracondylar Fractures

Another excellent method of skin traction as described by Dunlop may be used for handling difficult and complicated supracondylar fractures. This method is carried out with the patient in bed with adhesive traction applied to the skin of the forearm. The upper arm over-hangs the side of the bed and the forearm, which is in supination, is suspended in traction by a rope and pulley attached to a frame at the side of the bed. The direction of traction maintains the forearm in an angle of approximately 135° with the arm, i. e., it exerts traction in a distal and forward direction. A swathe and weight applied to the horizontal upper arm exerts pressure upon the shaft of the humerus in a posterior direction. Body weight acts as counter-traction, consequently the bed must be tilted towards the uninjured side. It will be seen that the purpose of traction by this method to gain and maintain

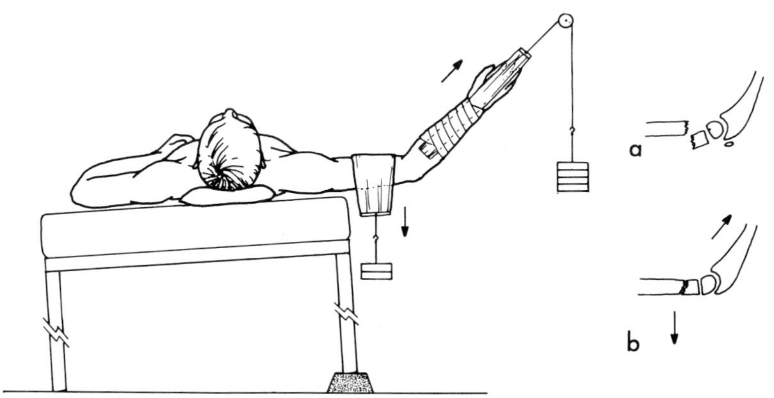

Fig. 29. Dunlop's method of applying skin traction for supracondylar fractures with displacement and/or circulatory impairment. Counter-traction is obtained by tilting bed to opposite side with shock blocks and utilizing body weight for this. Insets (a, b) show position of fragments before and after reduction by this method. (Smith, F. M.: Traction and suspension in the treatment of fractures. *Surg. Clin. North America,* Saunders, Philadelphia, April, 1951.)

reduction is the same as with over-head Kirschner wire traction. It also has many of the same advantages except that the injured elbow is not so highly elevated. It would seem to be just as safe a method and just as efficacious in avoiding the risk of Volkmann's ischaemia.

Immobilization for Supracondylar Fractures

In general it is necessary only to immobilize the elbow in acute flexion in order to maintain reduction of a supracondylar fracture, assuming that it has been possible to reduce the fragments prior to attempting flexion. It is this position of flexion utilizing the tensed triceps as a direct splint that maintains the reduction. Consequently, any method of immobilization that keeps the elbow flexed will likewise keep the fragments reduced. Some methods, however, are safe, while others are dangerous in the period of acute swelling.

Circular plaster-of-Paris casts and figure-of-8 adhesive dressings should never be used immediately after reduction to maintain flexion since they are non-elastic, constricting, and mask swelling to the point of permitting it to reach dangerous proportions. Besides these dangers neither of these two means offers any more efficient immobilization than do simpler and less dangerous ones.

Perfectly safe means for immobilization of an elbow in the flexed position are slings, neck halters, and the posterior molded plaster-of-Paris splint. Many supracondylar fractures without any displacement need no more fixation than that afforded by a simple sling made of muslin or a kerchief. Neck halters may be made by suspending the well padded wrist from the neck by means of a bandage or even by rubber tubing. A sling or halter will

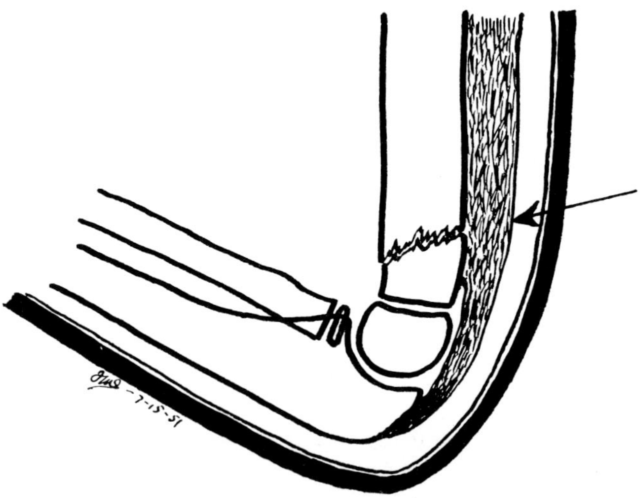

Fig. 30. Sketch showing triceps muscle (arrow) acting as a direct splint on posterior surface of humerus when the elbow is flexed *following* reduction of a supracondylar fracture.

permit the patient to practice a small amount of elbow flexion, but prevents extension of the joint beyond the position in which it is suspended. Active flexion by the patient will not disturb the reduced bone fragments. It is also possible for the surgeon to increase the amount of elbow flexion by shortening the sling or halter when swelling has decreased if he feels that by so doing the position of the fragments may be improved.

The Posterior Molded Splint

For the majority of supracondylar fractures requiring reduction and immobilization the posterior molded splint made of plaster-of-Paris is advisable. This type of splint has the advantage that it can be molded to fit any size patient before the plaster has "set." Therefore, if properly made (see below)

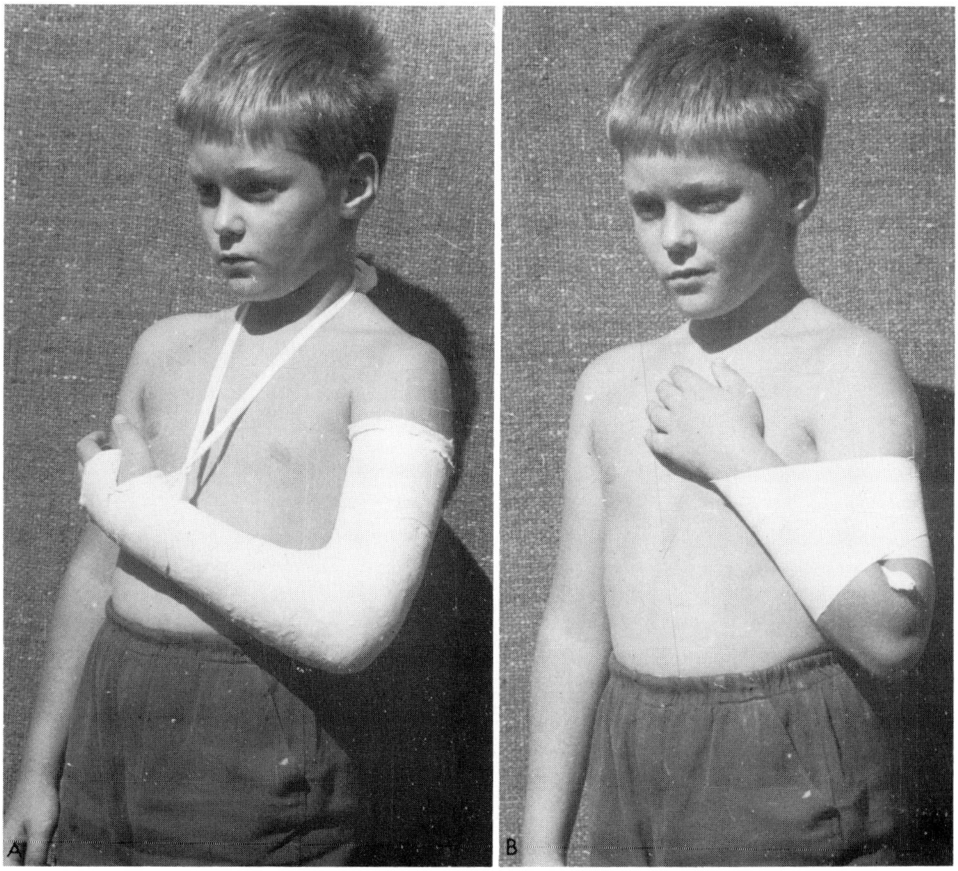

Fig. 31. "Splints" to be *avoided* after reduction of supracondylar fractures of the humerus or after other acute elbow injuries. (A) The circular plaster-of-Paris cast offers no "safety valve" for swelling which always continues to increase following reduction unless the elbow is highly elevated. It may increase congestion and help to cause ischaemia in spite of being well padded. It definitely hides the underlying pathology and delays early correction of complications by virtue of keeping the surgeon unaware that they are occurring. (B) The figure-of-8 adhesive strap dressing if not kept under close and frequent observation, because it is non-yielding and will increase congestion, swelling and bleb formation. It is difficult to remove because of pain.

it should have no rough edges or creases to irritate the skin or cause pressure sores over bony prominences. The splint is light in weight, may be easily removed for inspection of swelling, condition of the skin, and may be re-applied without altering its shape. The bandage holding the splint in place may be cut or loosened to accommodate for any increased or persistent swelling of the soft parts. The bandage may be applied in a figure-of-8 fashion over the splinted elbow so that it bridges the antecubital fossa, cannot cut into the swollen soft parts, or into the posterior aspect of the arm or forearm (see Fig. 25). The splint should extend from the posterior axillary fold to just proximal to the metacarpo-phalangeal joints. If it is made shorter so that it reaches only to the wrist joint, the weight of the hand will cause the latter to rest on the distal edge of the splint. Irritation of the skin from localized pressure will result. Prominence of the ulnar head resting on this same edge will likewise be uncomfortable and may cause a localized pressure area or even skin necrosis.

Preparation of the Posterior Molded Splint. The width of a molded splint will vary according to the size of the patient's arm. In young children up to six or seven years of age (unless very obese) a splint two inches wide is adequate; in larger children and in adults the splint is better if made from plaster three inches wide. Rarely is it ever necessary to use four inch plaster. The desired length of the splint is first determined by measurement of the flexed uninjured arm—posterior axillary fold to knuckles of hand. A layer of Canton flannel one inch wider than the plaster and three inches longer is cut and laid upon a board or other firm support with its fuzzy surface down. The plaster bandage is then rolled out dry, layering it back and forth the full length of the Canton flannel for a total of twelve to fourteen layers in thickness. (Plaster splints always shrink slightly when wet.) The plaster is then gathered up and dipped quickly and completely in luke-warm water; the excess water is quickly squeezed out, and the wet splint stretched out its full length on a board and rubbed back and forth to smooth it and rid it of air bubbles. It is then placed upon the Canton flannel and the edges of the latter folded over the edges of the wet plaster and pressed down.

Application of the Molded Splint. The splint is now ready for application. The soft (fuzzy) side of the flannel should be placed next to the skin. An assistant holds the splint at its upper and lower ends in its proper position upon the reduced elbow. The operator (or other assistant) should then bandage the splint smoothly and quickly to the entire arm, elbow, forearm and hand. In doing so it is important to keep the bandage flat where it passes over the wet splint. If it is necessary to twist or reverse the bandage, this should be done over the patient's skin so that it will mold the splint smoothly, evenly, and without any depressed creases in it. As soon as the plaster has "set" the splint must be rebandaged because the wet bandage will shrink upon drying and constrict the circulation. Rebandaging of the splint may be done by removing only a part of the original bandage at a time without fear of losing the reduction. After the arm and forearm portions are securely rebandaged, care being taken not to apply any circular layers of bandage in contact with the front of the elbow, a figure-of-8 may be made to bridge the front of the arm and forearm to act as a check-rein to prevent loss of flexion and to keep subsequent circular layers off the skin. By doing thus, dangerous constriction is avoided and subsequent swelling may occur without great risk of bleb formation. This will also permit inspection of the antecubital area for swelling, bleb formation if it occurs, and cleansing and powdering of the skin to prevent maceration from perspiration. If swelling should be discovered on the increase, the check-rein may be cut and re-applied with the elbow in slightly less flexion. Should swelling subside rapidly after three or four days allowing the splint to loosen, it may be re-bandaged more snugly and flexion increased by shortening the check-rein. If the patient is ambulatory the splinted arm should always be supported in a sling.

After-care for Supracondylar Fractures

The after-care for supracondylar fractures may be fairly well standardized so that it applies to those receiving closed reduction, reduction by traction and suspension, and open reduction for open (compound) fractures.

The milder forms of fracture with little or no displacement and not requiring manipulative reduction need not be kept immobilized for more than 10 to 14 days in a splint. Active exercises under guidance may be started certainly at the end of the first week. The patient should be seen and the splint and circulation inspected and evaluated the day after application. If no excess swelling or pain is present on this visit, he may not need to be seen again for two or three days. If swelling and pain are present, the dressing may have to be loosened, and the patient ought to be seen daily thereafter until his condition has definitely improved. An interval of a week between visits at this stage is too long (even if the patient is comfortable), because it may be advisable to snug up on the splint in order to prevent loss of elbow flexion.

It is a wise and safe rule to admit to the hospital every patient with a supracondylar fracture that has required manipulative reduction of the fragments even if no impairment of the circulation or excess swelling exists. The reason is that an increase in swelling always takes place during the first twelve to twenty-four hours following reduction. It may only be necessary to keep the patient in the hospital over-night for observation and elevation of the injured arm. With the patient in the hospital, his pulse, swelling, color, temperature and motion of his fingers can be *and should be* evaluated every hour and measures may be quickly taken to correct impairment if necessary before it is too late. If the patient has been allowed home, the parents cannot be expected to know when dangerous signs or symptoms present themselves. They may feel sorry for the child because of his suffering and loss of sleep and may fail to bring him back the following day, in order to give him some rest—not realizing that he may be developing a Volkmann's ischaemia and paralysis. A delay of six hours with a markedly impaired circulation may be all that is necessary to bring on such a condition. Had the child been in the hospital with such persistent pain, swelling, and weakened pulse, measures could have been taken to loosen constrictive bandages, decrease elbow flexion, give the arm higher elevation, or even to resort to Kirschner wire or Dunlop traction. If necessary through failure of any of these methods to bring back the pulse, operative exploration or splitting of the fascia might have to be performed.

The injured elbow should always be elevated upon a pillow so that it is higher than the patient's shoulder. At times suspension of the splinted elbow helps to keep down excessive swelling. Low intensity heat (goose-neck desk lamp) may be applied to the swollen area. The patient should be kept in the hospital until all danger from swelling has passed. He should then be given an appointment to the clinic or office at an early date for check-up.

The length of splinting necessary for supracondylar fractures with moderate displacement is approximately three weeks; for those with marked displacement splinting for four weeks to a full month is entirely adequate.

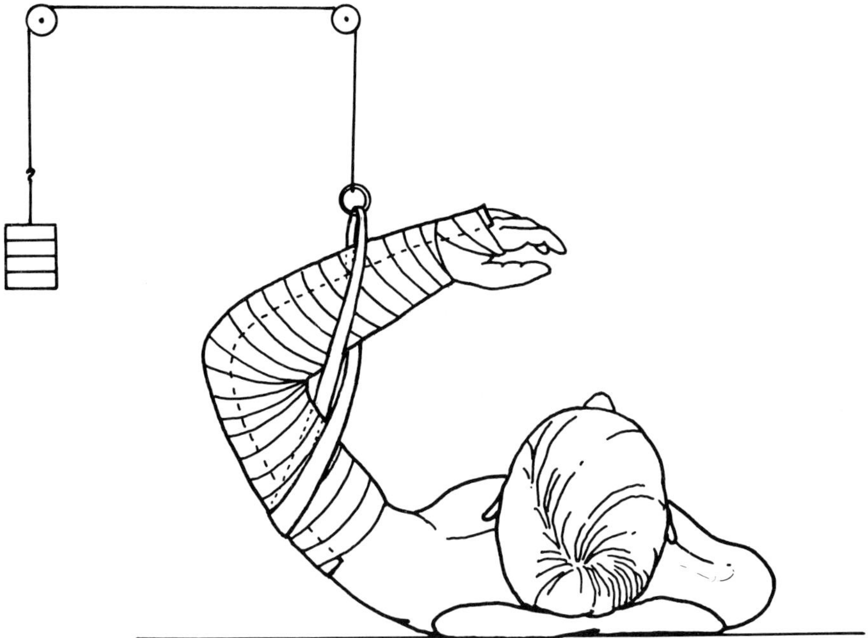

Fig. 32. Sketch showing method of obtaining *positive* elevation of a splinted elbow following reduction to reduce and/or prevent excessive swelling. The suspension sling is applied after the posterior molded plaster splint has hardened, so that its pressure is diffused and not concentrated in a small localized area. Therefore there results no pressure area or constricting band to cause pain or impede return circulation. This same sling entwines the splinted arm and forearm in a figure-of-8 fashion, consequently the extremity cannot fall out of it.

This applies as well to those cases treated by traction and suspension. To splint these cases for longer periods than mentioned permits much of the soft part thickening to become permanent through fibrosis and leads to delayed recovery or even permanent loss of function. (This is not merely the author's personal opinion; it is the opinion and experience resulting from a careful review of over 650 consecutive cases of supracondylar fracture treated on the Fracture Service of the Presbyterian Hospital, New York City.)

Active elbow motion should be instituted in these cases just as soon as the surgeon feels that there is no longer any danger of the fragments slipping. This is usually between the second and third week. The fragments may bend or "give" if allowed to go unprotected for prolonged periods, but they will not slip readily after two and one-half weeks, since children form callus early in this particular type of fracture. The best means of getting the patient to move his elbow actively is for the surgeon to sit down with him, carefully supporting the forearm portion of the splint after the bandage has been removed. The patient, at first apprehensive, will see that no harm is intended, and can be persuaded to flex his elbow slightly, especially if the wrist is supported while he does it. This is to prevent it from falling back suddenly into the splint and causing him pain. After this has been performed a half dozen times, the splint and sling should be re-applied. The patient should return every two or three days following this and have the same procedure repeated, with slightly increased range of motion encouraged each time. By the time the splint has been discarded the patient frequently will have an arc of active motion of at least forty-five degrees and will not be afraid to wear a sling only. While wearing the sling he may be permitted flexion exercises as often as desired and may be allowed to remove his arm from the sling half a dozen times a day to practice extension exercises.

Usually by the end of the fifth or sixth week the sling may be discarded and the patient permitted mild active use. He should not be put on a regular time schedule for exercises and should not be made to do exercises an exact number of times. The patient is his best judge as to how far he will exercise the elbow. Under no circumstances will he move it beyond the limits that cause pain. If the patient does not seem to be improving in his range of motion, passive motion (stretching, pump-handling, etc.) *should very definitely not be attempted,* since it will cause pain, over-stretching of infiltrated and inelastic muscle, and predisposes to the formation of myositis ossificans. The carrying of heavy weights (flat-iron, dumb-bell, or buckets of sand or water) should likewise be frowned upon as a method of gaining extension in the elbow. This is just another method of applying passive manipulation and causes pain and involuntary spasm on the part of the patient, thus delaying recovery of his active motion. Diathermy and massage are practically worthless following supracondylar fractures in children and very frequently cause harm and delayed recovery. If the child refuses to use his elbow or to regain active motion after eight to ten weeks, the one "trick" that may be tried with advantage is to tie up his good arm *inside his shirt* so that he cannot get it out and must use his injured arm for play and for eating. Some children, if seen often in the clinic or office, become impressed with the "seriousness" of their injury even after solid bony healing has taken place. They will permit themselves to take treatments (diathermy, etc.) regularly for months without showing the slightest improvement in function. It will be noted that in the intervals between treatments these patients do little or nothing to help themselves regain function. If such a stage is reached, it is often best to cancel all further visits to the clinic or office, put the patient on "follow-up" and give him an appointment not earlier than three months hence. In the meantime one must advise the parents to let the child play at will with others and not to caution him about his condition. It is a pleasant surprise to see how much improvement will be made more frequently than not by such a regime.

Operative Treatment

Except for open (compound) fractures open reduction in supracondylar fractures of the humerus in children is *rarely* indicated. It used to be common practice in many clinics to operate upon all badly displaced supracondylar fractures where there was impairment of the circulation. This was performed in the belief that the deep fascia could be left open in order to decompress it and get rid of the hemorrhage and edema beneath which was responsible for venous stasis; also for the purpose of relieving pressure of the proximal fragment upon the brachial vessels by reducing the fragments under direct vision; and because it was felt that this was one certain method of preventing Volkmann's ischaemic paralysis. It has since been learned that open reduction does not necessarily prevent Volkmann's ischaemia or even guarantee that the reduction of the fragments can be maintained. Besides, open reduction may predispose to growth disturbance in the lower epiphysis of the humerus, and, if performed a week or more after injury, it may very likely cause a myositis ossificans. With the increased usage of Kirschner wire skeletal traction and Dunlop skin traction in these serious fractures there is rarely any need for operative reduction. The circulatory embarrassment can be overcome by either form of traction and a reduction of satisfactory (if not perfect) quality can be obtained and maintained by traction.

Once in a great while a supracondylar fracture may be encountered which shows marked displacement which can be easily reduced and remains reduced as long as the elbow is kept acutely flexed and direct forward pressure with the thumbs is made continuously upon the lower fragment; however, when this pressure is removed, the distal fragment again slips posteriorly. These cases are rare, but the circumstances indicate that periosteum is interposed between the fragments, preventing the one from locking upon the other. If two or three immediate attempts to reduce such a fracture result in no success, it may be justified to perform open reduction. The surgeon should remember, however, that less than one percent of supracondylar fractures in children require open reduction. See Fig. 19 (A).

In cases of open (compound) supracondylar fracture the displacement of the fragments is usually great, circulation is often impaired and nerves are not infrequently involved. The wound of "compounding" is most often situated in the region of the anterior flexion crease of the elbow. Operation should be performed in these cases—not because of the fracture, but because of the contaminated wound communicating with it. This should be performed immediately and in a regular hospital operating room and not in the office or emergency clinic.

Very careful preparation of the skin surrounding the compound wound should be carried out by scrubbing with green soap and sterile water for five minutes, followed by alcohol and ether. The skin wound must be covered with a sterile compress while the above preparation is being performed. The extremity should then be painted with alcohol again or with a mild skin antiseptic and draped with sterile linen as for a perfectly clean operation. The operative technique consists first of excising the lacerated, contaminated, and devitalized skin edges in toto with a sharp scalpel. The instruments used for this must be discarded and the wound should be lavaged thoroughly and forcefully with normal saline solution, care being taken to wash from the center of the wound outwards and not to allow fluid to run from the adjacent skin into the wound. While the wound is thus being lavaged it is justifiable to sponge its surface gently with a wet compress in order to help loosen and remove particles of adherent dirt. The debridement must then be continued to include contaminated and devitalized bits of subcutaneous fat and deep fascia. Lavage with saline is again performed. Further debridement of torn and devitalized muscle tissue and periosteum is then performd and all tissue spaces (potential pockets for the collection of hematoma and bacteria) must be laid wide open. Careful hemostasis is important and careful removal of all devitalized tissue is likewise important; if hemostasis is poor and blood collects deep in the wound, or if devitalized tissue is left behind, both enhance the proliferation of pathogenic bacteria. Important nerves, blood vessels and tendons must of course be left, but the debridement should otherwise be complete. Lavage is again performed before reduction of the bony fragments is attempted. The fragments may now be manipulated into position under direct vision and the elbow flexed to hold this position. It is best not to suture the wound primarily. Sutures may be laid, but left untied while the wound is gently packed open with fine mesh gauze. A secondary closure may be carried out after five or six days. At the termination of the operation a Kirschner wire may be placed through the olecranon for skeletal traction when the patient is returned to his bed. Dunlop traction may be applied instead if the operator prefers.

Penicillin may be given intramuscularly after operation if desired, *but as an adjunct only* to lessen the risk of infection. Under no circumstances must the surgeon curtail his operative debridement in the belief that chemotherapy will make up for his lack of thoroughness. As a matter of fact it is rarely necessary to give chemotherapy in this type of upper extremity compound fracture, since with careful debridement and lavage they almost never become infected. This, of course, is quite the opposite of experience with compound fractures in the lower leg. Tetanus antitoxin ought to be given after first testing for skin sensitivity and if necessary after desensitization.

Supracondylar Fractures with Anterior Displacement of the Lower Fragment

Anterior displacement of the distal fragment in a supracondylar fracture of the humerus is extremely rare and occurs in less than two percent of such fractures. (See Fig. 20.) It usually results from a fall, striking directly upon the posterior aspect of the elbow and lower humerus. Several differences may be noted from those with posterior displacement. First, the deformity is different. The forearm appears slightly elongated and the elbow does not have the characteristic backward bulge as in posterior displacements. Second, there is never the serious threat to the circulation as in the usual type, because the brachial vessels become pushed forward and are not stretched over the sharp end of the shaft fragment or kinked between it and the distal one by flexion.

Treatment. This will depend upon the amount of actual displacement of the fragment. If this be slight, it is only necessary to immobilize the elbow in a posterior molded splint in extension rather than in flexion. If displacement be complete, manipulative reduction under anesthesia is indicated and should be accomplished by traction and counter-traction and by forcing the distal fragment posteriorly until it engages with the proximal one. The position for immobilization is usually in full extension. Very rarely it may be possible to utilize the flexed position for immobilization after reduction, but fluoroscopic check will best determine which position is the better. If by any chance, the surgeon should decide to immobilize the elbow in flexion, the radial pulse must be carefully and frequently checked for the next 24 hours. Patients upon whom reduction has been performed should be admitted to the hospital so that any complications may be watched for and given immediate care should they arise. If any rotation deformity is present this should be corrected at the same time as the anterior displacement.

The after-treatment is essentially the same as with other supracondylar fractures with a similar degree of displacement.

Unreduced Supracondylar Fractures

It is sometimes impossible to obtain anatomical reduction of the supracondylar fragments by any means, including open reduction. Other cases may be seen in which the original reduction was excellent, but owing to loosening of the splint as swelling recedes or because of over-activity of the patient in traction after pain has disappeared, the lower fragment of the humerus becomes angulated or even displaced again posteriorly. This is often very disturbing to the surgeon and to the parents of the child. If the recurrence of the deformity is discovered early, i. e., within four or five days after the initial injury, it may be corrected by another manipulation under anesthesia, or, if the case is having traction treatment, the amount of traction may be increased and the axis of pull directed in a more anterior direction while an increased pull in the posterior direction is placed upon the swathe applied to the humeral shaft. If correction is not readily obtained by either one of these means, undue force should not be used and further attempts should not be repeated over a period of several days. These will only cause harm and will almost certainly result in the formation of myositis ossificans in the brachialis anticus muscle. Even when the distal fragment becomes re-displaced as much as fifty percent, it may under these circumstances be advisable to leave it, provided the circulation to the forearm and hand are not compromised. It is certainly a much wiser decision for the surgeon to "leave well enough alone" than to insist upon obtaining complete anatomical restoration of the fragments at the highly probable price of incurring myositis ossificans. These fractures lay down callus early and heal rapidly and that is the reason for the inability to reduce them after five days to a week have passed. These children more often than not will tend to out-grow some of the deformity, and, if encouraged to begin active exercises of the elbow no later than three or four weeks, will often regain all but ten to fifteen degrees of flexion.

Should the loss of reduction be so great that the distal fragment completely over-rides the proximal and the circulation is seriously impaired, it would be far safer to perform open reduction three or four days after injury than to attempt further closed manipulation. It is important to check the position of the fragments at this time by roentgenograms, so that further corrective procedures may be done before it becomes too late and too risky. Should the loss of position not be discovered until ten days to two weeks following the original injury, it may be futile to attempt correction by closed methods; and, to perform open reduction at this stage when active new bone production is at its height, will result almost certainly in the formation of myositis ossificans. Should the deformity be discovered at this stage or later, it will be best to leave it entirely alone, and put the patient on a regime of active exercises and use as soon as possible in order to allow him to regain as much joint function as possible. If with growth and constant use marked limitation of function should result and give the patient a real disability, operative correction (osteotomy or ostectomy) can always be performed at a much later date (one year or more) without the risk of his developing this complication.

Late Deformities Following Supracondylar Fracture

Operative Correction. The deformities following supracondylar fracture may result from incomplete reduction or from growth disturbance in the lower epiphyseal plate of the humerus. Those from incomplete reduction are the cubitus varus ("gun-stock") deformity where the carrying angle is markedly reversed, or the flexion block deformity due to persistent posterior displacement of the distal fragment which was never reduced or which slipped following reduction. Cubitus varus deformity may result from incomplete correction of an original rotary displacement in which case the deformity is noted early. On the other hand a cubitus varus deformity may result from injury to the lower humeral epiphysis, which through subsequent growth allows the lateral condyle to grow more rapidly than the medial condyle. This deformity is likely to be progressive over a period of three or four years and may be detected by careful yearly measurements of the carrying angle with the elbow fully extended. It is extremely unlikely for a cubitus valgus deformity to occur following supracondylar fracture in

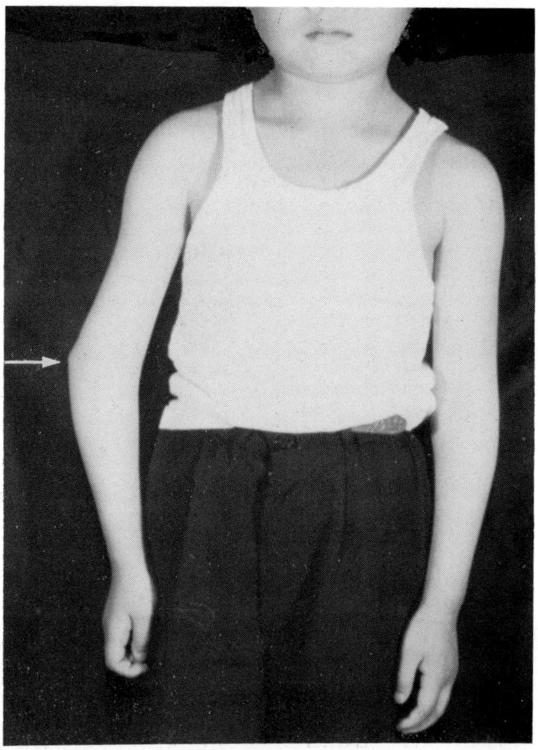

Fig. 33. Cubitus varus (gun-stock) deformity of right elbow following an incompletely reduced supracondylar fracture of the humerus.

contradistinction to its common occurrence following fracture of the lateral humeral condyle in children.

Treatment of Cubitus Varus Deformity. Should the deformity become so marked that the reversed carrying angle measures twenty-five degrees or greater, it may be wise to perform operative correction especially in girls, who desire a more perfect cosmetic result. Such a reversed carrying angle looks ugly and makes the patient appear awkward. It practically never interferes with elbow joint function.

Operative correction should consist of an osteotomy of the lower humerus with removal of a wedge of bone the base of which must line on the lateral side. To determine how wide the base of this wedge should be in order to correct and bring the axis of the lower humerus and forearm back to a normal carrying angle the operator will do well to make a tracing of the antero-posterior roentgenogram showing the deformity. This should be cut out with scissors to leave the mere outline of the bones on paper. A transverse cut is then made in this tracing just above the condyles of the humerus. By angulating the distal fragment and forearm laterally until the ideal correction is reached, it is a simple matter to measure the exact angle of the wedge of bone to be removed by osteotomy. Such a trial procedure may save the surgeon much worry and difficulty during the operative procedure and assure him of greater accuracy in his ultimate correction. The operation should not be performed in young children, but should be postponed (even in bad deformities) until the bones have reached or nearly reached full growth.

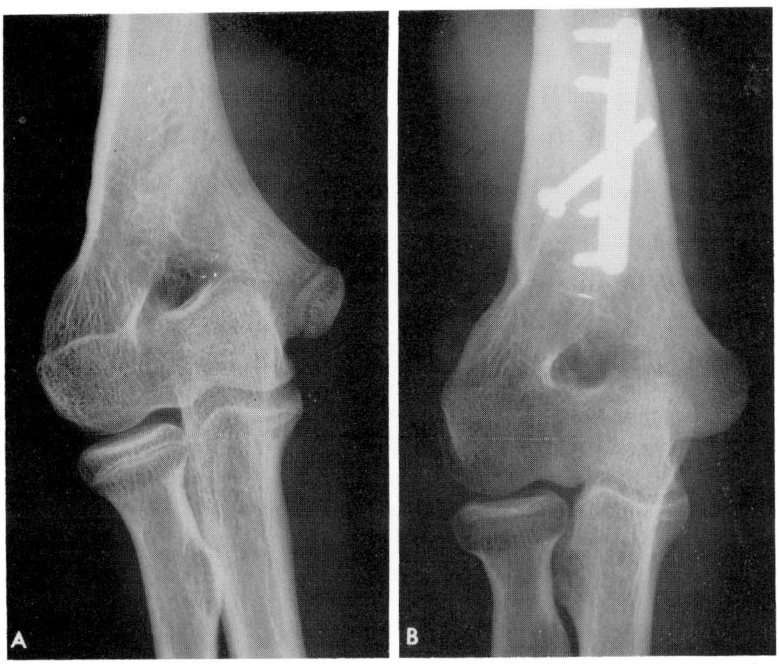

Fig. 34. Cubitus varus deformity. Roentgenograms, (A) before correction; and (B) after osteotomy and correction (see Fig. 35).

The technique of operation is carried out by making a posterior or postero-lateral incision. The triceps tendon and muscle may be split longitudinally and the two halves retracted to expose the posterior aspect of the lower humerus at its junction with the condyles. Should the operator prefer, he may use the Van Gorder type of incision which dissects a long tongue of triceps tendon downwards and splits the underlying muscle (Chapter XVII). The level for the osteotomy is then chosen which is at the junction of the shaft and condyles and which is sufficiently low to avoid the radial nerve. The periosteum should likewise be split, elevated and retracted to beyond the lateral and medial margins of the bone. The osteotomy wedge is then marked out on the posterior aspect of the bone with its angle on the medial side and with its base on the lateral side. The wedge may be marked by a sharp broad osteotome, after which drill holes should be made along the two sides, close together, and through the entire thickness of the bone. The osteotome is then used to complete the osteotomy and removal of the wedge. Any projecting spurs that might interfere with apposition of the raw ends in the corrected position may be cut off with a rongeur.

There will be some who will criticize the author for advising the use of internal fixation of the fragment following osteotomy, but it would seem to be highly advisable provided adequate and rigid fixation is to be employed. The reasons for this are: (1) the osteotomy is not performed in young children; (2) if the surgeon is to take the trouble to perform osteotomy for correction of a bad deformity and subjects the patient to such a

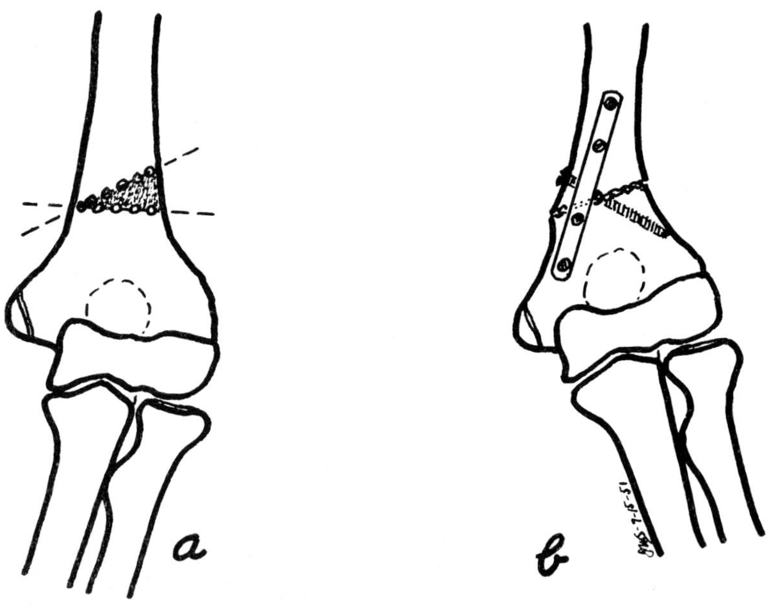

Fig. 35. Sketch showing: (a) cubitus varus deformity of elbow and site of wedge-shaped osteotomy of humerus; and (b) after correction and internal fixation of fragments.

risk, he ought to be able to assure the patient that the deformity is not only corrected, but will remain so; (3) with rigid internal fixation by plate and screws additional plaster immobilization for a long period of time is not necessary; and (4) gentle active exercises and motion may be begun after two weeks, with greatly increased chances of full functional recovery. The exposures advocated give adequate room for the application of a plate and screws and even an additional transfixation screw which will increase the rigidity of fixation and is thus highly advisable. Wire loops should not be used at this site for internal fixation, for the leverage is too great and may cause breakage or loosening and lead to non-union. Plaster-of-Paris immobilization alone is often used, but the results are frequently far from satisfactory.

Operative correction for gun-stock deformity is an operation not to be undertaken without due consideration of the hazards involved and the careful technique required for success.

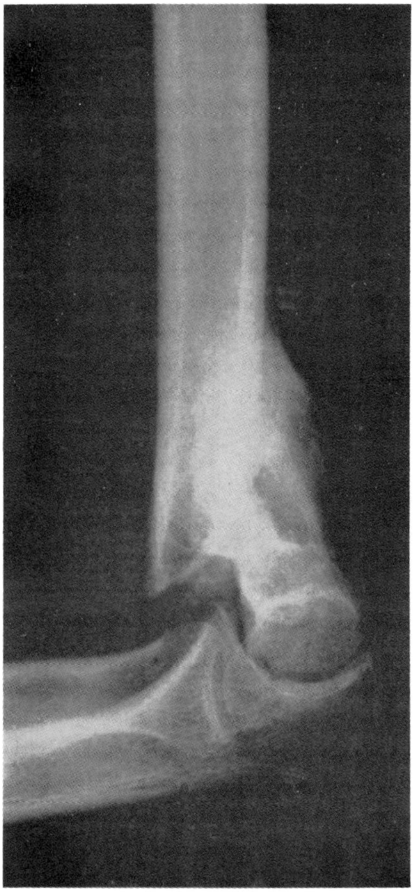

Fig. 36. Flexion block at elbow following fracture of lower extremity of humerus. Resection of the anterior projecting end of shaft may be indicated (see Fig. 37).

Treatment of Flexion Block Deformity. This deformity due to backward displacement of the distal humeral fragment allowing the lower end of the shaft fragment to project forward and interfere with flexion of the forearm may in very young children become corrected by growth and use. In older children or young adults the anterior projecting shaft may not be absorbed with growth and may cause a real mechanical block to flexion. It is in these latter cases chiefly that operation is indicated.

The operative approach should be anterior and may pass medial or lateral to the biceps tendon depending upon which side the bony prominence is more evident. If approached medially, the median nerve and brachial vessels must be identified and retracted further medially; if approached laterally, the interval between the brachioradialis and biceps muscle must be entered, the radial nerve identified and retracted laterally. In either case the prominence is felt and seen beneath the brachialis anticus muscle. The fibers of this muscle should be split and elevated to either side and the bony prominence or spur must be removed with a sharp osteotome.

Complications of Supracondylar Fractures

The complications following supracondylar fracture are so often serious, it is advisable to take precautions to avoid these, or, at least, to curtail their extent.

Bleb Formation. Following reduction of the fracture swelling often increases at the elbow. If the bandage holding the splint in place is applied with uneven pressure where it crosses the swollen elbow, the swelling will tend to bulge through or between turns of the bandage. The edges of the bandage, if tight, will cut into the skin and blebs will result. These may become large and require a decrease in the position of flexion. They may break and become infected, requiring dressings that interfere with maintenance of the desired position of flexion. The best treatment is prevention. This can usually be accomplished by the avoidance of too tight bandages across the anterior part of the elbow, by high elevation of the injured arm, and by the application of low intensity heat. (See Figs. 25 and 32.) Should blebs occur in spite of such care, the splint should be rebandaged but with no bandage touching the skin in the antecubital area. If the blebs be large, aspiration may be advisable to prevent rupture and possible infection. This should be done under strict aseptic precautions.

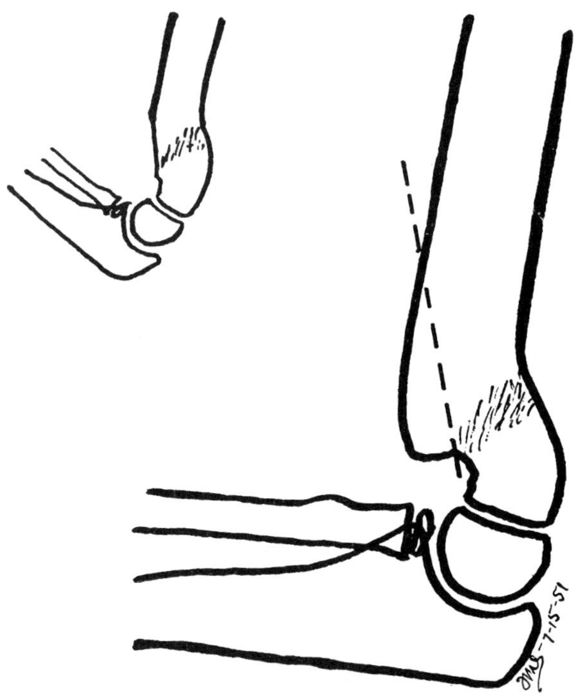

Fig. 37. Sketch showing flexion block deformity after incompletely reduced supracondylar fracture of humerus. Dotted line shows site for resection of anterior projecting mass of bone. Inset shows it after correction.

Skin Maceration of Antecubital Area. Due to the position of acute flexion used for immobilization after reduction, the skin of the forearm comes in contact with the skin of the lower arm. Moisture from perspiration collects between the two skin surfaces and evaporation cannot take place. As a result the skin develops surface maceration not unlike intertrigo, which may become annoying by burning or itching and be difficult to control without decreasing elbow flexion. To prevent this it is often wise to lay a thin compress of four layers of gauze across the antecubital area between the skin surfaces in order to keep them apart and to act as a wick to allow for evaporation of the moisture. If maceration has occurred, the area between the two skin surfaces may be carefully cleansed with soap and water, alcohol, dried thoroughly, powdered, and a wick placed in as described above. This can be done without the necessity of decreasing elbow flexion.

Myositis Ossificans. This is a late complication, but nevertheless one that may cause delayed recovery and permanent loss of function if not recognized and treated properly. (The etiology, pathology, prevention, and treatment of this condition has been described in detail in Chapter XIV.)

Volkmann's Ischaemia and Contracture. This is by far the most serious and most dreaded of all complications that may arise following supracondylar fracture. The ischaemia and paralysis may occur early before any treatment is instituted for the fracture, or it may occur within less than twelve to twenty-four hours after treatment has been started. Cases have been known to occur within six hours after the injury. (The condition is described fully in Chapter XIV.)

Prognosis of Supracondylar Fractures

The prognosis in the majority of supracondylar fractures in general is good, because these originally show only mild to moderate deformity, require no reduction or are fairly easily reduced, are not associated with serious circulatory disturbances, and the deformity, if any, is largely corrected by the child's growth. Functional return is usually very good if the patient's elbow has not been splinted for too long a time or otherwise overtreated. Carrying angle deformities may occur to a mild degree, but rarely to proportions that require later operative correction. In the more widely displaced supracondylar fractures and those with associated vascular and nerve lesions the prognosis is less good, but in general is not bad if they are treated with one of the traction methods which are highly successful in overcoming the risk of Volkmann's ischaemia. *These must be reduced early, must not have frequent repeated attempts at reduction, and must not subsequently be given other forms of injudicious treatment likely to cause myositis ossificans.*

SUPRACONDYLAR FRACTURE OF THE HUMERUS IN ADULTS

A fracture in the supracondylar region of the humerus in adults is much less common than in children. In general this fracture falls under the same classification as dicondylar (intercondylar) fractures in adults. If there is displacement of the fragment, this of course should be replaced, preferably by closed manipulation. If reduction is impossible to obtain, it is then advisable to suspend the arm in over-head Kirschner wire traction, and, if traction alone does not bring about replacement of the fragment, further manipulation may be attempted after 48 hours. Open reduction in adults with this injury is generally not indicated since it is impossible to use any form of internal fixation that will hold the fragments sufficiently rigid to permit early active motion in the elbow joint. The Kirschner wire traction method does allow early motion while the elbow is still in traction and suspension and functional recovery is more likely to be complete than if the elbow has been kept immobilized, or if the elbow has been operated upon and the fragment merely replaced without internal fixation. The after-treatment is the same as for dicondylar fractures. Complications are not common and should be treated as in dicondylar fractures.

The prognosis for supracondylar fractures in adults is in general fairly good provided marked comminution does not accompany the fracture.

FRACTURE (SEPARATION) OF THE MEDIAL EPICONDYLE (EPIPHYSIS) OF THE HUMERUS

In *adults* a fracture of the medial (internal) epicondyle of the humerus alone is so rare as to be almost a curiosity. In a series of 143 consecutive fractures of this epicondyle treated at the Presbyterian Hospital, New York City, only two cases unassociated with other fractures or dislocations were found occurring in adults. Both of these were due to direct force, one patient hitting his epicondyle against a window frame in a motor accident and the other being hit with a blunt object when she attempted to protect herself from an assailant. Neither case was accompanied by ulnar nerve injury. The displacement was moderate in each and the injury responded well to rest, heat and active exercises. The patients regained full function and use and were not afflicted with any late complications.

In *children* on the other hand fracture (separation of the epiphysis) of the medial epicondyle of the humerus is a common injury. The cause of the injury is in practically all instances due to indirect force; the epicondylar epiphysis becomes avulsed from its attachment to the medial condyle by the pull of the flexor-pronator group of muscles which take origin from it via a common tendon. The same manner of falling brings about this avulsion as causes a posterior dislocation at the elbow, i. e., a fall upon the hand with the wrist extended and supinated and with the elbow in extension. This puts the flexor-pronator group of muscles on the stretch and the suddenness of the force thus applied to the medial epicondyle separates it from the diaphysis of the humerus. This accounts for the frequent association of this fracture with posterior dislocation of the radius and ulna at the elbow. Depending somewhat upon the force of the fall and the duration of time that this force acts, the medial epicondyle epiphysis may show varying degrees of separation and displacement. There may be injury to the epiphyseal plate with definite separation being found on roentgenograms; or the epiphysis may be completely separated and displaced into the elbow joint proper.

There are in general five types of medial epicondyle fractures in children: (1) epiphyseal trauma without (visible) separation; (2) slight to moderate separation of the epiphysis; (3) marked separation with or without dislocation of the elbow joint; (4) marked separation with displacement of the epiphysis into the elbow joint; and (5) marked separation with displacement of the epiphysis into the dislocated elbow joint.

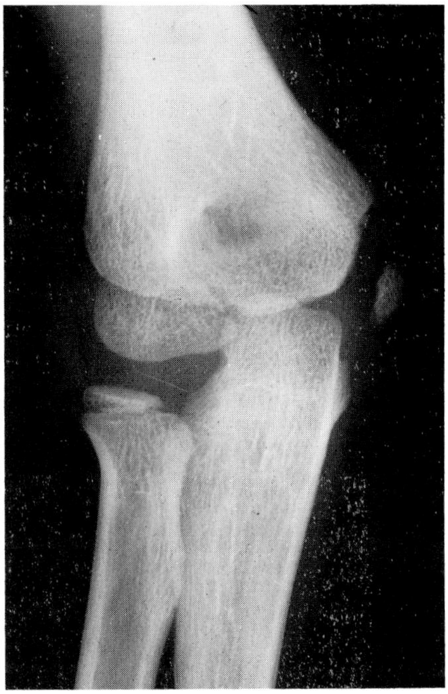

Fig. 38. Separation of epiphysis of medial (internal) epicondyle of humerus in boy seven years of age. Roentgenogram shows minimal displacement of the epicondyle fragment. Reduction is not necessary.

A. Epiphyseal Trauma without Separation

The diagnosis must be made on clinical grounds, i. e., by history of the fall followed by pain on the medial aspect of the elbow, tenderness in the region of the medial epicondyle, swelling, and the lack of visible or palpable deformity. The roentgenogram shows no abnormality when compared to the normal elbow. Pain is increased if the patient is made to pronate his forearm against resistance. The ulnar nerve is usually not involved unless direct contusion has followed the avulsion of the epicondyle.

Treatment. No splint is necessary. The patient should wear a sling for three or four days to permit rest and to relax the flexor-pronator muscles. Frequent soaks and active exercise of the elbow and wrist within pain limits are advisable and beneficial to the circulation and to the early return of full function. Pain and tenderness should last no longer than two to three weeks. The disability time is of the same duration.

The **prognosis** is excellent if the elbow is not over-treated by complete immobilization for three or more weeks. Growth disturbance may occur in the epiphysis of the medial epicondyle, but this rarely is manifested by more than slight irregularity or enlargement as noted on late follow-up roentgenograms. Such enlargement does not lead to loss of joint motion or to late ulnar nerve palsy.

B. Slight to Moderate Separation of the Epiphysis

The diagnosis is made on the same basis of pain and tenderness as in *A*. Swelling is likely to be greater and the medial epicondyle may be found to be movable and cause crepitus on palpation. Roentgenograms confirm the diagnosis and rule out or disclose other bone injuries. One should search for ulnar nerve disturbances.

Treatment. The elbow should be kept at rest and protected in a posterior molded splint and sling at right angles and in mid-rotation for four to five days. The splint should extend from the axilla to the base of the fingers. It is important *not* to wear this splint for longer than a week, and to urge the patient to practice active exercises at frequent intervals. A sling may be used for two weeks after discarding the splint. If immobilized in flexion for several weeks, it may take these children as much as a year to recover complete elbow extension. Active use may be permitted as soon as the patient is able to move his elbow well without pain. The disability time should not be greater than three to five weeks.

The **prognosis** is excellent if treatment is carried out as described above.

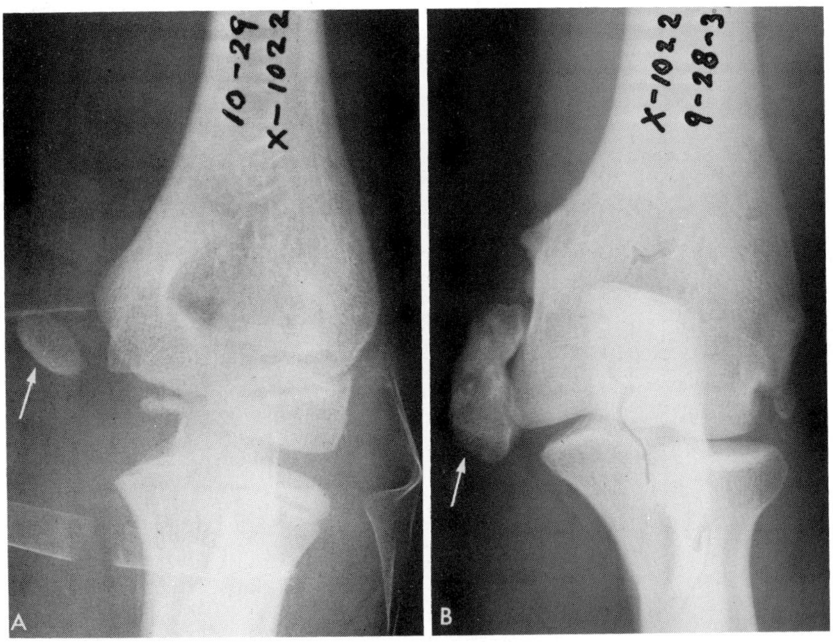

Fig. 39. Roentgenograms showing fracture and marked separation of the epiphysis of the medial (internal) epicondyle of the humerus in an eleven-year-old boy (A). The same elbow is seen (B) five years later. Note enlargement of the epicondyle which has remained displaced. No ulnar nerve signs had developed either from the residual displacement, enlargement, or from the fibrous union, and motion range had remained complete at the elbow joint. (SMITH, F. M.: Medial epicondyle injuries, *J.A.M.A.*, *142*:396, 1950.)

C. Marked Separation with or without Dislocation of the Elbow Joint

The diagnosis is based on pain and tenderness as in *A* and *B* plus greater swelling and possible ecchymosis although the latter is usually not seen in injuries of less than two or three hours duration. If swelling is not so excessive as to mask bony landmarks, the medial epicondyle may be found missing from its usual site and displaced a centimeter or more distally. (See Fig. 39.) It may be freely movable. If dislocation of the radius and ulna is present, it is much easier to detect separation of the medial epicondyle on palpation. Ulnar nerve injury should be carefully investigated. Roentgenograms will verify the separation of the epicondyle and comparative films of the uninjured elbow should likewise be taken in order to rule out the possible displacement of the epicondyle fragment into the joint cavity.

Treatment. This should be conservative. Even though it is rarely possible to reduce the displaced epicondyle by closed manipulation and maintain reduction, an attempt should be made to do so as follows: With the patient relaxed under general anesthesia, the operator's thumb and index finger are used to press and massage away the edema surrounding the displaced medial epicondyle until this fragment can be readily palpapted. Then with the forearm pronated and the elbow flexed to an angle of approximately seventy degrees the epicondyle fragment should be manipulated and pushed with the thumb and index finger in a proximal direction. The arm, forearm and elbow should then be immobilized in this position in a posterior molded splint extending from the axilla to the knuckles. The splint is for protection

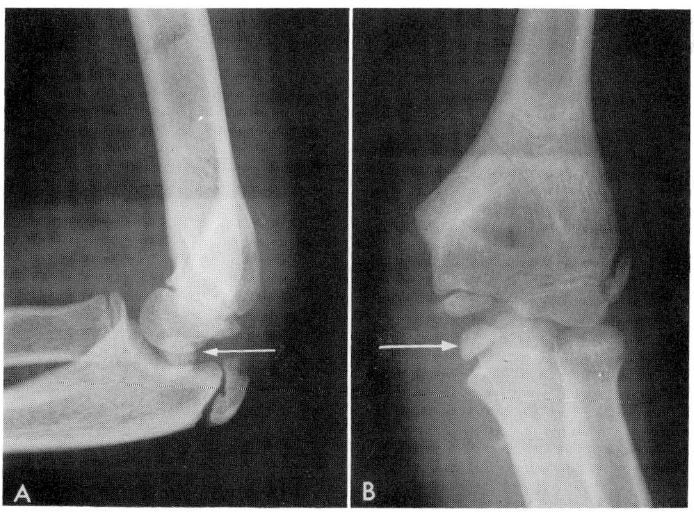

Fig. 40. Roentgenograms in lateral and antero-posterior projections showing avulsion of the epiphysis of the medial epicondyle and its displacement into the elbow joint. (Smith, F. M.: Medial epicondyle injuries, *J.A.M.A., 142*:396, 1950.)

and comfort only and should be dispensed with after seven days, followed by a sling and active exercises and use as described under *B*.

Open reduction for replacement and fixation of the displaced epicondyle fragment *per se* is advocated by some surgeons, but in the opinion of the author such an operation is definitely not indicated. The displacement alone of the epicondyle (provided the ulnar nerve is not affected by the original injury) causes no permanent disability, loss of elbow joint function, or weakness of the flexor-pronator group of muscles, even when displaced as much as two centimeters. To permit healing in its displaced position by fibrous rather than bony union (if unreduced) seems to cause some surgeons to worry concerning future function or possible growth disturbance, influencing them to advise operation in all such cases. (See Fig. 39B.) A well followed large series of this type of case shows that growth disturbance is certainly not lessened, bony union is not increased, and function is not improved by operative treatment. Regardless of the treatment the most important single factor in complete and early return of elbow joint function and use is the institution of early active exercises. This means that immobilization must be of brief duration.

If the ulnar nerve is affected at the time of the original injury or shows signs of impairment within the first two weeks after injury, operation should be performed and the ulnar nerve should be transposed to the anterior aspect of the medial condyle. If this is not performed early, the nerve may become extensively bound down or constricted by scar tissue in the process of soft tissue healing (Chapter XXI).

The disability time and prognosis for this type of epicondyle displacement should be approximately as in *B*.

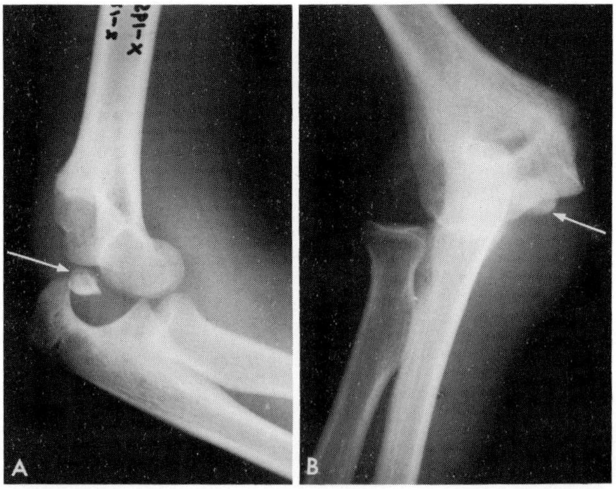

Fig. 41. Lateral and antero-posterior roentgenograms showing displacement of the avulsed medial epicondyle epiphysis into the dislocated elbow joint. (Smith, F. M.: Medial epicondyle injuries, *J.A.M.A.*, *142*:396, 1950.)

D. Marked Separation with Displacement of the Epiphysis into the Elbow Joint.

The clinical diagnosis is the same as in *C*. Roentgen examination is necessary to confirm displacement of the epicondyle epiphysis into the elbow joint. Its position in the joint is often over-looked unless one is in the habit of always searching for it in elbow injuries in children. This is because the fragment may lie at the level of the ossification centers of the trochlea and be mistaken for one of these. To leave such a fragment within the joint is to invite certain disaster. It is always safer to take roentgenograms of the normal elbow for comparison rather than attempt to rely upon memory alone as to degree of development and position of the numerous epiphyseal ossification centers in the growing child. The next most important point is to be aware that such intra-articular displacement may occur. The status of the ulnar nerve should of course be carefully checked before any treatment is begun.

Treatment. When the epicondyle has been displaced into and remains within the elbow joint, the treatment should *always* be operative. Although a few surgeons have described an occasional case in which it was possible to remove the fragment from the joint by closed manipulation (Schmier, Patrick), the majority of surgeons with extensive experience have had no such success. It therefore would appear wiser to operate immediately and make certain that the fragment was withdrawn from the joint and replaced. At the same time the ulnar nerve may be examined and transposed if necessary (Chapter XXI).

Operation. The elbow should be exposed by a slightly curved (concave anteriorly) three inch incision on the medial aspect. Towels should be clipped to the skin margins. When the subcutaneous tissue is incised and the deep fascia exposed, numerous blood clots will be found which must be wiped away. The epicondyle is not seen when the medial aspect of the joint is first exposed, but the operator will note the glistening white fibers of fascia overlying the upper portion of the flexor-pronator muscle group. (See *Frontispiece.*) On closer study he will see that these converge and curl into the joint through the torn capsule just below the medial margin of the articular surface of the trochlear process. By abducting the forearm slightly and applying traction to these converging fibers by means of mouse-toothed forceps, the epicondyle with conjoined tendon will be suddenly ejected from the joint. It may then be reduced and fastened to its normal position on the medial condyle by means of a mattress suture of heavy silk passed through a drill hole in the latter. Some surgeons prefer to excise the fragment and to re-attach the conjoined tendon of this muscle group to the condyle. Which method is preferable has not been settled, but the latter may have some advantage in that it does not leave an epiphysis that can become enlarged with growth.

Care should be taken to visualize the ulnar nerve before the epicondyle or conjoined tendon is replaced. If it appears contused, hemorrhagic or constricted, its sheath should be distended with saline solution introduced through a hypodermic needle of small caliber (hydrostatic neurolysis). If there is noted much hemorrhage surrounding the nerve where it lies in its groove on the posterior aspect of the epicondyle or any fibrous bands that might constrict it, the entire nerve for a distance of two inches above and below the elbow joint should be carefully freed and transposed to an anterior position.

Treatment following operation should be similar to that described under *B* and *C*. Immobilization must be brief and efforts should be made to obtain early active motion and use. Internal fixation of the fragment or conjoined tendon should hasten rather than delay the return of function.

The disability time is about six to eight weeks if thus treated. This longer disability time is due more to the extensive soft part damage in these injuries than to the fact that the epicondyle had been displaced into the elbow joint at the beginning. The prognosis is good to excellent, provided the original displacement has been recognized early and operated upon early. Late recognition and late operation are likely to give poor results. The ulnar nerve should recover full function if treated properly.

E. Marked Separation with Displacement of the Epiphysis into the Dislocated Elbow Joint

The only difference in the diagnosis in this instance is that there is an accompanying dislocation at the elbow joint. This may distort the anatomy, but at the same time it may make it easier to detect separation of the medial epicondyle from its normal location. Roentgenograms are necessary to determine the exact position of this fragment, and, if compared to films of the uninjured elbow, one should have no difficulty in spotting a displacement into the elbow joint before or after reduction of the dislocation. The condition of the ulnar nerve should be determined before any treatment is given.

Treatment

Operation is a necessity as in *D* and the elbow dislocation must be reduced at the same time. The ulnar nerve must likewise be treated in a similar manner if necessary. The author has seen one late case in which the nerve had been displaced along with the epicondyle and remained in the joint with it after closed manipulation had reduced the dislocation. Transposition of the nerve allowed it to recover full function.

The after-treatment, disability time, and prognosis are identical to those described under *D*.

FRACTURE OF THE MEDIAL CONDYLE OF THE HUMERUS

An isolated fracture of the medial condyle of the humerus is not a common injury. It occurs with much less frequency than fracture of the lateral

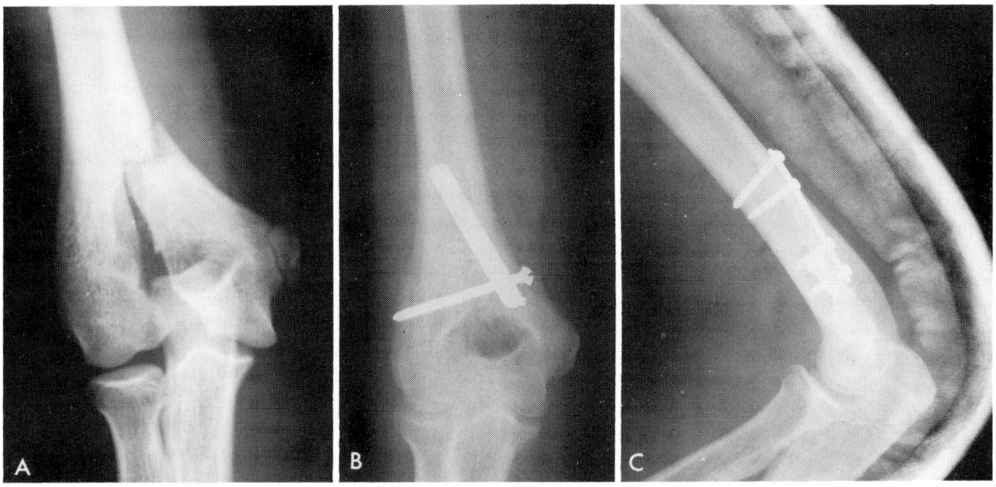

Fig. 42. Fracture of medial condyle of humerus in 15 year old boy. (A) Original antero-posterior view. It was impossible to obtain reduction by closed manipulation. Operation was performed the day after injury and the fragments were reduced and fixed internally with a four-screw plate and an additional transfixion screw. Active motion and exercises for this elbow were instituted one week after operation and continued throughout healing. (B and C) Antero-posterior and lateral roentgenograms taken after operation. *Result:* Normal anatomy and full function and use within four months.

condyle or both condyles (dicondylar). It is most likely to occur from a fall or from the patient being thrown against a hard object, as in a collision. The fracture line extends into the joint surface usually at about the middle of the trochlear process. From here it passes upwards and medially to emerge at the supracondylar ridge on this side. The fragment may not be displaced at all, in which case the chief symptom is pain in the joint which slowly increases as hemarthrosis becomes greater. Wide displacement of the medial condyle may occur, however, with separation from the lateral condyle and with angulation and possibly rotation. The medial condyle fragment may be comminuted or may remain as one single piece. Pain and disability are present from the onset.

Since the fracture line enters the articular surface the injury is a serious one, because displacement or incomplete reduction may cause restricted motion in the joint or even lead to the formation of traumatic arthritis.

Associated lesions are not common, but it is wise to check the function and sensation of the ulnar nerve for possible trouble, (contusion, stretching, or compression). The medial epicondyle may be fractured and become partially separated from the condyle by the pull of the attached flexor-pronator group of muscles.

Treatment

Closed Treatment. Where no displacement has occurred reduction is unnecessary. The joint should be aspirated to relieve hemarthrosis after which the elbow must be immobilized in a posterior molded splint and sling with flexion to approximately ninety degrees. Elevation, heat, and gentle massage may be given and are especially useful early in order to relieve swelling and induration. At the end of two weeks the splint must be removed four or five times daily for active exercises within the limits of pain, and hot soaks may be substituted for dry heat. The splint may be discarded at the end of three weeks and a sling only worn for two more weeks.

In growing children, although this injury is extremely rare, one must attempt reduction of a displaced fragment. If completely satisfactory reposition is not obtained, it would be wise to perform open reduction of the fragment. Closed reduction of a displaced fragment in adults is not very satisfactory from the standpoint of reduction and it is difficult to keep this in position without prolonged splinting unless the Kirschner wire method of skeletal traction is employed as in dicondylar fractures.

Open Reduction. In adults it is particularly important to obtain accurate reduction if considerable limitation of joint motion is not to be expected. This is especially true in young to middle-aged persons, who need a good functioning and strong elbow. In older individuals the same holds true, but resort to operative reduction should not necessarily be the first choice of treatment. Many of these older persons are in poor physical shape or are otherwise bad operative risks because of arthritis, comminution of the fracture, etc., and may better be treated by traction and early motion. Should the main fragment of the medial condyle be single, large, and widely displaced the treatment of choice is not only operative reduction, but this is also a necessity provided there exists no definite contra-indication on the part of the patient or upon the surgeon's experience and equipment to handle the situation properly.

The incision for exposure of the medial condyle may be made along the medial or postero-medial aspect of the elbow. (In the latter instance it is often more convenient to have the patient prone upon the table with the flexed elbow hanging over the end of a padded arm-board.) The ulnar nerve must be identified, retracted and protected. The fracture site is approached and only enough periosteum elevated to allow reposition of the main fragment. Any small loose fragments of bone or cartilage that may fall into the joint or cause interference with anatomical reduction should be removed. The main fragment should then be held firmly to the shaft and lateral condyle by a bone clamp. The best type of internal fixation that will give rigid immobilization should then be chosen and applied. This may be by nails, screws, bolt or plate or a combination of transfixion screw and plate (see Fig. 42 c, d). The periosteum is then sutured, the ulnar nerve replaced in its normal position (or transposed to the anterior surface of the condyle if this seems advisable) and the wound closed with interrupted silk sutures. If necessary to operate in children, internal fixation may be used, but it is inadvisable to place a nail or screw across the epiphyseal cartilage. Occasionally sutures must be used to fasten the periosteum of the fragment in place, but this at best is a poor substitute for internal fixation. Loops of wire are not much better than sutures and should be avoided if possible.

After-treatment. Cases treated by closed reduction and plaster fixation should be kept elevated and have constant low heat applied for the first few days. Massage (sedative only) may be given and with heat and elevation will assist with the reduction of swelling. At two weeks the splint should be removed four to five times a day for active exercises of the elbow short of causing pain. After three weeks the splint should be worn only at night for protection while sleeping, while a sling is used during the day. At four weeks the splint may be discarded. The exercises after the third week should be progressive and mild use may be permitted in addition after four weeks which should also be made progressive. Occupational therapy is useful and should be encouraged to assist in increasing joint motion and muscular strength and not solely for diversion.

Patients treated by operation and internal fixation (if rigid) may be started on active exercises within the first week. They need to be splinted for protection at night only after this time, whereas during the day they may be practising frequent active exercises. The treatment otherwise is similar to that in the closed cases, but recovery will be more rapid.

Complications

An early complication that must be watched for is a lesion of the ulnar nerve. Late complications are possible development of myositis ossificans (Chapter XIV); and epiphyseal growth disturbance with possible development of a reversed carrying angle (cubitus varus deformity) (Chapter XXI).

Prognosis

With none or minimal displacement of the medial condyle fragment the prognosis is good. With wide displacement the prognosis is only poor to fair unless this be reduced by open or closed means and motion started early. In a child there is always the possibility of growth disturbance against which the parents should be forewarned and advised that it may be corrected at a later date if the amount of deformity warrants it.

FRACTURE (SEPARATION) OF THE LOWER EPIPHYSIS OF THE HUMERUS

General Considerations

A fracture or separation of the entire lower humeral epiphysis is a rare injury. In the cases with no separation of the epiphyseal fragment the diagnosis may be completely missed. Where no separation is visible on roentgenographic films the diagnosis must be made entirely on the clinical finding of acute tenderness in the region of the epiphyseal line. This tenderness is usually situated at a somewhat lower level than is the tenderness in a supracondylar fracture without displacement. When the epiphysis is separated it is sometimes displaced in a forward direction or even angulated in this direction; more rarely it may be displaced or angulated somewhat posteriorly and it may be necessary to compare the films of the injured elbow with those of the normal elbow before the diagnosis can be made. On the other hand, the epiphysis may be displaced toward the lateral side and a diagnosis of dislocation of the elbow may be made until the roentgenograms are studied carefully when it will be noted that the ulna and radius along with the capitellar epiphysis are completely or partially displaced in a lateral direction. The mere fact that the capitellar epiphysis is displaced along with the radius and ulna means that the lower articular surface of the humerus (entire epiphysis) is displaced upon the diaphysis. Associated lesions are not common with this injury. It is possible, however, to have trauma to the ulnar nerve associated with the lesion. Again, hemarthrosis may accompany the injury and be an extremely painful symptom requiring aspiration in addition to reduction of the displaced epiphysis. There is of course a

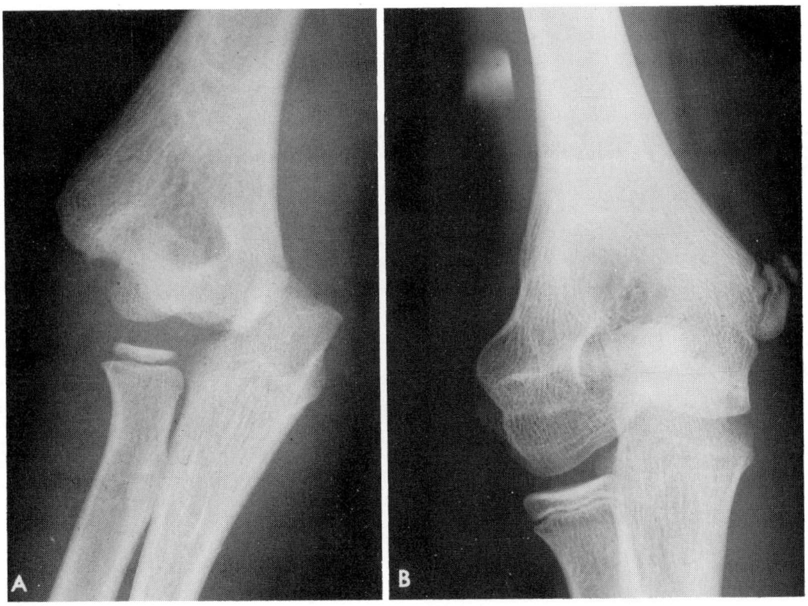

Fig. 43. Fracture-separation of lower humeral epiphysis in its entirety. This injury on antero-posterior roentgenograms is often mistaken for a dislocation of both forearm bones at the elbow joint. (A) Original antero-posterior roentgenogram in a boy seven years of age. Note that the radius continues to articulate with the ossification center of the capitellum which has been displaced medially and lies below the olecranon fossa instead of directly below the lateral aspect of the diaphysis of the humerus. The upper end of the ulna appears not to be articulating with anything, but it must be remembered that the ossification centers for the trochlear process are not as yet visible on roentgenograms taken at the age of seven years. (B) Same elbow four years, three months later. Note irregularity of lower humerus, i. e., lateral condyle, and trochlea, which has resulted from the original injury. Such irregularities never follow dislocation of the joint per se.

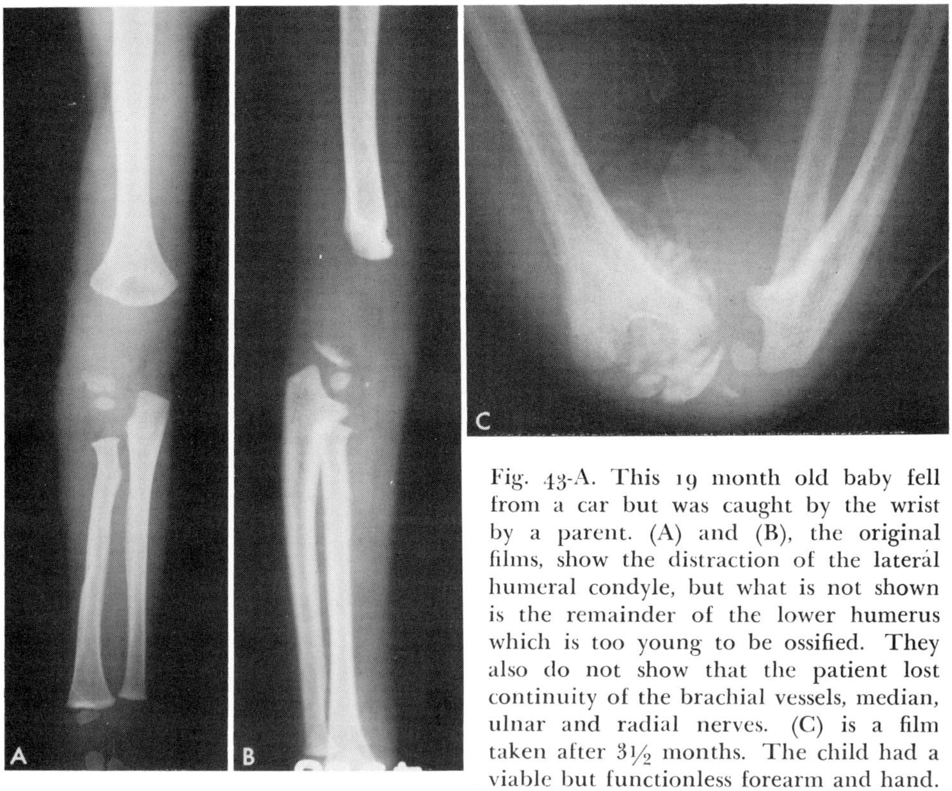

Fig. 43-A. This 19 month old baby fell from a car but was caught by the wrist by a parent. (A) and (B), the original films, show the distraction of the lateral humeral condyle, but what is not shown is the remainder of the lower humerus which is too young to be ossified. They also do not show that the patient lost continuity of the brachial vessels, median, ulnar and radial nerves. (C) is a film taken after 3½ months. The child had a viable but functionless forearm and hand. Neurological exploration revealed no possible chance of improvement.

chance of subsequent growth disturbance following the injury regardless of whether the epiphysis has been displaced or merely traumatized.

Treatment

Naturally, if displaced the epiphysis must be reduced very much as the lower fragment in a supracondylar fracture is reduced by direct manipulation in the proper direction under general anesthesia. The usual form of immobilization is moderate flexion in a posterior molded splint. Aspiration of the elbow may be advisable.

Open Treatment. Operation for replacement of the lower humeral epiphysis is not indicated unless a compound wound is associated with the lesion. All of these epiphyses can be replaced by closed manipulation and should be so reduced. To perform open reduction upon an epiphysis thus displaced is to further the chances of subsequent growth disturbance.

Complications

An early complication with this type of lesion is possible interference with the blood supply, but this is not common. If hemorrhage and edema have been extensive, immobilization should be in less flexion than ordinarily.

Late complications are usually the result of growth disturbance and consist of an increase in the carrying angle (cubitus valgus) or possible reversal of the carrying angle (cubitus varus). These do not require treatment unless the deformity becomes extremely marked. If such be the case, a subsequent osteotomy may be performed as recommended under similar deformities following a supracondylar fracture.

Prognosis

The prognosis in general is good. It is usually wise, however, to instruct the parents that a possible growth disturbance may result, but should not necessarily be expected. Return of full function is usually good and the disability time is rarely more than six to eight weeks at the most.

FRACTURE OF THE TROCHLEAR PROCESS OF THE HUMERUS

General Considerations

While a fracture of the medial condyle of the humerus is uncommon, a fracture involving only the trochlear process is still less common. It is usually sustained by a fall on the olecranon, which wedges and splits the trochlear process from the medial condyle. The fracture line may pass through the medial epicondyle as it emerges upon the inner side. These fractures are usually without displacement, but occasionally displacement may be great or even a fragment of the trochlear process may become loose within the joint. Loss of motion in the elbow joint will be great unless the fragment is replaced in its normal position; or, if completely loose, unless it be removed.

Associated Injuries. The ulnar nerve is sometimes damaged along with this injury and as mentioned above loose fragments are not uncommon within the joint. The fracture line may pass through the olecranon and coronoid fossae and both of these may become filled with organized connective tissue which may impair joint motion.

Treatment

Closed. If the fragment is not displaced, treatment should follow conservative methods and immobilization should be carried out by means of a posterior molded splint with the elbow held at right angles for a period of three weeks, followed by active exercises and hot soaks.

Operative Treatment. If the fragment is displaced and it is impossible to replace it by a closed manoeuvre, the joint should be opened. If it is possible to replace the fragment and fasten it with either a screw or Kirschner wire, this is advisable. If the fragment is too small for such fixation, it is best to remove it. If internal fixation has been used, the elbow should be immobilized for a period of approximately ten days only before active exercises are started.

After-treatment. Rest to begin with; later active exercises and physiotherapy in the form of hot soaks, light massage and occupational therapy.

Complications

Limited joint motion due to irregularity within the joint or possibly to aseptic necrosis following poor healing or even non-union as a result of a compromised blood supply.

Disability Time

The disability time is likely to run to three or four months before work requiring any particular strength is possible.

Prognosis

The prognosis in trochlear fractures is rather poor if there has been displacement.

FRACTURES OF THE CAPITELLUM OF THE HUMERUS IN ADULTS

General Considerations

Fracture of the capitellum of the humerus in adults is an injury which is not common, but is important because the fracture line separates the articular eminence from the lateral condyle. The line lies completely within the joint cavity so there no longer remains any capsular or ligamentous attachments to the broken off fragment. The importance lies in the fact that the fragment may later undergo aseptic necrosis and cause traumatic arthritis to develop in the elbow joint. It is also with great difficulty that such fragments can be replaced adequately by any closed manipulative procedure. As a result of this difficulty and of the great risk of late aseptic necrosis and traumatic arthritis the majority of surgeons advise that these fractures should be operated upon and the completely loose fragment removed. This procedure might appear radical to a person who has had little experience with such fractures, since removal of a large piece of the bone and articular surface from the elbow might seem to interfere with its function and stability. To the contrary it is better to be rid of the fragment so as to prevent its becoming irregular, rough and later interfering with joint motion especially flexion and extension. Late follow-up results on removal of the fragment show that functional recovery is more likely to be complete than if the fragment is reduced by closed methods and the patient's elbow immobilized for a period of four to six weeks while bone healing takes place.

The displacement of the capitellar fragment may be only in a proximal direction and may be shifted as much as one to possibly two centimeters without any evidence of rotation. The displacement is best seen on lateral roentgenograms, and, if displaced widely, it may likewise be seen on anteroposterior films, but it is never seen so well on these. Other cases may show

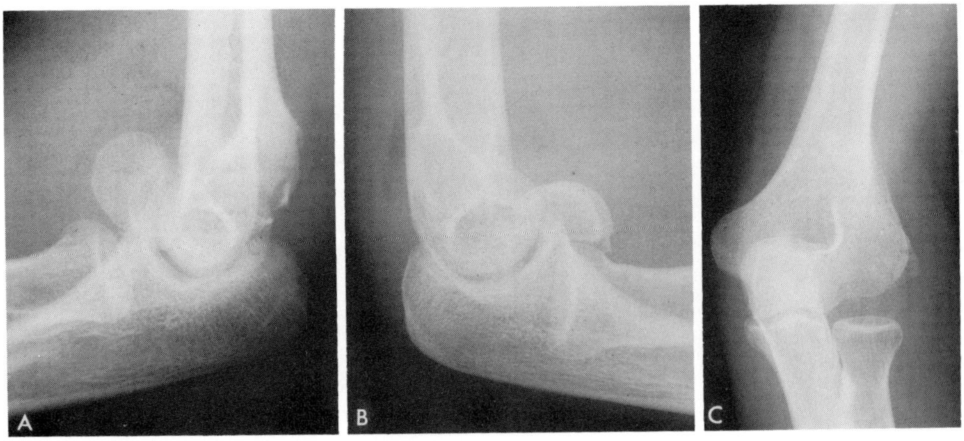

Fig. 44. Fracture of capitellum of humerus in adult. (A) Original lateral view showing capitellar fragment displaced in a proximal direction. This patient was a woman 30 years of age. The elbow was operated upon and the fragment was excised. (B) Original lateral view of elbow in a 22 year old woman showing capitellar fragment displaced in a proximal direction and rotated 90 degrees forward as well so that the articular surface faces in a proximal direction. This fragment as in *A* was removed at operation, because it was situated entirely within the joint and was devoid of soft tissue attachments and blood supply. (C) Antero-posterior view of elbow seen in *B* two years and six months after operative removal of fractured capitellum. *Function:* excellent; no pain; full use.

not only displacement in a proximal direction, but a forward rotation of the articular fragment of ninety degrees. In other words the articular surface of the fragment faces not anteriorly, but proximally toward the head of the humerus. Occasionally it becomes so firmly wedged in this position as to interfere greatly with elbow joint motion.

Treatment

Closed treatment for articular fractures of the capitellum in adults is not as a rule good when the fragment has been definitely displaced to a moderate degree. In very young adults or in children, whose epiphyseal centers are closed, but, in whom there is also a greater tendency for rapid and more complete bone healing to take place than in adults, it may be justified to attempt closed reduction of the fragment under anesthesia by direct manipulation with the operator's thumbs in an attempt to replace it in its normal position. This may be checked by fluoroscopic and subsequent roentgenographic examination. Following manipulation the elbow should be placed in moderately acute flexion in order to maintain the reduction, and then immobilize it in a posterior molded splint. Undisplaced fractures should be immobilized similarly for a period of four weeks.

Open Operation. In adults open operation seems to be the best form of treatment for these fractures, because, it not only gets rid of the completely loose and avascular fragment, but it cuts down on the risk of development of traumatic arthritis at a later date. The patients seem to do very much

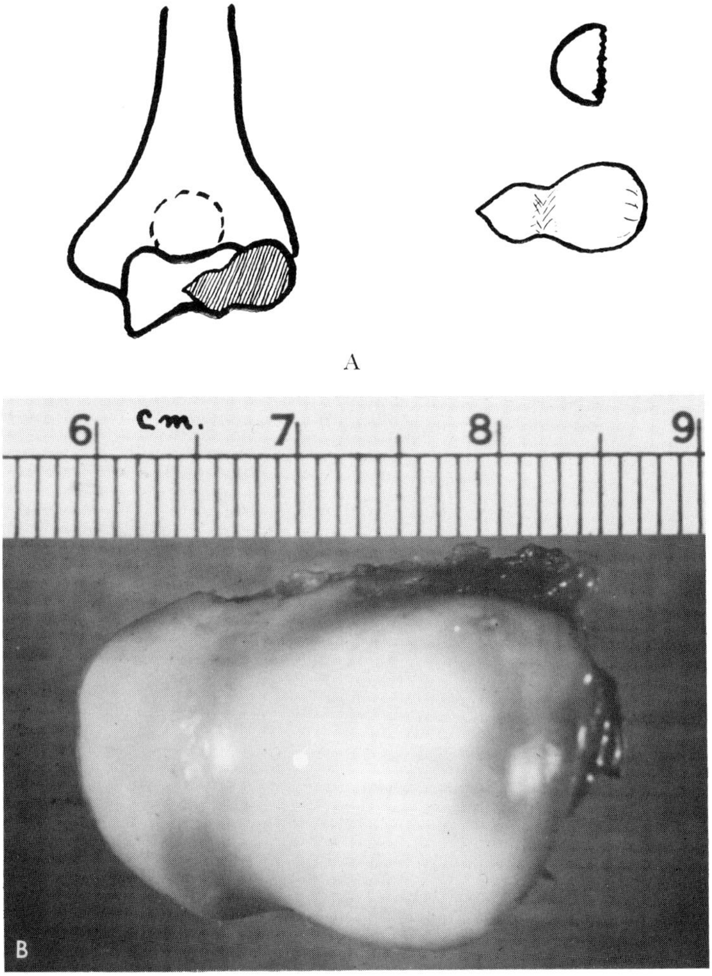

Fig. 45. (A) Sketch showing size, shape, and extent, and location of fracture of capitellum of humerus. Note how the fracture line extends into the outer, anterior aspect of the trochlear articular surface. (B) Photograph of actual fragment of capitellum removed from patient whose elbow was seen in Figure 44B.

better without the fragment and are not likely to develop more than a very small amount of lateral instability at the joint. Ordinarily they do not develop any disturbance in the inferior radio-ulnar joint. The entire range of motion should be greater and more likely painless than if the fragment were replaced and the elbow immobilized.

If the fragment is to be removed, the operation of course should be at an *early* date, preferably the day of the injury rather than four to five days later when the hemorrhage and exudate have begun to organize. Immediate operation is not only easier while the tissues are soft and before fibrosis has set in, but it also permits removal of the collected blood from the joint which of course causes pain due to the intense hemarthrosis. Immediate removal of the fragment followed by splinting for two to three days to permit the patient to recover from the immediate post-operative reaction and pain is the ideal treatment. Following this the patient should of course be started on active exercises within pain limits and these should be increased as rapidly as the patient can take them. It is not unusual to find that such a patient one week after operation is able to move his elbow through an arc of seventy to one hundred and fifty degrees and at the same time be able to perform full rotation.

Disability Time

The disability time in closed reduction naturally is very much greater than if the elbow is operated upon and the loose fragment removed. This is because it is necessary to immobilize the elbow for a period of at least four to six weeks and it will probably take at least an equal length of time if not double, to recover the maximum range of motion. If the fragment is removed at operation, the patient is started on a regime of exercises within three or four days after operation. The disability time for light work should not be greater than six weeks at the most. For heavy work it may run up to as high as eight to ten weeks.

Prognosis

The prognosis would depend more or less on the treatment given the particular individual. If a large fragment is broken off and replaced there is always chance of development of traumatic arthritis. If the same fragment were to have been removed at operation, there is no longer any likelihood of impingement between the radial head and the capitellum and therefore no possibility of articular roughening or spur formation which can interfere with motion and cause pain. The interval between the raw surface of the humerus and the radial head (where the capitellum has been removed) usually becomes glazed over with a thin layer of scar tissue. A few patients develop a slight increase in the carrying angle, but it is extremely rare that this becomes great enough to cause any late disturbance such as neuritis in the ulnar nerve.

FRACTURE OF THE LATERAL CONDYLE OF THE HUMERUS IN ADULTS

General Considerations

Fracture of the lateral condyle of the humerus in adults is not a frequent injury, but is more common than the isolated fracture of the capitellum. The lesion is often associated with a fracture of the capitellum and the two may be in separate fragments. Not infrequently the fracture line through the lateral condyle may extend downward and medially to include the outer half of the trochlear process. When this fracture involves the deep portion of the trochlear notch, there may be associated a lateral subluxation of the forearm bones upon the humerus due to the fact that the radial ridge of the trochlea has been displaced and there is nothing to hold the ulna in place, since the medial collateral ligament is frequently torn at the same time. When such a lesion is present, the ulnar nerve may likewise be involved. These fractures are extremely difficult to reduce when they are widely displaced and are difficult to hold reduced, even when treated by open reduction and internal fixation. The resulting loss of motion may be great because of the persistent tendency of the ulna to sublux towards the lateral side. Fracture of the olecranon process is occasionally seen with this fracture.

Treatment

Closed Treatment. For undisplaced fractures the lesion should be treated by closed methods and immobilization in a posterior molded splint for a period of four weeks. The splint may be removed periodically at the end of two weeks for early active exercises and soaks in hot water at frequent intervals. If the fragment has been displaced, reduction should be attempted and the fragment molded back into position by thumb pressure in the required direction, followed by immobilization as described above. It is extremely important to obtain accurate anatomic reduction of the condyle otherwise any change in its normal vertical or transverse axes will interfere with full hinge joint motion at the elbow. Should there be an additional fracture with separation of the capitellar process, closed reduction will probably not be satisfactory and functional return will also be poor. Open reduction should then be performed.

Open Reduction. When there is marked displacement of the lateral condyle fragment or if there is displacement of an additional capitellar fragment, neither of which can be replaced accurately by closed manipulation, the fracture should be opened and the lateral condyle fragment replaced and held by internal fixation. If the capitellar fragment is completely loose and displaced, this had best be removed so that it will not interfere with motion and also remain to undergo aseptic necrosis due to lack of blood supply. If, as mentioned under general considerations, the capitellar fracture line passes through the middle of the trochlear process so that the upper ulna is allowed to sublux laterally and it is impossible to keep this from doing so, it might be justified to replace the capitellar fragment to act as a prop to maintain the position of the ulna. In addition to fixation of the fragments by nails, screws, or even Kirschner wires, a second incision should be made upon the medial aspect of the elbow and the torn medial collateral ligament should be repaired with mattress sutures of silk. Following operation the elbow should be immobilized in a posterior molded splint for ten days to two weeks and then active exercises should be started. Swelling and pain may be alleviated and motion increased by hot soaks in conjunction with the exercises. Every possible attempt should be made to regain early

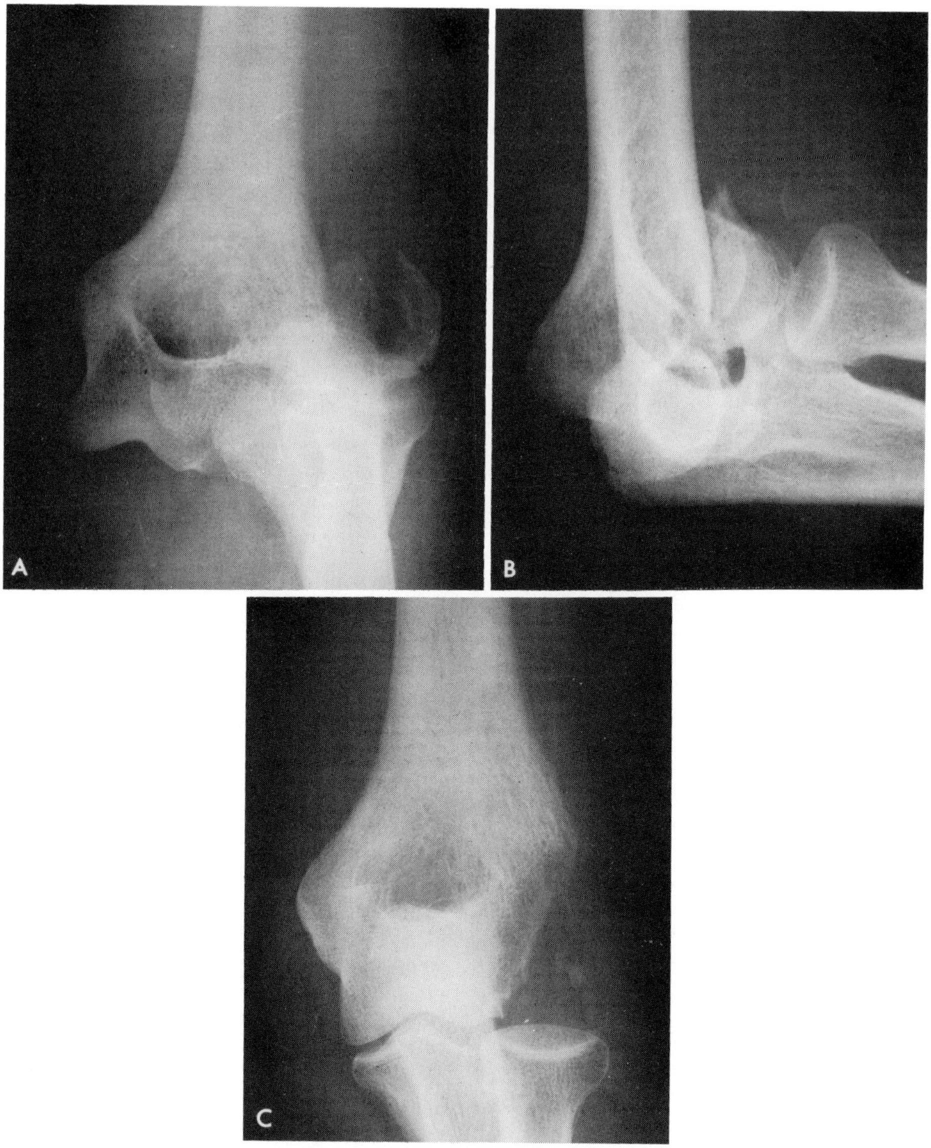

Fig. 46. Roentgenograms of elbow of 50 year old woman showing dislocation of joint and an associated fracture of the lateral condyle of the humerus. (A) Antero-posterior, and (B) lateral views. The elbow was operated upon, the dislocation was reduced, and the fragments of the fractured and displaced lateral condyle were excised. (C) Antero-posterior view five years after operation. *Result:* excellent; motion range full; very slight lateral instability.

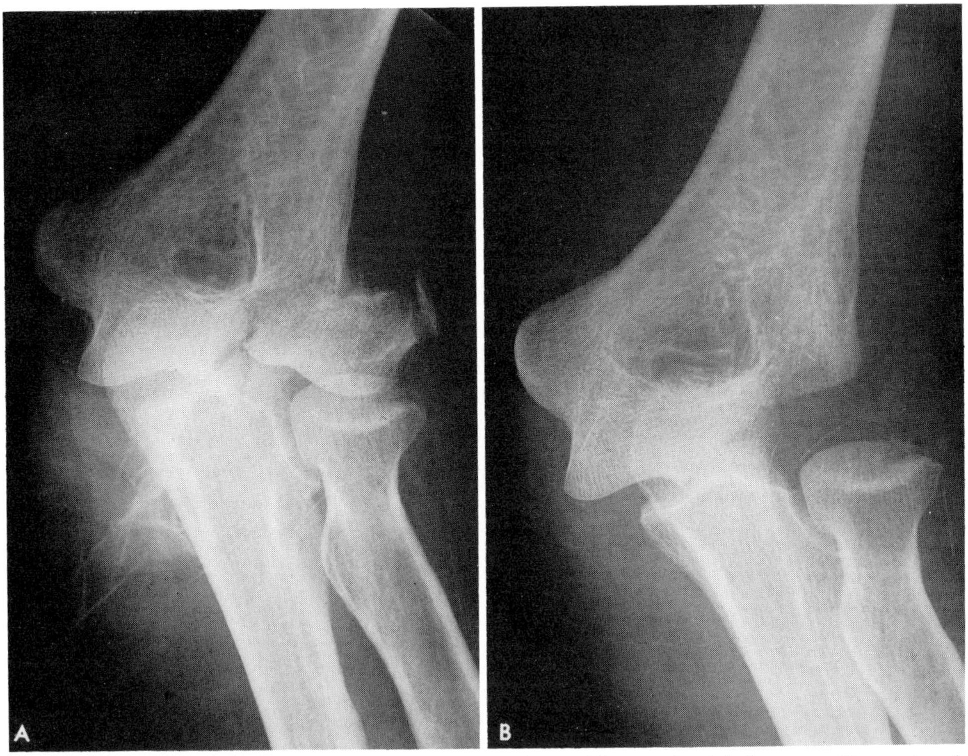

Fig. 47. Fracture of lateral condyle of humerus (unstable type) with fracture line extending into trochlea and with tendency towards subluxation of radius and ulna lateralward. (A) Original antero-posterior view in 48 year old woman. (B) Same elbow after operative removal of the lateral condyle fragment (which contained capitellum and outer lip of trochlear process) and repair of medial collateral ligament. Note that subluxation persists. *Result:* poor anatomically and only fair from functional standpoint.

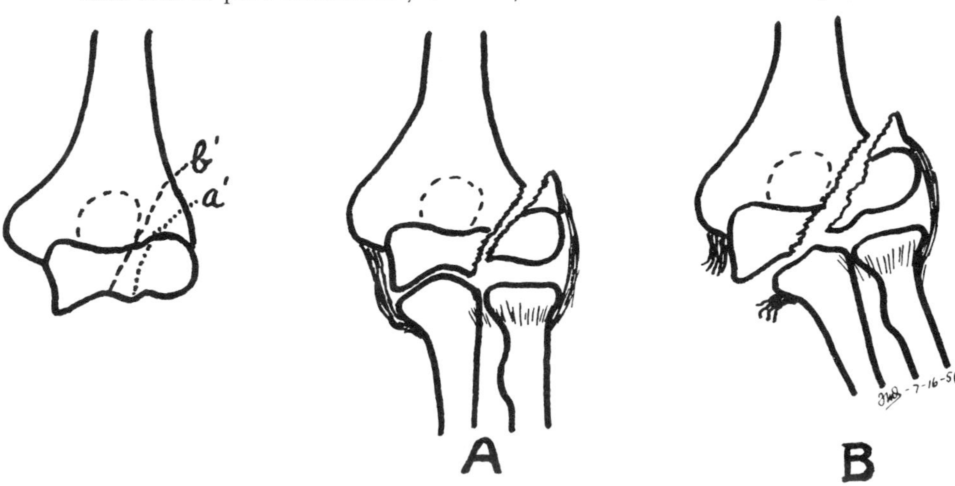

Fig. 48. Sketch showing types of fracture of lateral condyle of humerus in adults. (A) and (B) These represent the stable and unstable types with the fracture lines passing through *a'* and *b'* respectively. The stability of *A* depends upon the lateral lip of the trochlea being intact. If the lateral lip of the trochlea is a part of the lateral condyle fragment, the ulna and radius both shift in a lateral direction and the medial collateral ligament must rupture as in *B*.

motion, particularly flexion at the elbow joint. Operation should be performed at an *early* date, preferably on the day of the injury, since hemorrhage and induration undergo organization after a few days and will make the operation more difficult. There is also a greater likelihood of extraosseous and extracapsular bone formation if operation is postponed until a week or later.

After-treatment. After either the closed reduction or open reduction with internal fixation treatment should consist of immobilization in a posterior molded splint, followed by the institution of early active exercises within pain limits and at frequent intervals. As motions increase exercises should be likewise increased, but never to the point where they cause pain and fatigue, since either one will retard the patient's progress. Whirlpool baths are beneficial as is also occupational therapy after four weeks have passed in order to strengthen muscles as well as to help increase motion in the joint.

Complications

Complications are rather frequent. One of these is ulnar nerve disability, and, if it persists, transplantation of the ulnar nerve should be performed. There is also the persistent tendency of the ulna to sublux in a lateral direction when the fracture line passes through the center of the trochlea and when it has been necessary to remove a large, loose capitellar fragment. Myositis ossificans is a complication that is to be feared, and this may be prevented or at least minimized by *early* operation.

Disability Time

The disability time is likely to be prolonged in these injuries and it is rare that these patients can get back to anything but light work short of four to five months.

Prognosis

In general the prognosis is good if there is one large fragment embracing the lateral condyle and capitellum together. If there is a separate fracture between these two portions, the prognosis is not good, since it is more difficult to obtain and hold reduction even by the employment of internal fixation. In other words, without comminution the prognosis is good if satisfactory reduction has been obtained either by closed or open methods and followed by early active exercises. If comminution is present, the prognosis is only fair as to functional recovery. If there is a persistance of lateral subluxation of the ulna, the prognosis for functional recovery is very likely to be poor.

FRACTURE OF THE LATERAL CONDYLE OR SEPARATION OF THE EPIPHYSIS OF THE CAPITELLUM IN CHILDREN

General Considerations

An injury through the lateral condyle of the humerus or epiphysis of the capitellum in children though not nearly so common as the supracondylar fracture in children is often of a more serious nature. This is because of the ultimate prognosis as to function and subsequent anatomical deformity. The fracture line can be seen to run medially and distally in the lower humerus beginning just above the lateral epicondyle and extending into the joint surface. On roentgenograms its lower limit is visible only in the diaphysis. The lower fragment consists of the capitellar epiphysis with a variable size portion of the humeral diaphysis attached to it. The lesion, being close to the epiphyseal line is essentially an epiphyseal fracture in spite of the fact that the fracture line does not pass along the epiphyseal plate.

Growth disturbance frequently follows this lesion and is due to impairment of the blood supply of the distal fragment or damage to the epiphyseal

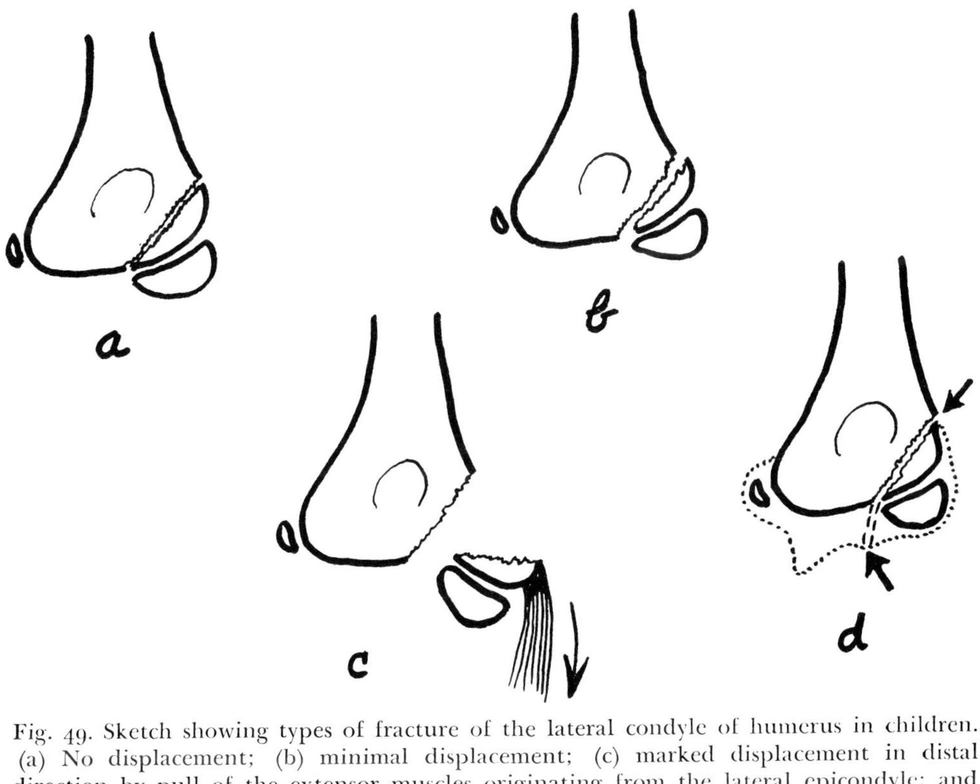

Fig. 49. Sketch showing types of fracture of the lateral condyle of humerus in children. (a) No displacement; (b) minimal displacement; (c) marked displacement in distal direction by pull of the extensor muscles originating from the lateral epicondyle; and (d) fracture line shown passing through the cartilagenous lower end of the humerus (designated by dotted line) but not visible on roentgenograms. The visible part of the displaced fragment always consists of the ossification center of the capitellum plus a variable sized portion of the diaphysis of the lower humerus which together make up the lateral condyle.

plate from the original trauma, to undue force used in manipulative reduction, or to repeated attempts at manipulative reduction. Displacement of the lower fragment varies from nothing to complete downward, forward and lateral displacement and in those cases with marked displacement there is almost always rotation of the fragment to as much as one hundred and eighty degrees in some instances. The cause of the displacement results from the degree of tear in the periosteum and overlying fascia and is brought about by the pull of the extensor muscles of the wrist which have their common origin on the lateral epicondyle.

It is obvious in the cases with displacement requiring a reduction that reduction be done *early* before the surrounding tissues become completely infiltrated and inelastic and that the reduction be anatomically accurate, otherwise there will result an irregularity in the lower articular surface of the humerus. Also, if the fragment is not replaced in direct apposition in its anatomical position, healing may result in either a non-union or fibrous union. It is likewise important that after reduction is accomplished, the fragment must be maintained in this position if bone healing is to be expected, subsequent deformity avoided and if full function is to be restored in the elbow joint.

Very often it is impossible by closed methods to bring about a reduction owing to the amount of displacement and rotation of the displaced fragment. It is also difficult to maintain such a reduction. For these reasons many surgeons prefer to perform open reduction on all such fractures with marked displacement and fasten the fragments internally.

Subsequent growth disturbance is a common sequel because of the difficulty in the re-establishment of the blood supply to the displaced fragment, which loses most or all of it when torn completely away from the diaphysis. Therefore, realizing the difficulties of obtaining adequate reduction by closed methods and the ability to maintain the reduction, one should keep in mind the probable *necessity* for performing open reduction.

It is in general advisable in displaced epiphyses not to operate unless absolutely necessary since open reduction predisposes to epiphyseal growth disturbance. How-

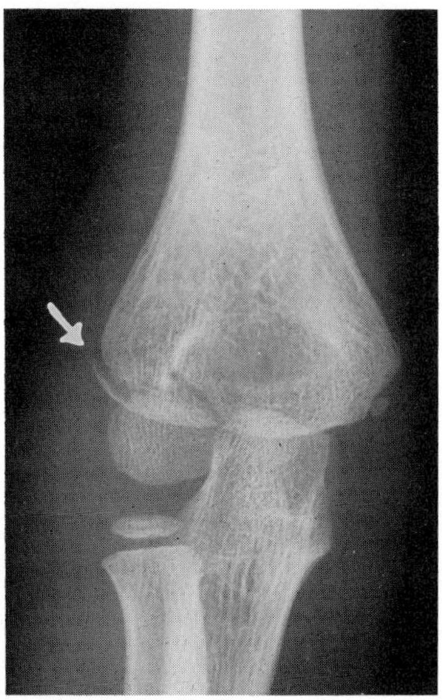

Fig. 50. Fracture of lateral condyle of humerus in a child. Antero-posterior roentgenogram of six year old child's elbow showing no displacement of the lateral condyle fragment which consists of the capitellar ossification center plus a thin shell of the diaphysis of the humerus.

ever, in this particular lesion the importance of obtaining accurate reduction (for the reasons stated above) may make open reduction imperative if closed manipulation fails to give a *completely* satisfactory reduction of the fragment. It might seem advisable to make one attempt at a closed reduction, warning the parents beforehand that this may not be successful; and, if not, then resort to open reduction and internal fixation rather than to repeated forceful attempts to gain reduction by closed manipulation.

Such repeated attempts at closed reduction are definitely harmful, cause additional damage to an already traumatized epiphysis, and pre-dispose not only to an increased probability of subsequent growth disturbance and non-union, but also to the formation of myositis ossificans in the brachialis anticus muscle.

Treatment

Closed Treatment. For those cases without displacement there is absolutely no necessity for manipulation. If the patient is suffering considerable pain as a result of hemarthrosis within the elbow joint, this can be relieved by aspiration. The elbow should be gently flexed to slightly less than a right angle and should be immobilized in a posterior molded splint extending from the axilla to the knuckles. A sling should also be applied.

In those cases requiring reduction the child should be given a general anesthetic to relieve pain and to obtain complete muscular relaxation. Traction is then applied to the partly flexed forearm with counter-traction to the upper arm. While maintaining the pull the forearm should be slightly *adducted* in order to widen the space on the outer aspect of the joint. While traction and adduction is being continued by an assistant the operator should manipulate the displaced fragment with his thumb and fingers and rotate it as well to correct lateral or angular shift and bring it into proper contact with the humerus. This is one lesion where actual visualization of the movements of the fragment during reduction may be advantageously watched under fluoroscopic control. If the reduction has been successful, the forearm should then be flexed at the elbow to an angle of approximately 60 to 70 degrees following which traction may be discontinued and the elbow immobilized in a posterior molded splint as stated above. The splint should be worn for approximately four weeks until good healing of the fragments is evident on roentgenograms. The treatment otherwise as far as sling, elevation, etc., is essentially the same as described under supracondylar fractures. Following removal of the splint a sling should be worn for approximately two weeks more, during which time the patient is encouraged to exercise the elbow for a few minutes every hour, and, as motion begins to increase, to begin mild active use.

Open Reduction. Operative reduction may be carried out as a primary procedure or after reduction has failed with an adequate attempt by closed

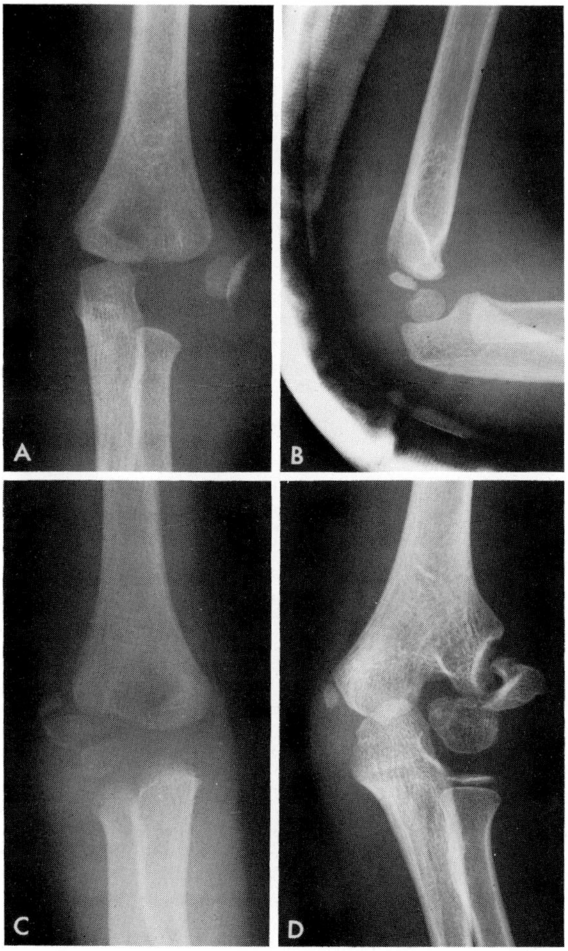

Fig. 51. Fracture of lateral condyle of humerus in a child aged three years six months showing marked displacement of fragment downwards, outwards, and extensively rotated. (A) Original antero-posterior view. Open reduction was performed and the fragment was fastened internally with a single suture. (B) Lateral view with elbow in plaster splint after operation. (C) Antero-posterior view four weeks after operation showing loss of fixation and lateral displacement of the fragment. (D) Same elbow two years later showing non-union of the fragment and growth disturbance.

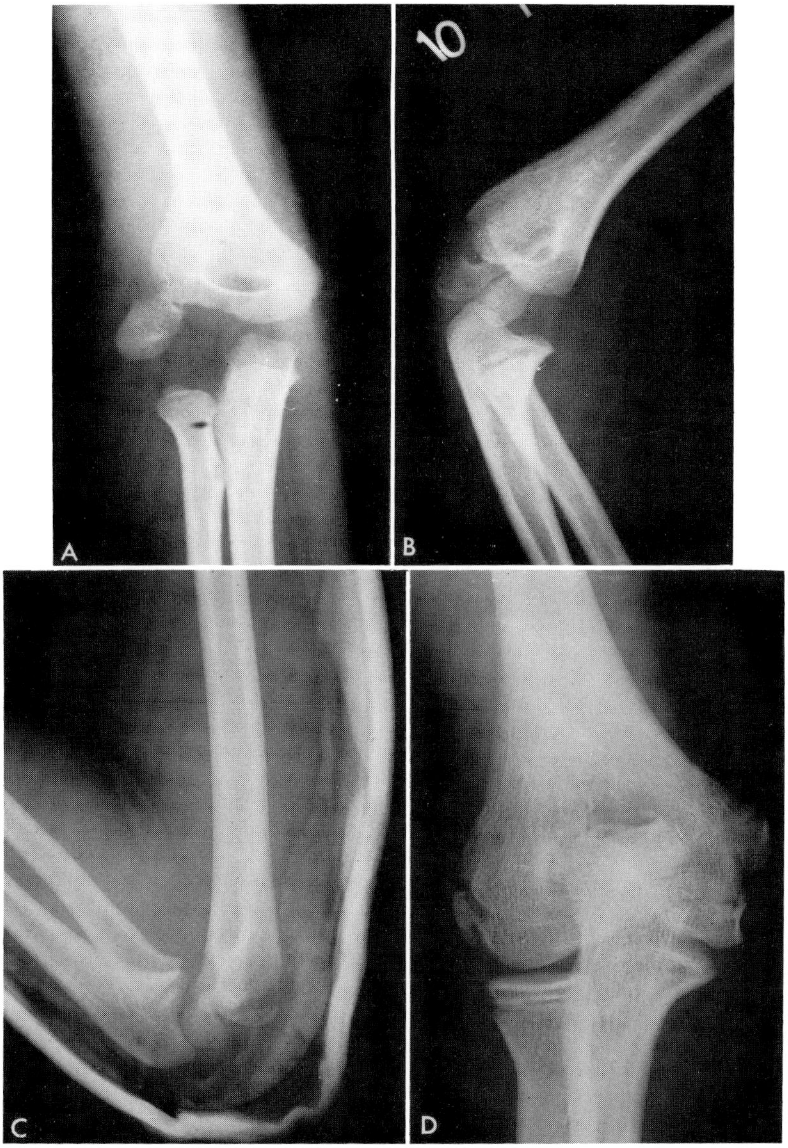

Fig. 52. Fracture of lateral condyle of humerus in a seven year old boy with marked displacement. (A) and (B) Original antero-posterior and lateral views. (C) Lateral view after closed reduction and immobilization in posterior plaster splint. (D) Antero-posterior view of same elbow nine and one-half years later. *Result:* anatomy and function normal.

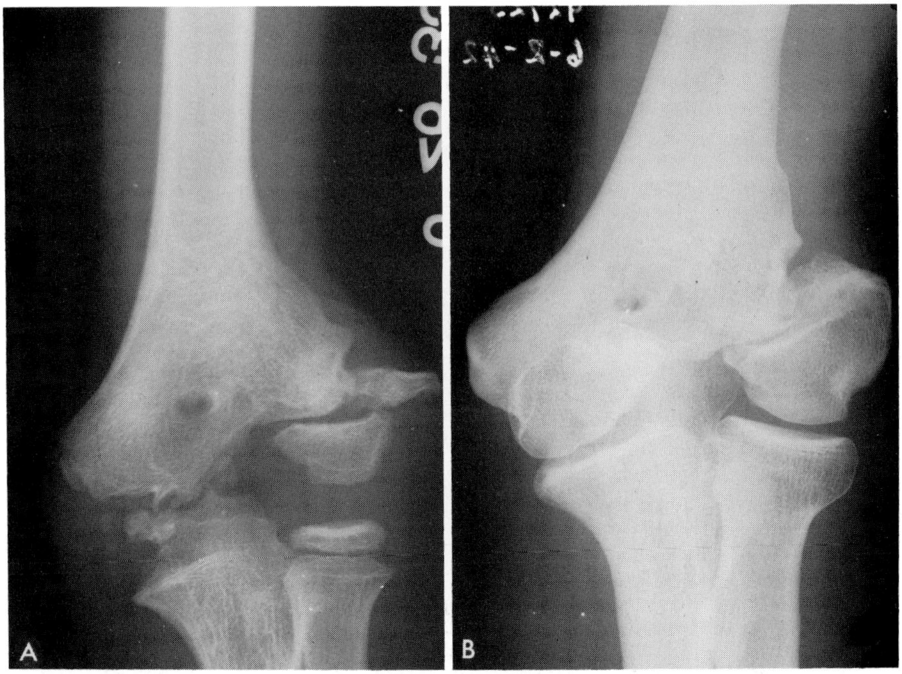

Fig. 53. Fracture of lateral condyle of humerus in eight year old boy showing, (A) growth disturbance one and a half years after injury. (B) Non-union nine years later in same elbow.

manipulation. If operation is to be performed, this should be done *early* preferably within the first twenty-four hours following injury. If put off for as long as two or three weeks, such a procedure may not only be extremely difficult and unsatisfactory, but it predisposes to the formation of myositis ossificans.

At open reduction when the fragment is replaced anatomically, it should be fastened to the diaphysis of the humerus with some form of rigid formation, such as a nail or screw. Attempts to suture this fragment in position do not give firm enough fixation and often result in subsequent displacement or growth disturbance. If the portion of the diaphysis fractured and displaced along with the capitellar epiphysis is so small or thin that it is impossible to use screws or nails for fixation, a Kirschner wire (s) may be drilled directly through the capitellum and epiphyseal plate upward into the main diaphysis; the excess wire may be permitted to project externally and the skin wound may be covered with a sterile dressing. At the end of three weeks the wire or wires may be withdrawn.

Theoretically, such a procedure might be considered as unsound, i. e., to cross the epiphyseal plate with a wire, but actually the caliber of the wire is so small that very little additional damage can be done to the epiphysis

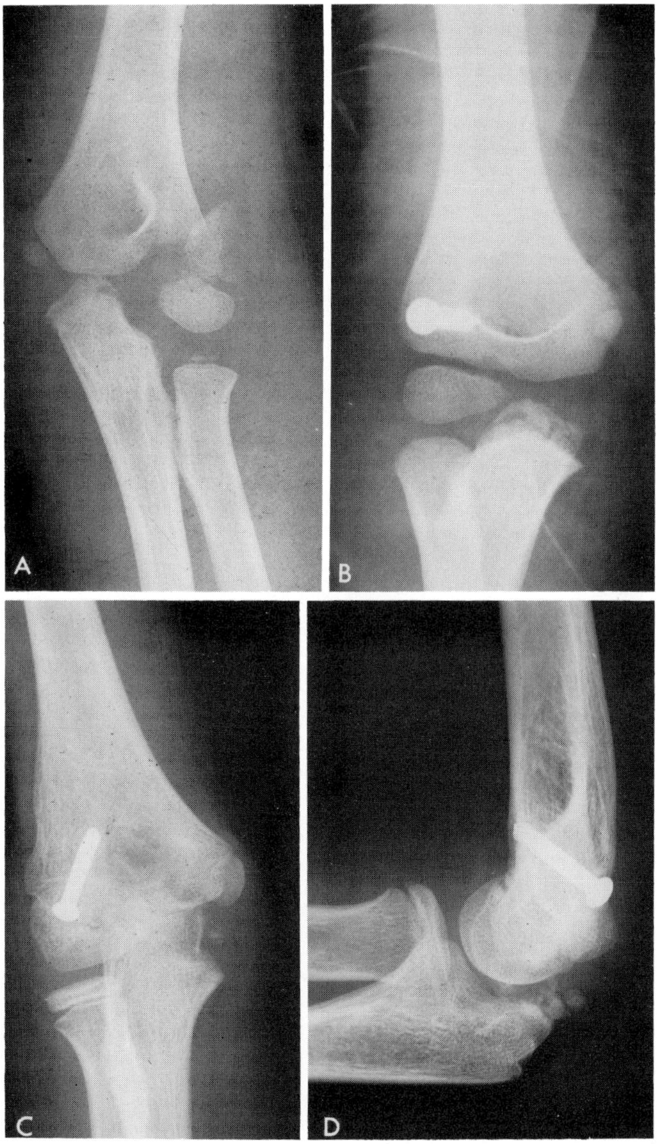

Fig. 54. Fracture of lateral condyle of humerus in five year old girl with marked displacement of the fragment. (A) Original antero-posterior view. (B) Same view after open reduction and internal fixation of fragment to diaphysis with a single screw. (C) and (D) Antero-posterior and lateral views five years later. *Result:* excellent.

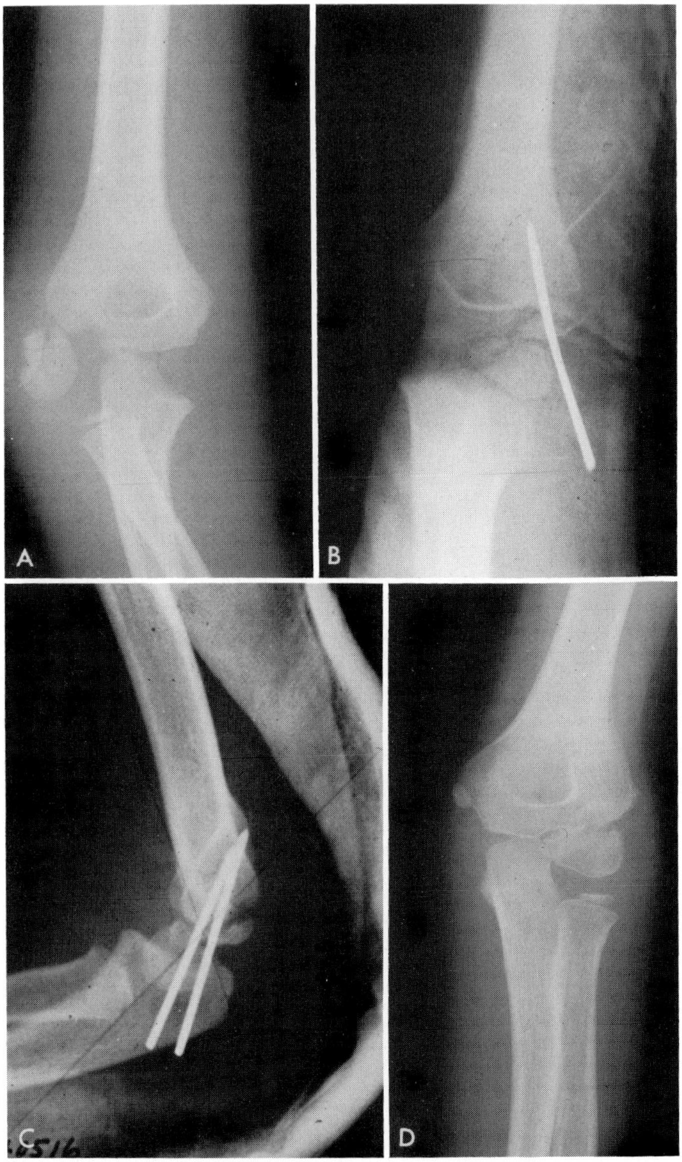

Fig. 55. Fracture of lateral condyle of humerus in seven year old boy with marked displacement of the fragment. (A) Original antero-posterior view. Open reduction was performed and the fragment was fastened (pinned) to the shaft by means of two Kirschner wires passed through the small fragment of diaphysis. The outer ends of these wires were left in the subcutaneous position and they were subsquently removed five weeks later. (B) and (C) Antero-posterior and lateral views of elbow after operation showing wire fixation in place and the posterior molded plaster spint used for additional protection. (D) Antero-posterior view eight weeks after injury. *Result:* excellent.

and the advantages of obtaining rigid fixation of the fragment at least temporarily would seem to far out-weigh any slight theoretical disadvantage.

In *late* cases where the fragment has not been reduced for one reason or another and the patient has come to the surgeon after several months with marked deformity and impairment of function, it is necessary to operate. At this time the fragment should be removed completely rather than attempt to replace it and fix it internally. The advantage of excision at this stage versus late open reduction is that there is less likelihood of slight malposition of the fragment or of excess bone formation causing interference with flexion and extension of the joint. Increased range of motion following late open reduction has not been very impressive in reported cases. One warning should be given, however, in such late cases, namely, that if there is present any evidence of myositis ossificans on roentgenographic examination, no operation should be done for at least one year or at least until three months have elapsed since the bone formation in the brachialis anticus muscle has been shown to have completely disappeared on the roentgenograms.

Prognosis

The prognosis depends upon the amount of the original trauma and displacement, the accuracy and maintenance of the reduction, and upon the question of possible later growth disturbance. Incomplete reduction or failure to maintain reduction leads to a broadened lateral condyle of the humerus even if bony union takes place and will almost certainly lead to limited elbow joint function, especially flexion and extension. If the loss of function becomes considerable or if there is marked displacement, it may be necessary at a later date to remove the lateral condyle at operation. It must be remembered, however, that late removal rarely gives any marked improvement in function.

Late Complications

As a result of retardation of the growth in the lateral humeral condyle and development of an increased carrying angle (cubitus valgus deformity) late ulnar neuritis often develops. This is caused by stretching of the ulnar nerve which takes a longer course to reach the forearm as it passes behind the medial epicondyle of the humerus. Another cause of late neuritis with an increased carrying angle is that the tip of the olecranon is tilted further medially than normal in full extension of the elbow. This tends to "crowd" the ulnar nerve each time the elbow is fully extended, thus setting up an inflammatory thickening in the sheath overlying it.

Late ulnar neuritis often does not develop for ten years or more following injury. Cases have been known to develop this complication as late as 30 years after injury. The parents of the child should always be warned concerning this possibility, and this may be done without alarming them unduly. The symptoms consist of numbness or tingling in the ulnar nerve sensory distribution in the hand or fingers. If the nerve lesion becomes progressive, there will be subsequent impairment of its motor function with either weakness or complete paralysis with atrophy of the intrinsic muscles in the hand. The importance of warning the patient or his parents concerning the possibility of a late neuritis is necessary, because, when it develops, the patient rarely connects it with the previous injury and may do nothing about it until it is too late. Something can be done to relieve it, namely, transposition of the ulnar nerve, but this should always be done before the motor function of the nerve becomes involved and before intrinsic muscular atrophy develops, otherwise there is little hope for return of this function. If transposition is performed early, the chances of complete recovery are excellent (Chapter XXI).

"SIDE-SWIPE" FRACTURES OF THE LOWER EXTREMITY OF THE HUMERUS

The injury known as a "truck-swipe," "side-swipe," or "car-window" elbow is the most serious type of fracture with which we have to deal in this region. It is a shattering type of injury which occurs when the driver of an automobile passes too closely another car or truck with an over-hanging body and his elbow is struck while resting upon the window-sill or when he skids into another object. The blow upon the elbow is a direct injury and is delivered at high-speed. The elbow and lower humerus are driven violently against the window-frame and the shattering force thus delivered practically causes the elbow to "explode."

Unfortunately, the injury is fairly common. It is almost always a compound (open) fracture and there may be extensive loss of substance including skin, muscles, vessels, portions of nerves, and even bone fragments. Contamination of the wound is likely to be great from portions of clothing ground into it. The elbow joint as well as the bones is extensively smashed. Some mild forms of the injury are seen, but the majority are very serious and some even require primary amputation due to loss of blood supply to the lower forearm and hand or to other irreparable damage. It is frequently impossible to do very much for the extremity owing to the damage, poor blood supply, and contamination and often the most that can be expected as a result is a flail elbow. The chance of infection of course is great and this may even be so serious as to result in gas gangrene.

The associated lesions are compound fracture of the upper extremity of the radius and ulna that frequently accompany the humeral fracture. Hemorrhage and shock may be severe and requires the administration of blood transfusions.

Treatment

Closed Treatment. The amount of injury of course determines the type of treatment to be given. Fractures which are not compounded, but show comminution of the fragments may be treated by over-head traction and

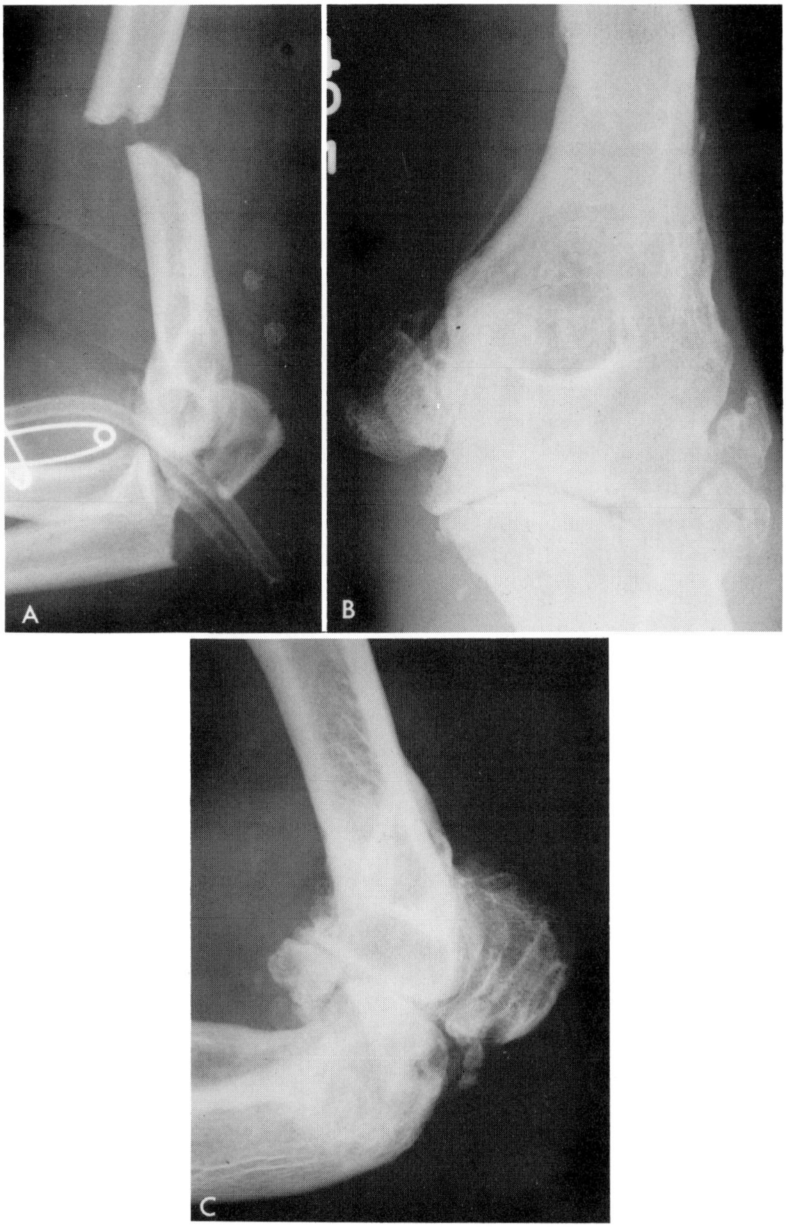

Fig. 56. Truck swipe ("side swipe") fracture of elbow region. (A) Lateral view two days after operation (debridement). Note drainage tubes. The fracture was treated by suspension. This patient was a 30 year old man. (B) and (C) Antero-posterior and lateral views of the same elbow 17 years later. Note narrowing of joint space and the extra-articular bone formation. Motion was limited 60 per cent, but pain was minimal. Patient works as draftsman.

suspension with a Kirschner wire plus gentle manipulation of the fragments with an attempt to obtain the best possible function without attempting to regain perfect anatomical position of these. Active motion should be instituted early for the purpose of obtaining elbow joint motion. It is practically never possible to perform open reduction and internal fixation of these fragments owing to their large number. If they should be few in amount, it may be advisable to perform open reduction, but of course this must be done only by surgeons experienced in this type of work. The best functional results are usually obtained by conservative treatment rather than by the ill-advised attempts at open reduction and internal fixation.

Open Treatment. Operative debridement must be done when the fracture is compounded, but this should not be so thorough as in the ordinary compound fracture owing to the very extensive comminution and extreme degree of soft part damage. In other words the debridement should be somewhat on the conservative side because more thorough debridement may devitalize bone fragments and cause extensive muscle damage. Large quantities of normal saline solution should be used to lavage the wound, but no chemical irritants should thus be employed. The compound wound should be packed open loosely with fine-mesh plain or vaselined gauze. Sutures may be laid for secondary closure, provided no infection has set in after five or six days. Immobilization is best carried out by the over-head Kirschner wire skeletal traction which maintains the fragments in the best position possible and also allows for changes of dressings or inspection of the wound. Tetanus-antitoxin should be given and penicillin or sulfa drugs may and probably should be given in view of the extensive soft part damage accompanying the bone lesion.

A careful check should be made of the patient's temperature, pulse and general reaction, and, if there is any indication that infection is occurring in the wound, this should be inspected. Should infection be present, it is necessary to drain by opening the wound completely and using counter-drainage if necessary. The wound should then be thoroughly irrigated with normal saline solution, rather than with such a solution as Dakin's since the former is physiological and less irritating to the soft parts, the bones and joint lining. Even though the acute infection clears up there may possibly remain dead fragments of bone that require removal by sequestrectomy. The chance of ankylosis taking place is great if the joint has become infected. If one suspects that ankylosis is going to occur, he should place the joint in the position that he feels is optimum for the particular patient according to his daily needs and occupation.

After-treatment. The primary purpose of the treatment is of course to obtain a closed and clean wound. If it is possible to close the original wound which has been packed open at operation by secondary suture five days later, this may be advantageous and may help to prevent secondary infection. It is usually advisable to avoid further operative procedure, however, except for necessary drainage or sequestrectomy. As soon as the wound has become closed active exercise is in order to assist the patient in regaining as much motion as he can. Some form of brace may be necessary to lend stability to the elbow since many of these become flail as a result of the extensive original damage to the bones. A brace makes it easier for the patient to flex his elbow actively without assistance of his other hand.

Disability Time

The disability time is likely to be very great and may extend to a year or even longer.

Prognosis

The prognosis is always serious because of the extent of the primary injury and the possibility of infection or gangrene. The deformity may be so great that the patient has practically a useless arm. Since all treatment, however, is directed towards saving the arm and obtaining active motion and strength, these patients may recover a useful arm for light or sedentary work, but rarely one that is good for hard labor or in skilled occupations. Disability for such work may become complete.

GUN-SHOT WOUNDS OF THE ELBOW

It is impossible to advise specific therapy for gun-shot wounds in the elbow region since the pathology, contamination and time element may be so variable. A complete and thorough examination must be carried out to determine the extent of the injury not only to bone and joint but to all of the soft parts, checking especially for vascular or nerve damage. Even in the presence of severe damage, loss of substance (bone and soft parts), and extensive contamination an attempt should be made to save the extremity if arterial circulation to the forearm and hand is good. Loss of circulation due to arterial laceration can only be restored by early surgical repair by a surgical team trained in this particular type of work. Extensive damage, loss of substance, and contamination followed by infection would mitigate against any possible success with such a procedure even in the presence of chemotherapy. Gangrene would result and subsequent amputation would be necessary, possibly at a higher level and at greater risk to the patient because of the dangers of pathogenic organisms, especially of the gas forming group.

Minor gun-shot wounds should be explored under strict aseptic technique in the operating room, the wounds of entry and exit debrided, explored for foreign material (clothing, etc.) and thoroughly irrigated. Hemostasis must be obtained and hematomas must be evacuated. If the arterial circulation is impaired, the artery must be explored and decision made as to repair or amputation if found divided. If the artery is in spasm or is thrombosed, it may be advisable to perform arterial sympathectomy or sympathetic nerve block (Chapter XVIII). Any injured nerves must likewise be explored. It is not so important to repair divided nerve trunks early, but the exact pathology should be determined and if found divided their ends should be anchored and marked with black silk, stainless steel or tantulum wire suture for later identification. In general, the wound must be treated much the same as in compound fractures from other causes, i. e., an attempt made to save the extremity, preserve as much function as possible, and to convert a contaminated wound into one that is surgically clean. Early wound healing without or with minimal infection is to be desired if a successful result is to be achieved.

Severe gun-shot wounds with associated marked loss of substance may seem hopeless to begin with, but if the circulation is not irreparably damaged, considerable restoration of function may be obtained by adequate debridement, strict adherence to aseptic technique at the time and in the after-care, early skin grafting and by reconstructive bone and nerve surgery at a later date. There is some hope in the future of utilizing internal metal or plastic prostheses to replace loss of bone or joint surfaces, but as yet such procedures have been attempted only in isolated instances. Where damage and contamination to the joint surfaces has been extreme it is sometimes advisable to perform primary excision of all the fragments. This would give the patient the equivalent of a primary arthroplasty which, if not satisfactory from a functional standpoint, could be followed by subsequent reconstructive procedures, or, if inadvisable by arthrodesis in a useful position. An upper extremity should be saved if possible unless its circulatory status is completely hopeless or unless spreading infection presents an immediate and serious threat to the patient's life.

DOOR-HANDLE INJURIES

Pedestrians formerly were not infrequent sufferers from a peculiar type of injury inflicted by the door handle of an automobile that brushed them in passing. The long ends of the handles not only pointed forward, but often turned outward at their tips, making an ideal hook to catch the clothing or actual flesh of the victim's arm or elbow. The injury though often trivial sometimes was of a severe nature. A protruding door handle of a rapidly moving car could penetrate skin and muscles, fracture the underlying bone and cause avulsion of large amounts of soft tissue. Many serious compound fractures with loss of substance thus resulted, including severely or irreparably damaged radial nerves.

Much credit must be given to the National Safety Council for bringing this type of injury to the attention of automobile manufacturers and for persuading them to alter the design of door handles which they have done, thereby eliminating the possibility of this particular type of injury. The injury may still occur from an old-fashioned car, but fortunately few of these are still able to be driven. Confronted with a patient thus injured, treatment must be according to the damage sustained and whether the injury is a clean or contaminated one (Chapter XV).

Chapter XI

The Upper Extremity of the Ulna

FRACTURES OF THE OLECRANON

FRACTURE OF the olecranon process of the ulna is a common injury in adults, but less so in children. It is also not so serious or so important in this latter group. The fracture line may be transversely placed due mainly to indirect violence as in attempting to break a fall by landing on the hand with the elbow partially flexed. Such fractures may or may not show separation of the fragments, depending upon the presence or absence of tear of the periosteum and triceps expansion. The injury is analogous to transverse fractures of the patella with or without separation and depending upon the degree of tear in the quadriceps expansion. The level of the fracture is usually located at the middle portion of the greater sigmoid fossa, but it may be higher or lower. If at a lower level, the fracture may permit anterior displacement of the distal ulnar fragment. In children the fracture is commonly of the greenstick variety, but a type is occasionally seen in which some separation of the fragments may occur. The fractures with separation may be of the transverse variety with the upper fragment displaced in a proximal direction or oblique with its line coursing in a distal and posterior direction, the lower fragment being displaced anteriorly. In children roentgenograms may fail to reveal the fracture line in the diaphysis of the ulna and the diagnosis must be made from the clinical signs of swelling and acute tenderness over the olecranon epiphysis. It is important to keep this in mind because of the slight possibility that growth disturbance may occur at a later date. Very rarely it may later become necessary to operate to remove a portion of the enlarged olecranon process if this reaches sufficient size to cause symptoms or loss of elbow joint extension.

One must be careful not to make an erroneous diagnosis of fracture of the olecranon in children by mistaking multiple ossification centers for fracture lines. The center or centers of ossification in the olecranon epiphysis usually appear (on films) at about the tenth year. If doubt exists in the surgeon's mind as to whether or not this ossification center is fractured or is one with multiple centers, he should make a comparative roentgenogram of the uninjured olecranon.

Comminuted fractures of the olecranon are less common than transverse fractures and are usually caused by direct violence. These may show little or no separation. They are sometimes associated with an open (compound)

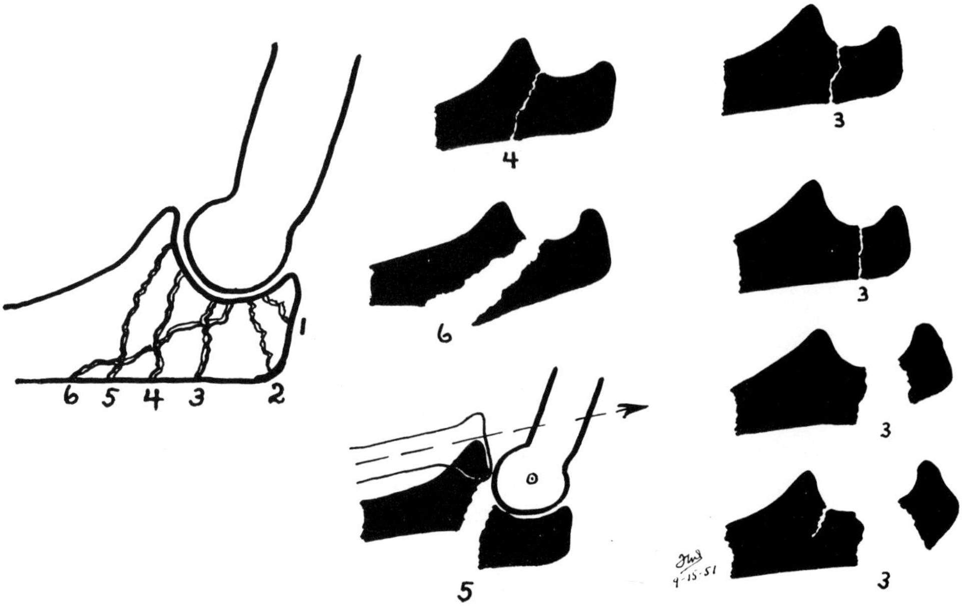

Fig. 57. Sketch showing common sites of fracture of olecranon in adults with characteristic types of displacement when present.

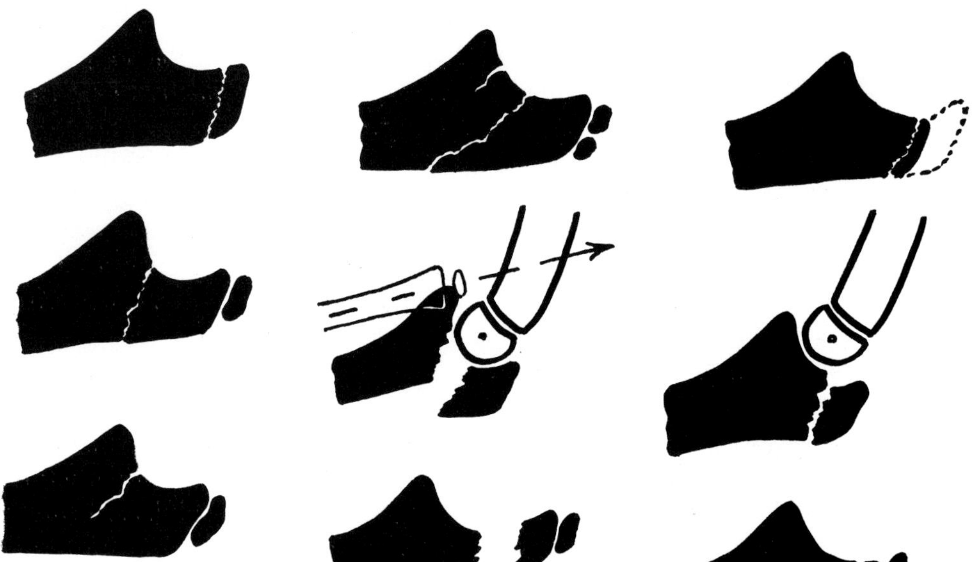

Fig. 58. Sketch of olecranon fractures in children showing characteristic sites and displacements. It should be remembered that the ossification center for the olecranon appears on roentgenograms at about the age of 10 years and one must not mistake a normal epiphyseal line for a fracture.

wound, which of course is serious because such contamination will involve the elbow joint proper.

Associated Lesions. Ulnar nerve injury may accompany olecranon fractures especially those with comminution due to direct force. Anterior dislocation of the proximal end of the shaft of the ulna may occur if the fracture through the olecranon is situated just above the level of the coronoid process; and anterior dislocation of the radial head may be associated with such displacement of the shaft.

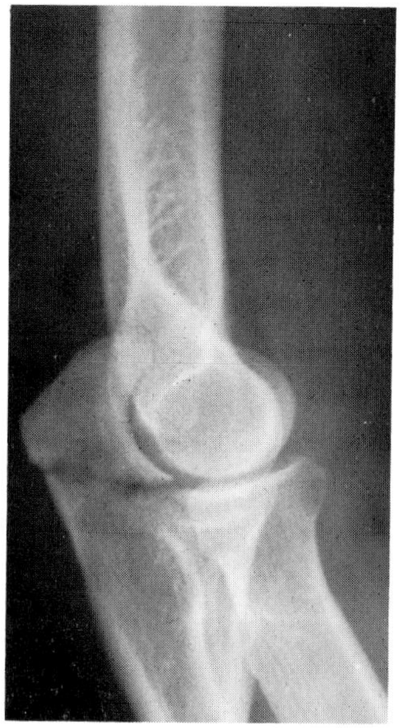

Fig. 59. Lateral roentgenogram showing fracture of olecranon process without displacement. The lack of bony displacement is due to the fact that the triceps tendon expansions have remained intact. No operative repair is indicated in such a case. Treatment should be conservative and active elbow motion may be started in 10 days after the injury.

Treatment

In general, treatment of olecranon fractures depends largely upon separation of the fragments (see Fig. 57). Should the fragments show less than 0.5 centimeter separation on the lateral roentgenogram, and this does not increase with flexion of the elbow to a right angle, or, if the patient is able to extend his elbow joint actively against gravity, the treatment may be conservative. If wide separation of the fragments exists and this increases upon flexion of the elbow, or, if the patient is unable to extend his elbow actively against gravity, operation is usually indicated. If the patient is elderly or some other definite contra-indication exists such as an infected laceration or abrasion overlying the fracture site, treatment should be of a conservative nature.

Operation is a *necessity* in the opinion of the author as well as many other surgeons when there is separation of the fragments and when the fracture is compounded. Operation is usually advisable in simple cases with separation provided this can be performed by a qualified surgeon in a hospital properly equipped for bone surgery. Such an operation is not a difficult procedure, but strict aseptic technique must be followed, because an infection will almost certainly result in suppurative arthritis of the elbow joint, possible ankylosis and marked permanent disability. The reason for advising operation in these fractures is that: (1) irregularity of the joint surfaces if not corrected will later cause pain, restricted motion, and the development of traumatic arthritis; (2) loss of strength in the triceps tendon, which has been elongated by the separation of the proximal fragment from the distal; and (3) in young and middle aged individuals, who need a strong and movable elbow, operative repair offers them a more certain and a more rapid chance of obtaining a good result. In elderly individuals, who do not have to do hard work, and in growing children operation is usually not indicated unless the fracture is compounded.

Treatment in Adults

Conservative Treatment. When little or no separation of the olecranon fragment exists, the elbow should be immobilized at ninety degrees in a posterior molded splint from the shoulder to the knuckles and the splint should be worn for one week in order to permit pain, swelling and muscle spasm to disappear. Following this a sling is worn for another two to three weeks and the patient should be put on a regime of frequent active exercises, hot soaks and mild massage in order to restore elbow joint function as quickly as possible. Bony union is usually complete in six to eight weeks. Some surgeons advise the use of a splint for as long as three or four weeks, but prolonged immobilization is unnecessary and inadvisable (when the triceps fascia is intact), because it allows the formation of intra-articular adhesions and permanent limitation of joint motion. It may be advisable not to immobilize the elbow in more than a sling from the beginning, particularly in individuals with a tendency towards arthritis.

With wide separation of the olecranon fragments the fracture, if treated

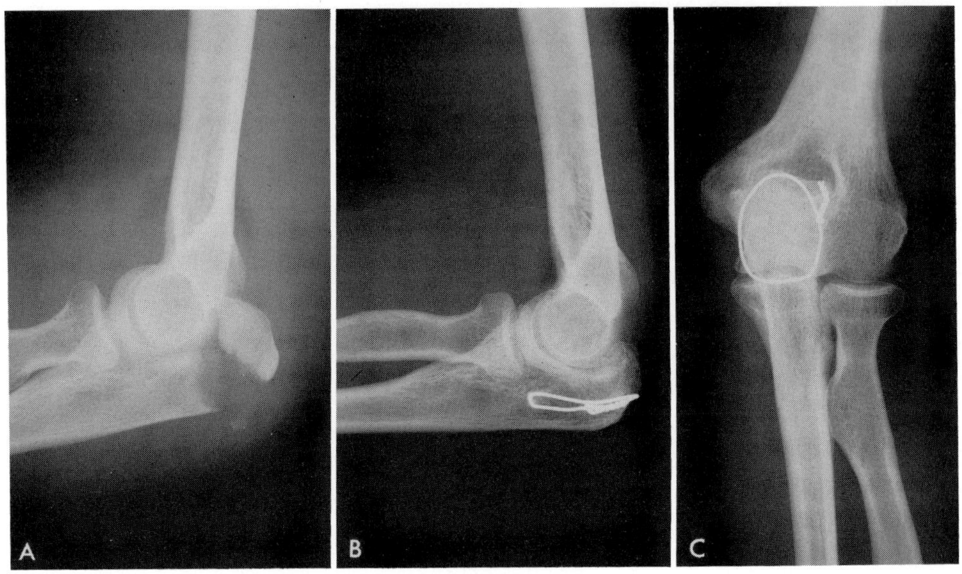

Fig. 60. (A) Lateral roentgenograms of elbow of woman 34 years of age showing fracture of olecranon with displacement of the fragment. The expansions of the triceps tendon must be torn to permit such displacement. Treatment consisted of immediate operative repair of the bone by wire loop passed through distal fragment and through insertion of triceps tendon on proximal end of the olecranon fragment. The torn triceps expansions were repaired by interrupted silk sutures. Active exercises were started within one week after operation. (B) and (C) lateral and antero-posterior views of same elbow four years later showing solid bone union. *Result:* excellent.

conservatively, should have an attempt at manual reduction and the elbow should then be immobilized in a posterior molded splint in full extension in order to relax the triceps pull upon the proximal fragment. Some authors advise the use of criss-cross adhesive strapping placed over felt padding to maintain approximation of the fragments, but such strapping may interfere with circulation and besides is extremely inefficient for the purpose intended, owing to the extensive edema of the overlying subcutaneous tissues. Closed reduction and splinting in extension should be used *only* where it is impossible to operate in otherwise healthy individuals.

Operative Treatment. Open reduction and internal fixation of an olecranon fracture with separation may be accomplished by the use of a wire loop of stainless steel or tantulum and of good strength (18 gauge) plus repair of the triceps tendon and periosteum. This method will permit early active motion in the elbow joint and thereby assure quicker and more complete return of function and strength. Fixation with plate and screws is not so satisfactory in this particular region as with a wire loop or a single large screw. A Steinman pin driven down through the olecranon process into the distal ulna has been advocated, but the proximal end of this pin either has to project from the skin, or, if cut off and buried beneath the skin, may cause pressure upon it with some chance of infection developing. Fascial repair after the method described by Rhombold may be useful when the fracture is comminuted and other forms of internal fixation are not possible.

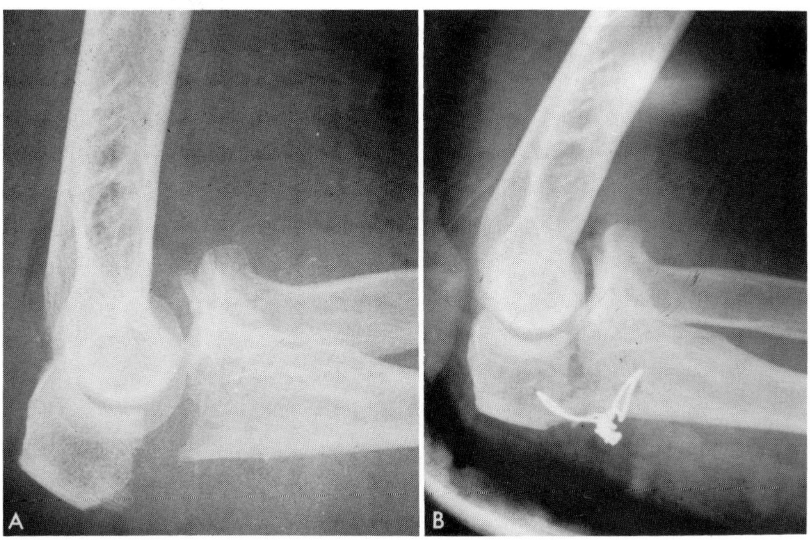

Fig. 61. (A) Lateral roentgenogram showing fracture of olecranon with anterior subluxation of radius and distal ulnar fragment upon the humerus. (B) Lateral view after operative repair with wire loop and suture of triceps expansions. Owing to the fracture line being situated in the distal part of the olecranon (permitting forward subluxation), wire loop fixation was inadequate. This fracture should have had intramedullary screw fixation alone or in addition to the wire loop to counteract the forward subluxation tendency.

In some fractures with extensive comminution it may be wise and simpler to excise the olecranon as advised by Watson-Jones and MeKeever and as is frequently done with comminuted fractures of the patella. This method has been reserved for comminuted fractures high in the olecranon area in elderly individuals. It is extremely important that the triceps tendon and its expansions be repaired if the olecranon has to be excised. In order to obtain a stronger repair it may be necessary to weave a strip of fascia lata through the lower triceps tendon and anchor it through a drill hole in the proximal end of the ulnar shaft.

If operation is to be performed, the best results are to be obtained when

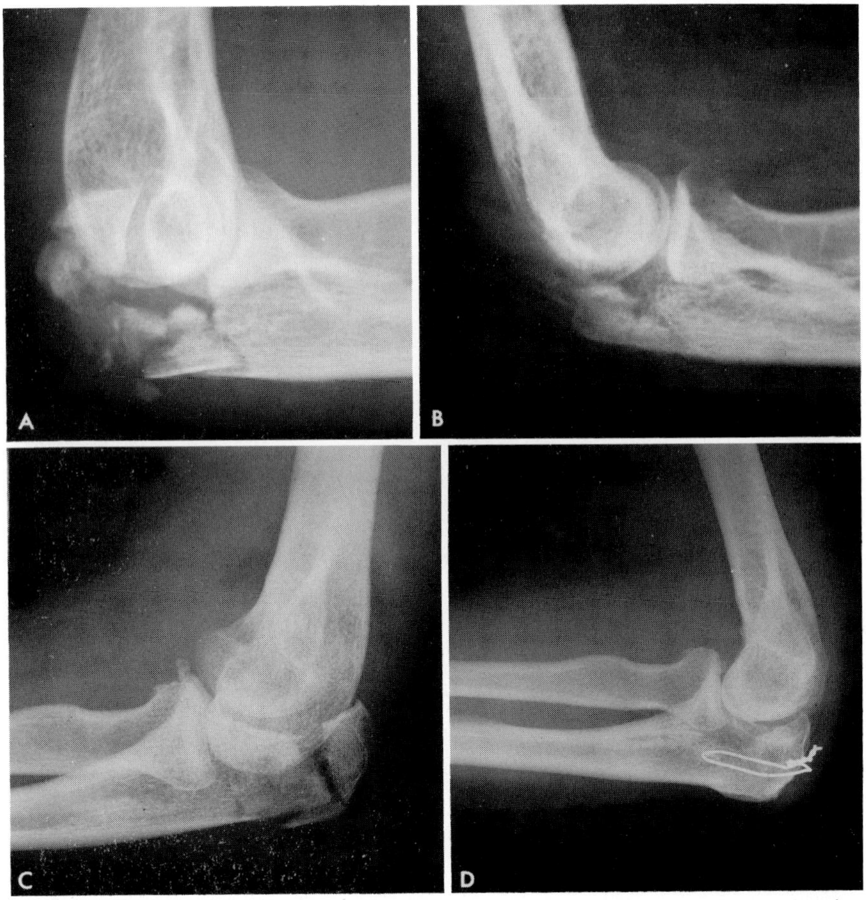

Fig. 62. (A) Lateral view showing fracture of olecranon with marked comminution resulting from fall on tip of elbow, i. e., by direct force. (B) Same elbow two weeks after operative removal of the comminuted fragments and reattachment of the triceps tendon to distal periosteum. This patient was operated upon two weeks after original injury. The result was good, but by no means perfect. (C) Lateral view of another patient with an open (compound) comminuted fracture of the olecranon. Immediate debridement was performed. It was not necessary to excise the fragments in this case and internal fixation was possible with a wire loop. Active exercises were commenced as soon as the wound healed. (D) Lateral view one year six months after operation. The wire loop was subsequently removed. *Result:* excellent.

this is performed *immediately or within the first two days after injury.* Regardless of what type of internal fixation is used or what type of repair is carried out, it is extremely important to lavage the elbow joint thoroughly with saline solution in order to remove clots of blood or fibrin and to search for and remove any loose fragments of bone and cartilage that may tend to fall into the joint cavity and act as loose bodies and cause irritation.

Technique of Operation. Open reduction is easily performed through a lateral incision beginning just above the tip of the olecranon and curving slightly laterally and then medially in the distal portion until it crosses the posterior crest of the ulna about two inches below the fracture. Care should be taken to avoid the ulnar nerve on the medial aspect. The skin flap is dissected medially and the periosteum is incised longitudinally and elevated from both sides of the olecranon and ulnar shaft. After lavaging the joint and removing any completely loose fragments, the main olecranon fragment should be approximated to the upper shaft with a bone hook to test its reduction. The most satisfactory means of internal fixation should then be chosen which will give firm fixation. If a wire loop is to be used, it should be of sufficient strength (22 or 18 gauge) and should be passed through a transverse drill hole situated at least 1.5 centimeters below the proximal end of the distal fragment. The purchase of the wire loop upon the proximal fragment may be obtained by a transverse drill hole in the proximal fragment, if this fragment is sufficiently large and not comminuted and if the bone is not unduly soft. It is often better to pass the proximal end of the loop through the insertion of the triceps tendon into the olecranon since this gives a stronger grip and shows less tendency to pull out of or split the fragment. While the main fragment is again held approximated to the distal with the bone hook, the wire loop is then snugged up and twisted, care being taken not to twist the ends more than is necessary to bring the twist

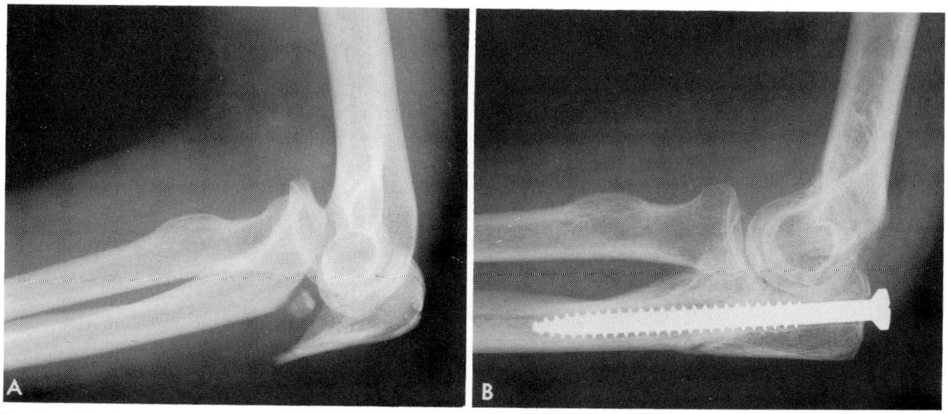

Fig. 63. (A) Lateral view showing oblique fracture of olecranon with forward displacement of distal fragment (not a good type for wire loop fixation). (B) Post-reduction lateral view after open reduction and internal fixation with an intramedullary wood-type screw. The torn triceps expansions were repaired by suture. This type of fixation permits early active joint motion and helps in its speedy recovery.

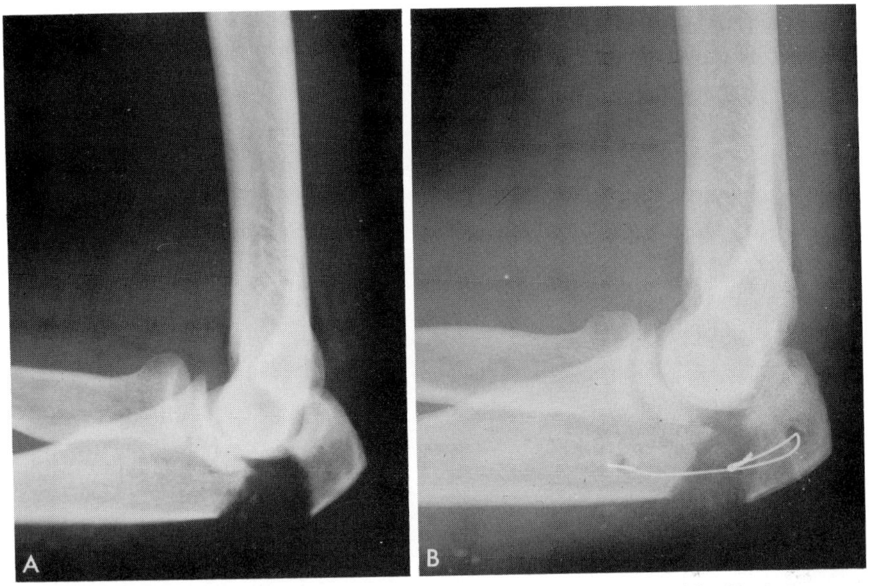

Fig. 64. (A) Original lateral view showing fracture of olecranon with displacement in a 50 year old woman. (B) Same elbow three weeks after operative repair with inadequate sized wire loop. Sufficiently strong wire must be used for such fixation or the patient is subjected to all the risks of open reduction without receiving any of its benefits.

in contact with the surface of the bone. Any further twisting is very apt to cause the wire to break. The excess portion of the twisted wire should be cut off and the short, twisted end turned downwards alongside the bone to lie beneath the periosteum so that it cannot project and cause irritation of the skin. The elbow should then be gently manipulated to make certain

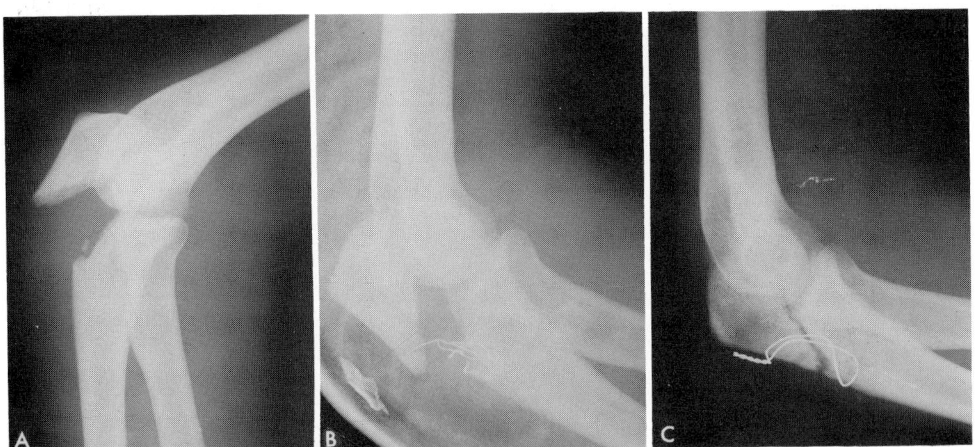

Fig. 65. (A) Lateral view of fracture of olecranon with displacement. (B) Same elbow the day following open reduction and internal fixation with wire loop of too small caliber. Wire has broken and the fragments have again separated. A second operation was required to reduce and re-wire the fragments. (C) Same elbow three months after second operation showing excellent position. Healing of the fracture is occurring though somewhat slow. (Case of Dr. R. Diefendorf.)

that the wire fixation is adequate and allows no motion of one fragment upon the other. Repair of the periosteum and triceps tendon should then be carried out with interrupted sutures of fine silk. The skin and subcutaneous tissue may be closed by whatever sutures the surgeon prefers.

There is no single method of internal fixation for olecranon fractures that is entirely satisfactory in every case. *Regardless of the type of internal fixation used there must be adequate fixation followed by early active motion if good results are to be uniformally obtained.*

As has been mentioned before one may use screws, plates or pins, but in general a wire loop is the most satisfactory form of internal fixation in this particular type of fracture. Under no circumstances should extremely fine wire be used since this will break more readily than not or tend to cut through the bone, and in either case loss of fixation will result. The gauge of the wire should be No. 22 or preferably stronger, i. e., No. 18. Either a stainless steel or tantulum wire may be employed. Repair of an olecranon fracture with silk or catgut sutures or by means of Kangaroo tendon is a very unsatisfactory method and will not permit early active exercises.

Screw Fixation. The proximal olecranon fragment is held in apposition with the distal by a bone hook and a large drill hole is made after splitting the triceps insertion. A wood type screw three inches in length and of sufficient caliber is then passed down through this fragment and made to engage the shaft. As this is tightened, it snugs the two fragments together (Fig. 66c). The periosteum and triceps expansion is repaired as described above. This method often gives excellent fixation and permits early active motion. Screw fixation may be utilized in addition to a wire loop when the fracture line is oblique or slightly comminuted and gives better fixation than with either one alone.

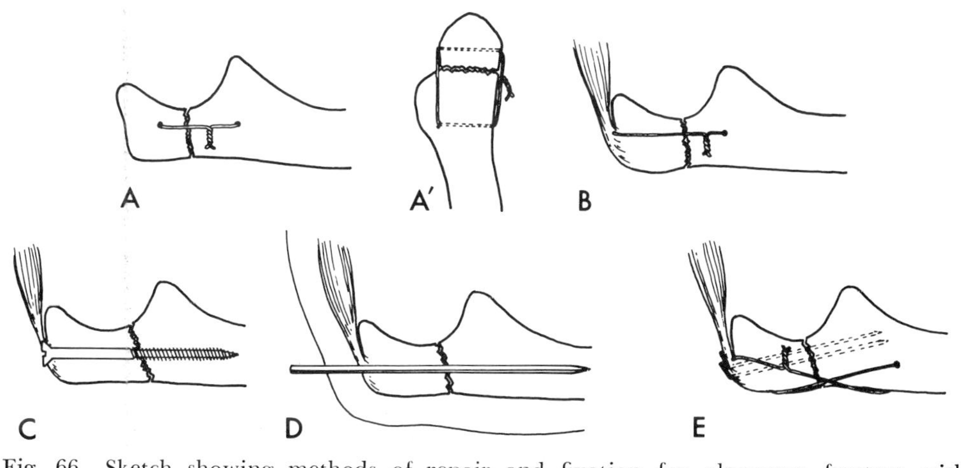

Fig. 66. Sketch showing methods of repair and fixation for olecranon fracture with displacement; (A) wire loop through both fragments twisted or knotted on lateral side; (B) wire loop passing through triceps insertion so as not to split the fragment; (C) wood type screw alone; (D) intramedullary pin with Proximal end projecting from skin; and (E) fixation with two Kirschner wires and an additional figure of 8 wire loop.

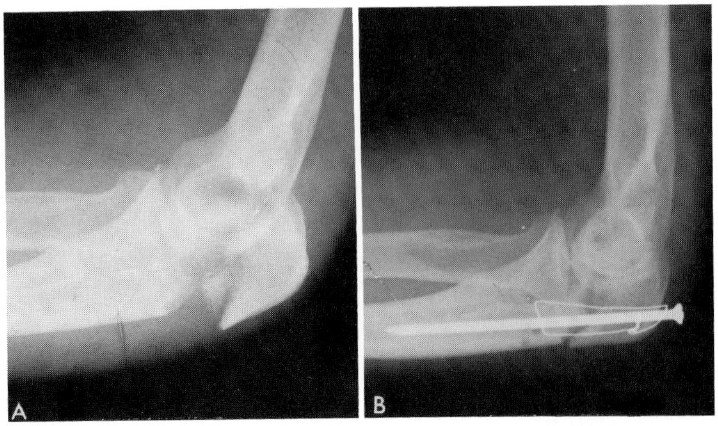

Fig. 67. Fracture of olecranon with displacement. (A) Original lateral view. (B) After internal fixation with long screw and wire loop. Note lack of anterior subluxation of distal fragment.

Rhombold's Method of Fascial Repair. This technique utilizes the triceps tendon which tends to force the olecranon fragments together when the triceps muscle contracts. It is useful in some comminuted fractures or where other means of internal fixation cannot be used, but is not a simple procedure and it does not give the rigid fixation that may be obtained by a strong wire loop. The procedure is carried out by turning down a strip of the triceps tendon approximately four inches long by one-half inch wide. The lower end of this strip is left attached to the olecranon. A large hole is drilled through the posterior crest of the distal fragment and connected with a hole on each side of the ulna slightly more distally placed. The strip of tendon is then split longitudinally and inserted through this proximal hole and each half is brought out on its corresponding side. While the fragments are maintained in apposition by means of a bone hook, these strips are drawn upwards and sutured to the periosteum and to each other and to the triceps fascia by interrupted silk sutures. It is also necessary, of course, to repair any tear in the triceps expansion.

Excision of Olecranon Fragment(s). In fractures situated high in the olecranon and severely comminuted it is often justified to excise the fragment (s) rather than attempt to repair them with wire or screw fixation. Another instance in which excision is justifiable is in old olecranon fractures that have not been reduced. The triceps tendon and expansions must be repaired at the same time if strong elbow extension is to be regained.

The author feels quite strongly that excision of the olecranon fragments should not be adopted as a routine operative procedure in early cases.

Treatment in Children

Conservative treatment is usually advisable in fractures of the olecranon in children since most of these show no separation. Even with separation

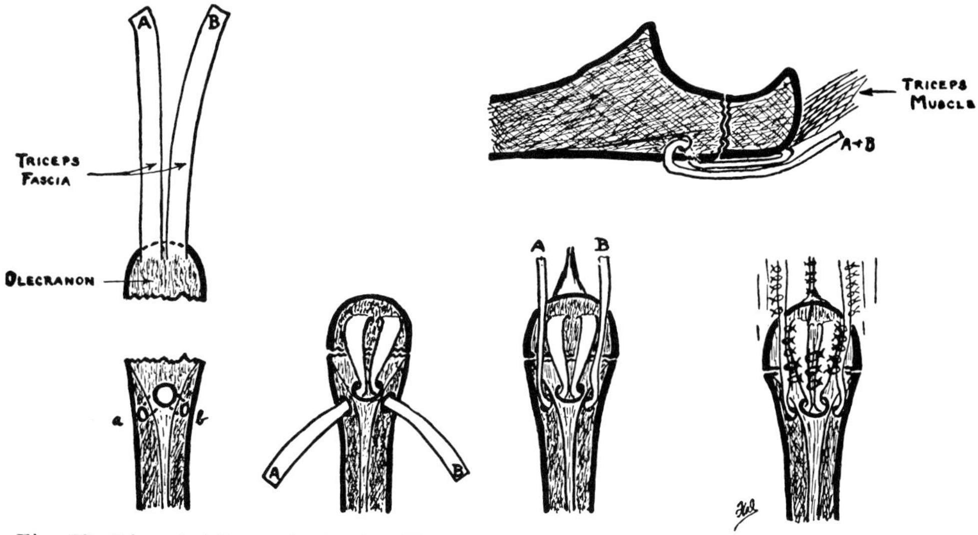

Fig. 68. Rhombold's method of utilizing the triceps fascia to repair a fracture of the olecranon. (Bancroft and Marble: *Surgery of the Motor Skeletal System*. 2nd Ed. Chapter 32, Lippincott, Philadelphia, 1951.)

three or four weeks of immobilization in extension is sufficient, for these fractures heal rapidly and one need not fear subsequent joint stiffness. Active exercises may be started in the unseparated cases in two weeks and in those with separation in four weeks. No massage should be given in these children. Where the olecranon fracture is oblique, beginning just above the coronoid process, and the distal fragment tends to dislocate in an anterior direction, a reduction must be obtained by manipulation or suspension and held by plaster else marked functional impairment may result in the joint.

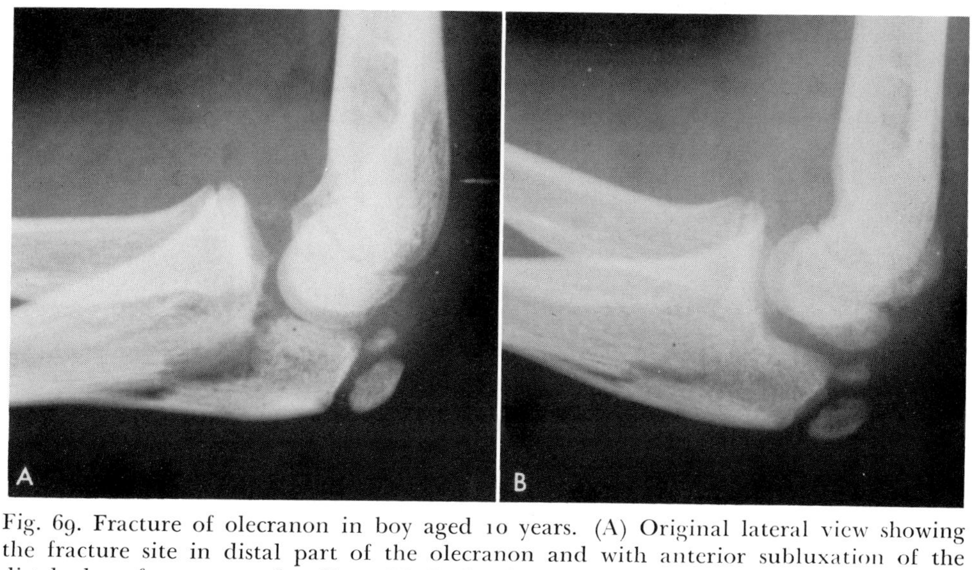

Fig. 69. Fracture of olecranon in boy aged 10 years. (A) Original lateral view showing the fracture site in distal part of the olecranon and with anterior subluxation of the distal ulnar fragment and radius. (B) Reduction affected by suspension method shown in Figure 70. *Result:* excellent. (Case of Dr. A. Pappas.)

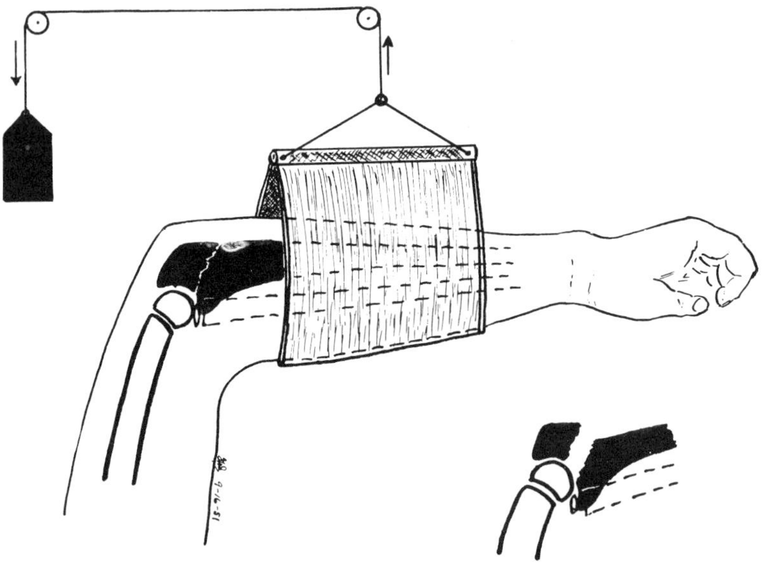

Fig. 70. Sketch showing method of suspension by which it is sometimes possible to reduce the forwardly displaced distal fragment in a fracture of the olecranon in a child. (See insert for type of displacement.) The suspension sling forces the proximal end of the distal ulna in a dorsal direction.

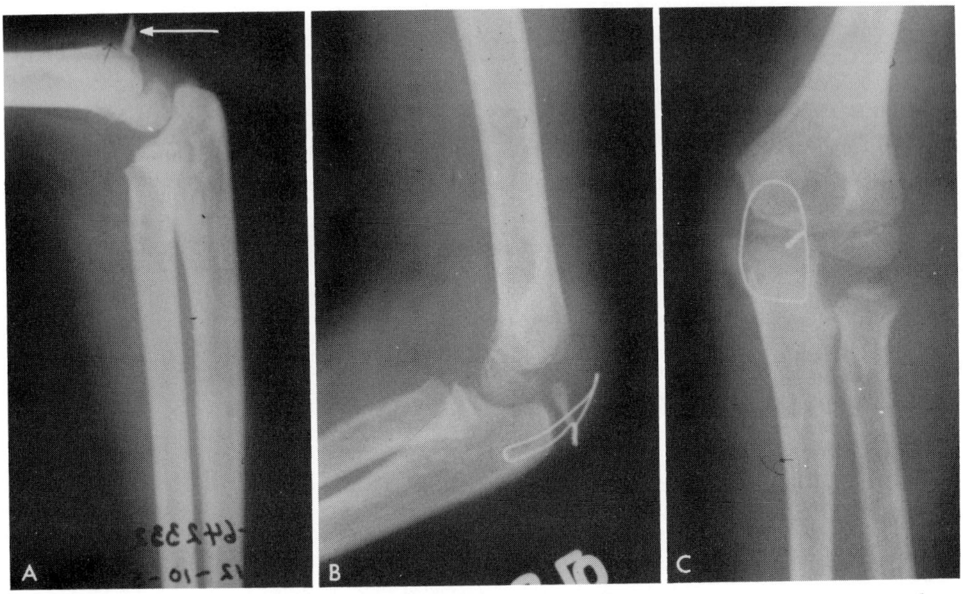

Fig. 70-A. (A) Lateral view of elbow of a 7 year old boy showing what appears to be a small chip of bone (arrow) from olecranon. This actually is just a thin shell of the diaphysis and the main olecranon, being cartilagenous at this age, does not appear on the film. A definite palpable defect could be felt where the tip of the olecranon normally should be and he was definitely *unable* to extend this elbow against gravity. (B) and (C) lateral and antero-posterior views after open reduction show the fragment reduced and held in position with a wire loop. The upper part of the loop was passed through the triceps tendon insertion into the cartilagenous olecranon.

Operative treatment in children should be limited to cases with open (compound) wounds or cases which have some other associated complication requiring it. However, operation should be avoided if possible since it predisposes to growth disturbance by adding additional trauma to the epiphyseal cartilage. Should growth disturbance subsequently develop regardless of the original treatment and the olecranon becomes so irregular or elongated that disability and pain result, corrective operation may then be performed.

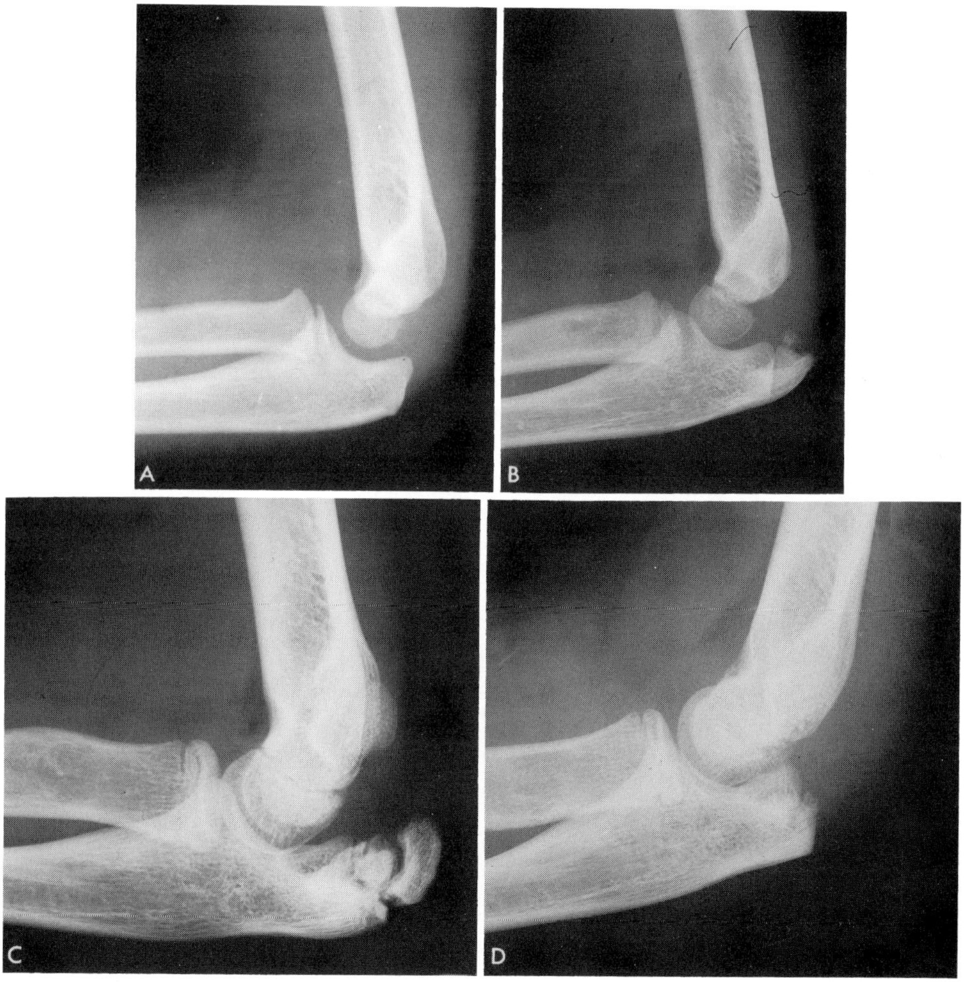

Fig. 71. Lateral roentgenograms of seven year old boy showing evidence of progressive growth disturbance (over-growth) of olecranon following injury to its epiphysis. (A) Original film showing no evidence of bony injury. Clinically there was acute tenderness over the olecranon epiphysis which persisted for one month. (B) Same elbow five and one-half months after injury. Note irregularity, early ossification, and beginning elongation of the olecranon. (C) Same elbow six and one-half years after injury. Note overgrowth of olecranon and persistence of its epiphyseal cartilage. (D) Same elbow after removal of excess olecranon to permit better extension of the forearm.

After-care in Operative Cases

If good internal fixation has been obtained, a splint is necessary for only three or four days or until the operative reaction has subsided. A sling should be worn for two to three weeks to rest the elbow between exercises. It is imperative to institute early active exercises at frequent intervals, but these should be performed always within the limits of pain. As soon as motion has shown good recovery, the patient should be encouraged to use the elbow for light work. Warm soaks and massage are soothing and help the circulation, but the latter should be omitted in children. No passive manipulations either in flexion or extension should be permitted at any time since these will only cause pain, add injury, and retard the rapidity of functional recovery.

Complications

The main complications following fracture of the olecranon are some limitation of complete elbow extension or loss of strength in performing extension. These complications are not so apt to occur if motion is started early regardless of whether the patient is operated upon or not. If for any reason operation is not performed in the cases with wide separation, extension of the elbow is very likely to be both limited and weak. Pain is not as a rule a late complication unless traumatic arthritis develops following the injury. Early or late ulnar nerve impairment should be investigated and treated as soon as noted. It may be necessary to transpose the ulnar nerve to the anterior surface of the elbow.

Disability Time

The disability time following olecranon fractures is usually about six weeks for light work. For heavy laboring work this may be prolonged to eight to ten weeks.

Prognosis

In olecranon fractures with little or no separation the prognosis for excellent function and strength is usually good provided the elbow has not been subjected to prolonged immobilization in splints and the patient has been made to carry out early active exercises and use. In fractures with marked separation the prognosis is good if early operation is performed and good internal fixation obtained followed by early motion and use. If it has been impossible to operate and these cases have been treated conservatively, the prognosis is never good for full function and a strong elbow.

FRACTURE OF THE CORONOID PROCESS

Fracture of the coronoid process of the ulna is most commonly associated with a posterior dislocation of the radius and ulna upon the humerus. The injury may be found alone, however. It should be remembered that the tip of the coronoid process is intra-articular in position and that a fracture near its tip may cause the broken off fragment to become a loose body within the elbow joint. The fracture occurs most commonly about six to ten millimeters from the tip of the process, so that the fragment has attached to it joint capsule or a portion of the brachialis muscle which furnishes some blood supply. Hence this latter type offers a much better chance of bony union.

Dislocation of both bones at the elbow with an associated fracture of the coronoid process shows a greater tendency to recurrence and therefore requires more prolonged immobilization in flexion and a delay in active exercise especially in the direction of extension (Chapter XIX).

With a simple fracture of the coronoid process *without* elbow dislocation and without extensive tearing of the collateral ligaments one must expect hemarthrosis to develop in the joint. This may become extensive enough to distend the joint capsule, and give severe pain and loss of motion.

Treatment

The majority of coronoid fractures show little displacement and require as treatment merely rest, protection and relief of pain. Those with displacement may require an attempt to better their position to permit improved chances of bony healing, or they may require removal of the fragment. In either event the surgeon should strive to regain motion in the elbow joint as quickly as is safely consistent with the pathology in the particular case.

The diagnosis of coronoid fracture may be suspected on clinical examination, but can only be made with certainty on roentgen examination. The status of the surrounding soft part swelling, hemorrhage and hemarthrosis may best be determined on careful clinical findings and this is frequently of more importance from the standpoint of the treatment to be chosen than are the films.

Closed Treatment. When little or no separation of the fragment exists the first step in treatment must be to relieve pain. If the hemarthrosis is mild and the joint capsule is not tense and exquisitely tender, aspiration is not necessary. The elbow should be immobilized in a posterior molded plaster splint from the axilla to the base of the fingers with the elbow in a position of approximately 80 to 90 degrees for rest and temporary protection. Elevation and mild heat will assist in relieving swelling and pain. The splint should not be worn for longer than five to seven days and may be removed four or five times daily for soaks in warm water, massage, and mild active exercises. A sling should be utilized for an additional two weeks for rest intermittent with the soaks and exercises. Light active use may be allowed after two to three weeks following the initial injury.

If hemarthrosis is severe, recovery will be slower because of pain on attempting exercises. Early aspiration of the joint is therefore indicated, first to relieve pain, second to overcome the necessity of absorbing the blood (a slow process at best), and third to permit early exercise which will hasten the recovery of joint function and shorten the disability time (Chapter XIII).

Following aspiration the elbow should be immobilized in a posterior molded splint and subsequently treated as described above under cases not requiring aspiration. If separation of the coronoid fracture is considerable, the elbow should be immobilized in more acute flexion in order to bring the main ulna in closer proximity with the displaced fragment.

Operative Treatment. Ordinarily it is unnecessary to operate upon freshly fractured coronoid processes per se unless the fragment is widely displaced and completely loose within the joint. If an associated radial head fracture with displacement is present and removal of this is necessary, the detached coronoid fragment may be removed at the same time. Some coronoid fractures heal in the displaced position and cause a prominence that interferes with elbow flexion. These may be operated upon subsequently (after all fear of possible development of myositis ossificans has passed) and the prominence removed (Chapter XXI).

Complications

Early. The main complication that may be encountered early is an increased tendency for recurrence of the elbow dislocation. This can best be prevented by immobilization of the elbow after reduction in more acute flexion and in not allowing extension exercises beyond 120 degrees for at least three to four weeks.

Late. Myositis ossificans occasionally occurs with this injury especially when an elbow joint dislocation has been present and when there has been extensive laceration of the brachialis anticus muscle. (For causes and prevention of the condition see Chapter XIV.) A loose body in the elbow joint

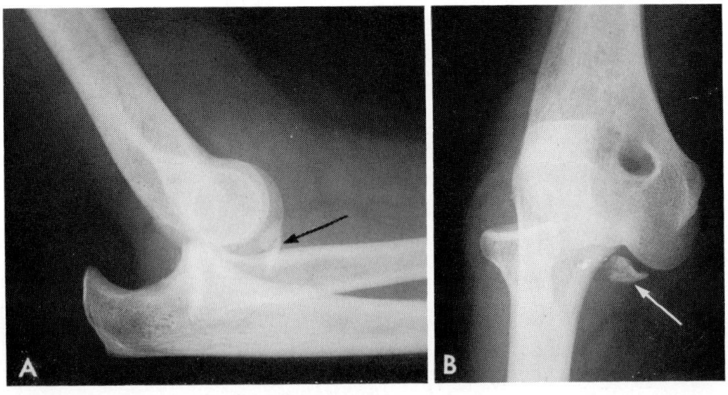

Fig. 72. Fracture of coronoid process of ulna. (A) Lateral, and (B) antero-posterior roentgenograms showing fracture of the coronoid process accompanying a posterior dislocation of the elbow joint.

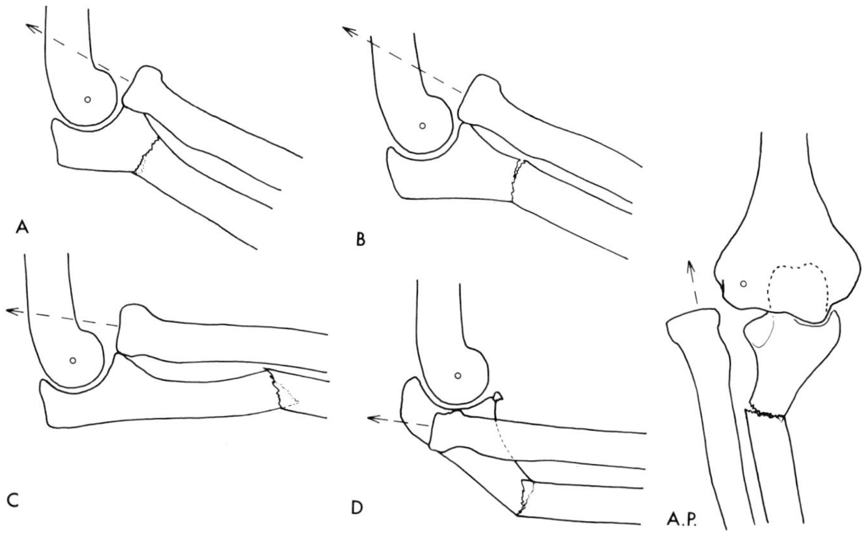

Fig. 73. Monteggia fracture deformities; a, b, and c show extension types and d, the flexion type (after Watson-Jones). Arrow shows failure of the axis of the radius to pass through the center of the capitellum when the ulnar fracture fragments are angulated. The displacement of the upper radius is *always* in the direction pointed to by the apex of the angle formed by the ulnar fragments.

may result from a broken off tip of the coronoid. If this causes irritation, pain, or obstruction to motion, it should be removed by operation. Mechanical obstruction to flexion resulting from an enlarged healed coronoid process after fracture may occasionally be found. If this causes pain and disability, operation should be performed and the enlarged tip of the process should be removed.

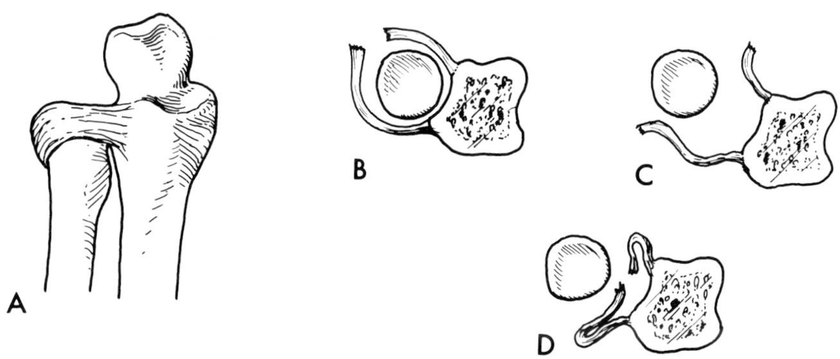

Fig. 74. Sketch of upper extremities of radius and ulna. (a) Normal relations. (b), (c) and (d) Cross-sections at level of radioulnar joint showing torn orbicular ligament and its possible relations to the radial head after dislocation of latter.

Prognosis

In general the prognosis following fracture of the coronoid is good if early motion is instituted after a brief period of rest and protection. The disability time should not exceed two to three months. If complications arise, the prognosis will be less favorable for full and painless function.

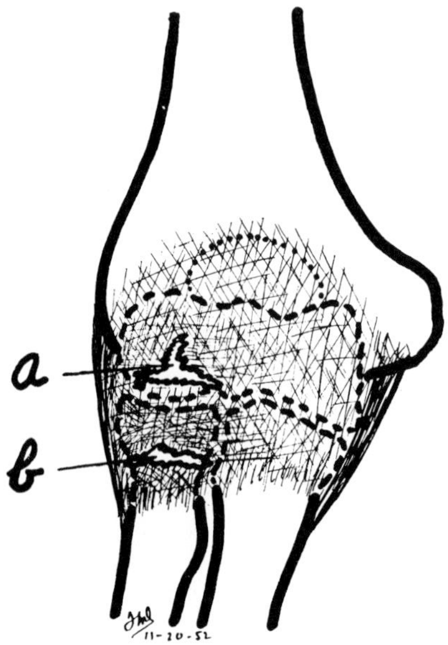

Fig. 75. Sketch of anterior aspect of elbow joint showing possible sites of tear in capsule which allows the radial head to dislocate: (a) through main capsule; (b) distal to orbicular ligament.

FRACTURE OF THE CORONOID PROCESS IN CHILDREN

An isolated fracture of the coronoid process of the ulna in children is an extremely rare injury. It may accompany a posterior dislocation. If such a fracture is encountered the treatment would be identical to that described under treatment for similar fractures in adults. Bony healing is less of a problem in children and the majority of these fractures heal well. They are not so likely to form loose bodies within the joint requiring subsequent operative removal. Early active motion is indicated and should lead to early restoration of function.

MONTEGGIA FRACTURE

(Fracture of shaft of ulna associated with dislocation of head of radius)

General

This combination of injuries is not uncommon. It was originally described by Monteggia in 1814 and since that time the lesion has been known by his name. The injury occurs most frequently in children, but can occur as well in adults. It is an extremely important type of injury because a complete diagnosis is often over-looked and only the obvious fracture of the ulna receives treatment. If the associated radial head dislocation is not recognized, it will lead to deformity, restricted motion and disability. In view of the fact that the radius and ulna are attached at their two extremities by strong ligaments and along their shafts by an interosseus membrane, if either bone becomes fractured and angulated, the distance between the extremities of this bone must become shortened. If the second bone fails to fracture, *something else* must happen to it, i. e., dislocation of one of its extremities. This occurs in a Monteggia fracture. The shaft of the ulna may be fractured at any level from the lower third to just below the olecranon process. If its fragments become angulated the radial head is almost always displaced from its articulation with the lesser sigmoid notch of the ulna and the capitellum of the humerus. The direction of the radial head dislocation corresponds in general to the axis of the distal ulnar fragment which it tends to follow.

Pathology

The mechanism of the injury in these cases is due almost always to direct force upon the ulna, such as a fall upon its posterior aspect. This force fractures and displaces the fragments in a forward direction. The orbicular ligament usually ruptures since it is less strong than the interosseus membrane and allows dislocation of the radial head. Cases have been found at operation in which the torn orbicular ligament had folded in behind the dislocated radial head making it impossible to keep the latter in place after closed reduction. Other cases have been found in which the orbicular ligament has remained intact, but the radial head had pulled out through the thin capsule distal to the ligament and in which the ligament had fallen in behind the radial head, thus preventing any attempt at closed reduction. Since the injury is usually due to direct force the ulnar fracture is frequently associated with an open (compound) wound on the dorsum of the forearm.

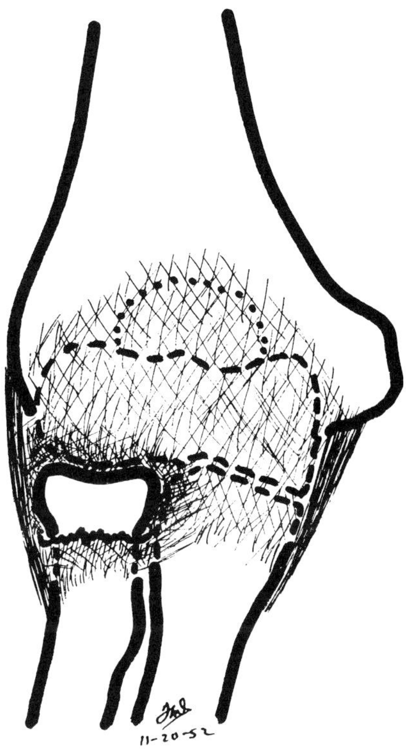

Fig. 76. Sketch of anterior aspect of elbow joint showing how radial head may become dislocated in anterior direction by tearing capsule below orbicular ligament and pulling out from beneath it. The radial head then comes to lie upon the intact portion of the ligament. To bring about reduction of the radial head the orbicular ligament must be incised.

Diagnosis

There is often a depression over the posterior aspect of the shaft of the ulna at the site of the fracture. Palpation of the radial head reveals this not to be in its normal position. The patient usually holds his elbow in partial flexion and in approximately mid-rotation. Examination for posterior interosseus nerve palsy should be made since this is found in about one-fourth of the cases. Roentgenographic examination which shows the angulated fragments of the ulna only and does not include the elbow joint in lateral projection is inadequate therefore to rule out dislocation of the radial head. It is very easy to determine on a lateral view of the elbow whether the radial head is dislocated or not. A line drawn through the long axis of the radius and projected upwards past the humerus normally

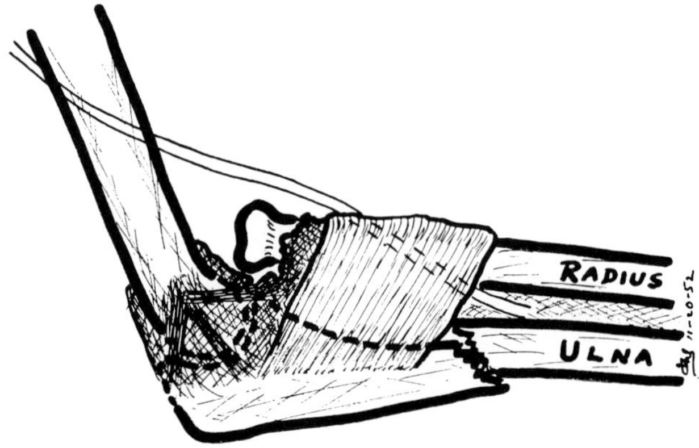

Fig. 77. Sketch of lateral aspect of elbow joint showing anterior dislocation of radial head (with Monteggia fracture). The radial head may lie anterior to an intact or partially intact orbicular ligament. The posterior (dorsal) interosseus nerve may be pressed upon or stretched by the displaced radial head before it enters the supinator muscle.

passes through the center of the capitellum. If it does not, there is dislocation of the radial head.

Types of Displacement

There are in general two types of deformity; (1) anterior angulation of the ulnar fragments associated with anterior dislocation of radial head; (2) lateral angulation of the ulnar fragments associated with lateral dislocation of the radial head. Some authors have described a third type in which the ulnar fragments were angulated posteriorly and the radial head was dis-

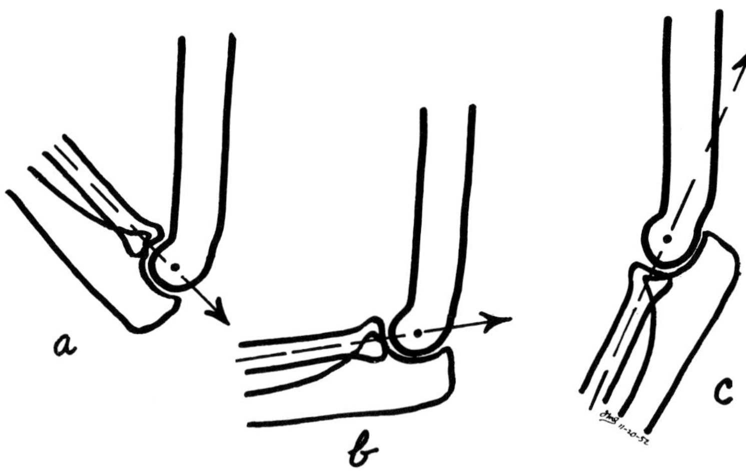

Fig. 78. Sketches of lateral roentgenograms of the elbow in: (a) acute flexion; (b) at 90 degrees; and (c) in full extension to show how the longitudinal axis of the radius normally passes through the center of the capitellum or the capitellar epiphysis.

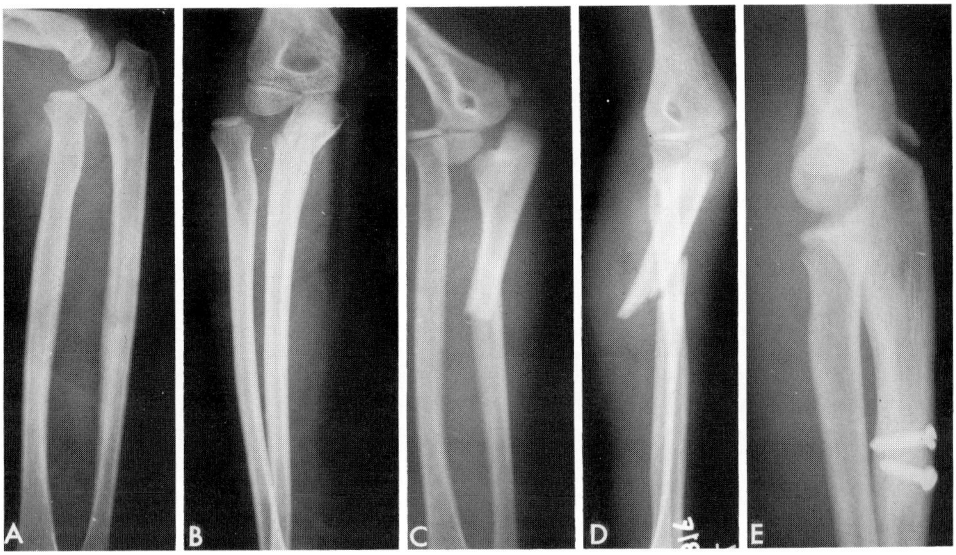

Fig. 79. Roentgenograms showing types of Monteggia fracture. (A) and (B) Lateral and antero-posterior views of eight year old patient with fracture of ulna high in shaft just below coronoid process and with antero-lateral dislocation of the head of the radius. Closed reduction successful. (C) and (D) Lateral and antero-posterior views of nine year old patient's forearm showing fracture of ulna just above its middle. Note displacement of head of radius. Closed reduction was performed, but two days later open reduction was carried out. The torn orbicular ligament was found folded in behind the radial head. The ulnar fragments after being reduced openly were fixed with two screws. Supplementary plaster fixation was necessary as the screws alone were inadequate. Today fixation of the ulna would be better carried out by a plate and screws. An intramedullary nail would give excellent fixation in an adult, but might damage the epiphysis of the olecranon in a child and lead to growth disturbance. (E) Same elbow one and one-half years after operation.

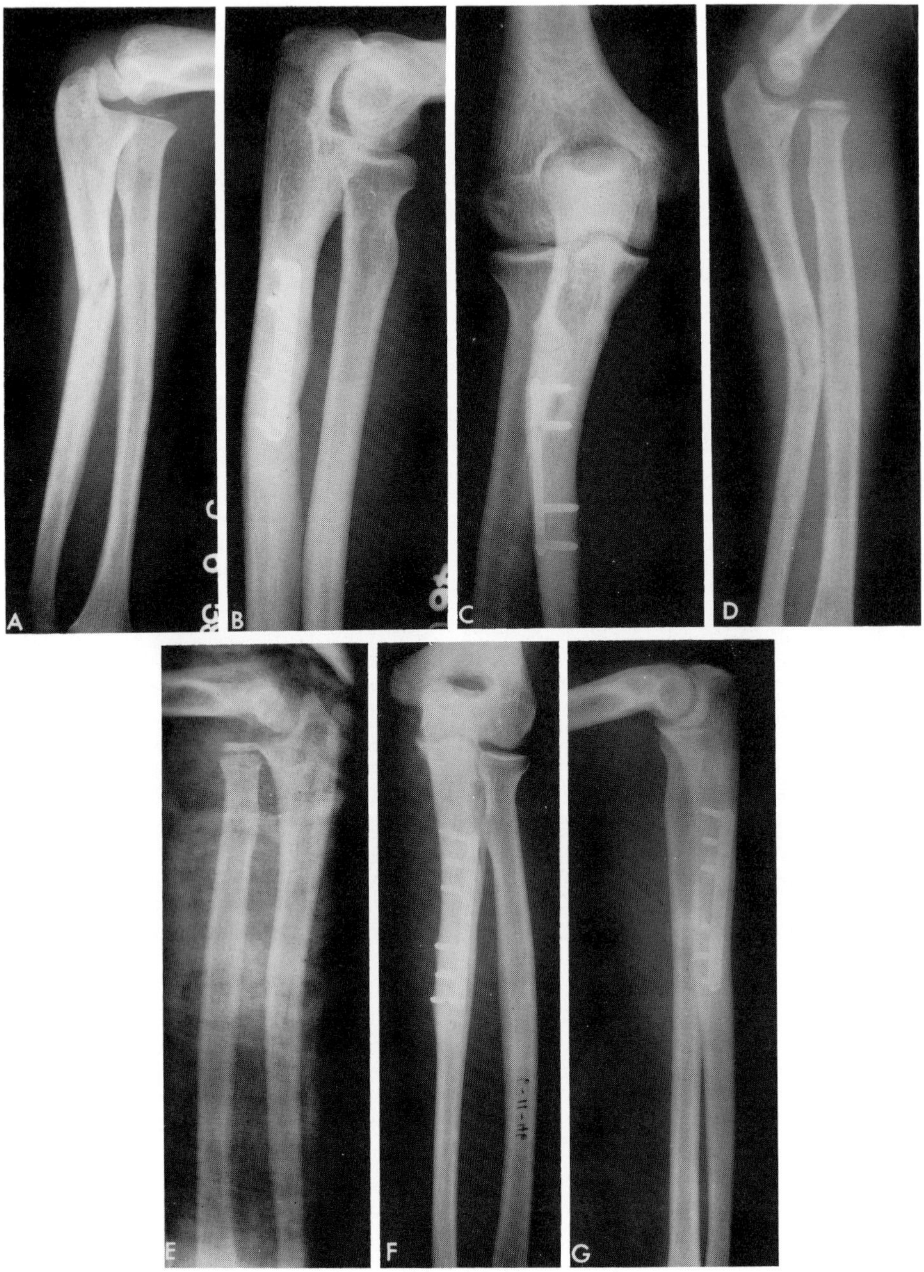

Fig. 80. Monteggia fractures. (A) Lateral view showing greenstick type fracture of ulna but with anterior dislocation of head of radius in nine year old boy. This patient also had paralysis of the posterior interosseus nerve. Open reduction was performed one week after injury upon the ulna and a four screw plate was used for internal fixation. Full recovery of the nerve resulted after one month. (B) and (C) Lateral and antero-posterior views of same elbow seven and one-half years after operation. (D) Lateral view of forearm and elbow in eight year old girl with greenstick type fracture of ulna. The radial head dislocation was originally missed. Closed reduction was performed upon the ulna, but view (E) shows the radial head still dislocated anterior to capitellum. Open reduction was performed the following day and the ulna was fixed internally with a six screw plate. The orbicular ligament was sutured after reducing the radial head. (F) and (G) Antero-posterior and lateral views of same arm four and one-half years later. *Result:* excellent.

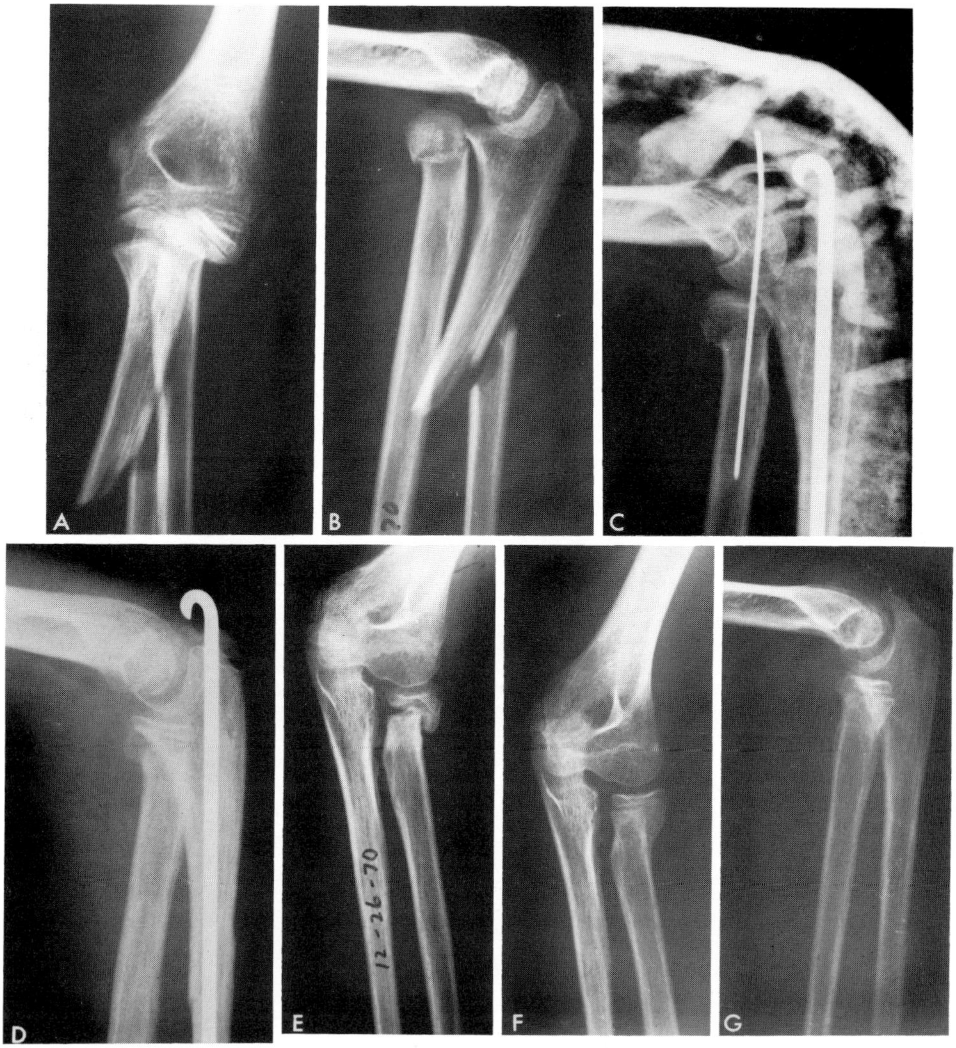

Fig. 80-A. (A) and (B) show front and lateral views of the elbow of an 11½ year old girl with a Monteggia fracture-dislocation. Note that the radial head besides being dislocated also has a fracture through its neck with considerable tilt and displacement. Closed reduction was unsuccessful and open reduction was carried out through a Boyd incision. [See Fig. 101 (f)]. The ulna was readily reduced by traction and manipulation and fixed internally with a Rush intramedullary pin. The orbicular ligament was torn. It was not only difficult to reduce the radial head but impossible to hold it in anatomical position until a Kirschner wire was drilled from the posterior aspect through the capitellum, radial head and into the shaft of the radius as seen in the postoperative film in (C). The proximal end of this wire was cut off and allowed to remain subcutaneous. The elbow was immobilized in a posterior molded plaster splint. The wire was removed 3½ weeks after operation (D). The Rush pin was removed 3 months after operation. (E) shows the elbow at 4 months and (F) and (G) at 8 months. On this last date she lacked only ten degrees each of elbow extension and supination.

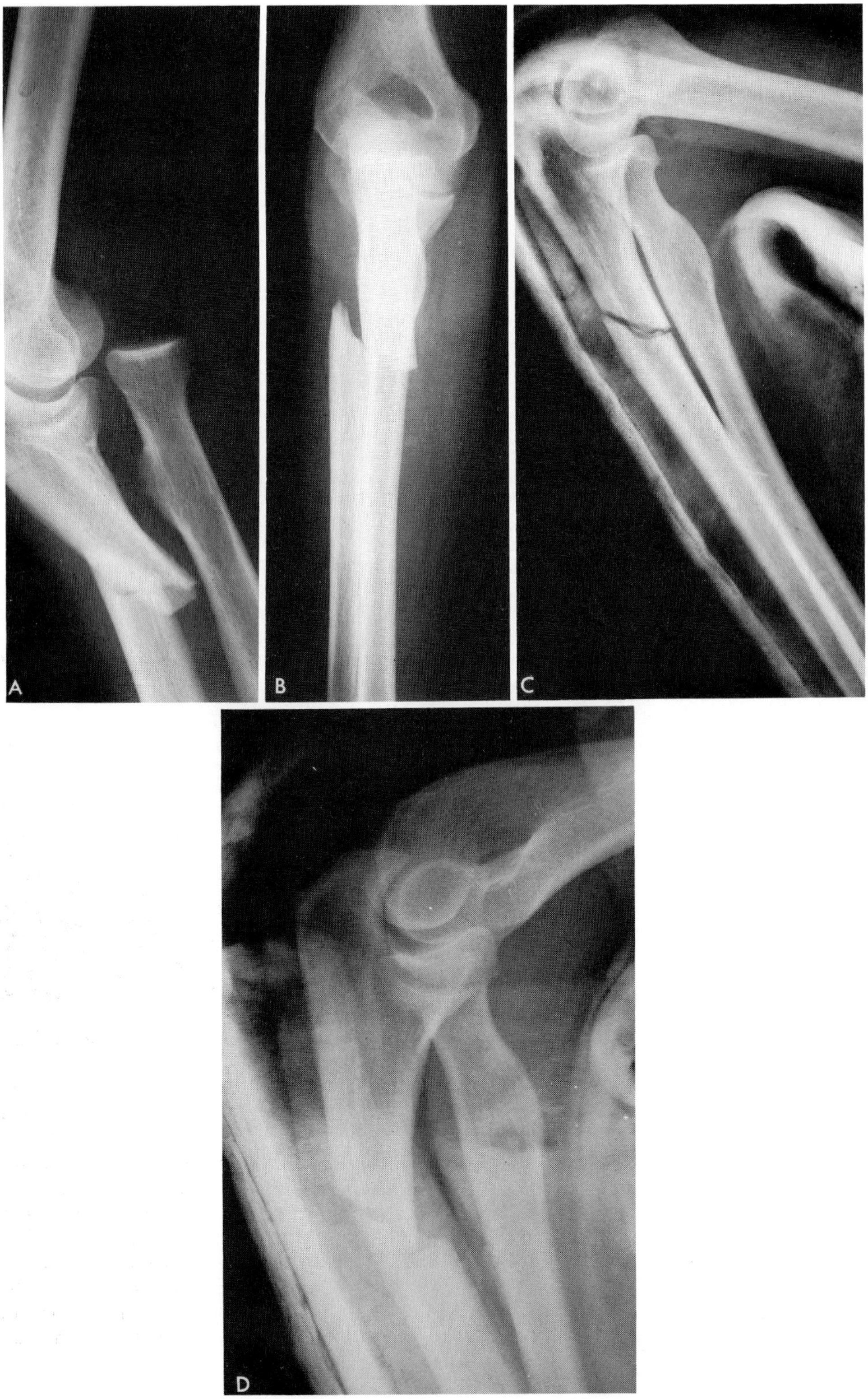
A
B
C
D

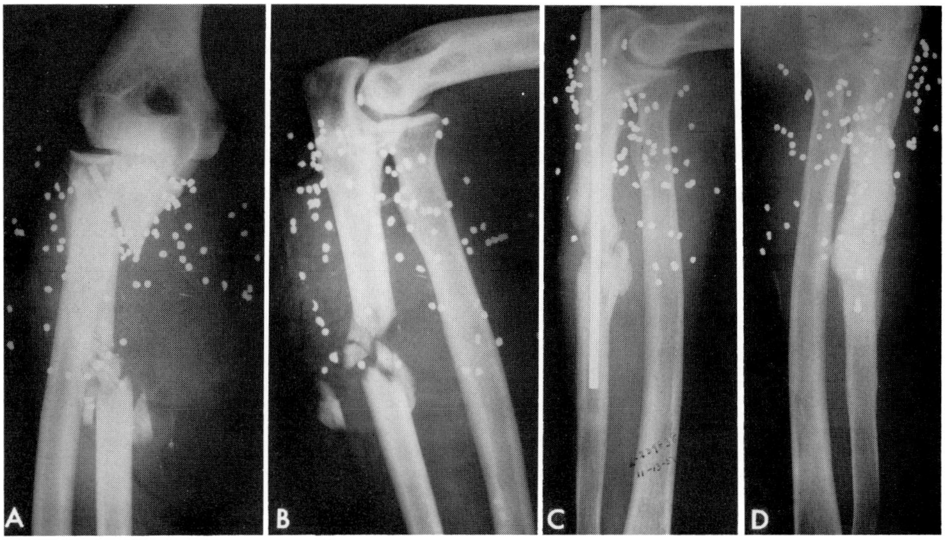

Fig. 81-A. (A) and (B) antero-posterior and lateral view of a 38 year old man's elbow after a shot-gun blast which took away skin, muscles, ulnar artery, veins and ulnar nerve. He was treated first by debridement since his radial pulse was good and the ulna was fixed with an intramedullary Kirschner wire. Superficial infection only resulted and subsequently the wound was skin grafted. The wire was then changed to a Rush pin (C) and bone grafts applied. After one year an onlay bone graft was fastened to the lower united ulnar fracture site and this healed well (D). At the end of two years the patient had an obvious ulnar nerve paralysis, but his wrist and rotary motions were approximately fifty per cent normal.

located in the same direction. Although such dislocations are possible, it is much more likely in this type for the radial head to be fractured rather than simply dislocated.

The level of the fracture in the ulna is usually in the upper third of the shaft, but it may occur in the lower third or even between the coronoid and olecranon processes. The fracture may be transverse, oblique, comminuted or of the greenstick variety. The commonest angulation of the ulna is with the apex of the angle pointing forward and with a similar dislocation of the radial head.

Treatment

There is no single method of treatment which can be used in all cases. Many of these fractures may be reduced by closed methods, remain reduced, and show excellent results.

←

Fig. 81. Monteggia fracture in a 63 year old man. (A) and (B) Lateral and antero-posterior views of original fracture showing displacement and dislocation. (C) Lateral view after closed reduction and plaster immobilization showing good replacement of fracture fragments and radial head. (D) Shows angulation of ulnar fragments while in plaster five weeks after injury. This fracture would have been better treated and the position of the ulnar fragments maintained had open reduction with internal fixation been performed. Loss of reduction of the ulnar fragments will almost certainly lead to re-dislocation of the radial head and a bad elbow.

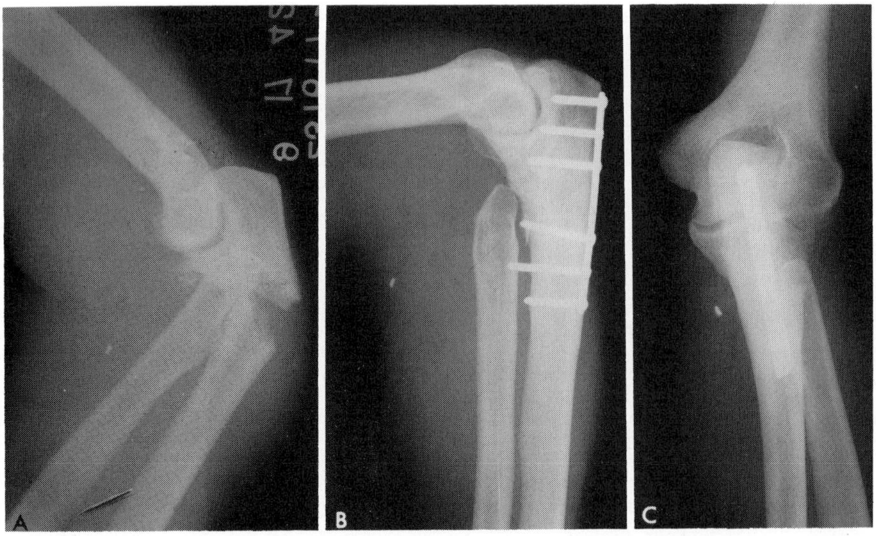

Fig. 82. Monteggia fracture of the "flexion type." The fracture is situated high in the ulna. The apex of the angulation points posteriorly and the dislocation of the radius is likewise in a posterior direction. In this particular type of displacement the radial head is nearly always fractured as well as dislocated. A large fragment of the radial head can be seen lying just distal to the capitellum while the main axis of the radius passes posterior to it. Immediate open reduction was performed in this man (aged 40 years) and the ulna was internally fixed with a six screw plate after excising the radial head and its fragments in toto. Active exercises were started one week after operation and at two months he was performing moderately heavy manual labor. (B) and (C) Lateral and antero-posterior views of same elbow five years after operation.

Closed reduction should be tried under general anesthesia with traction upon the extended forearm. While making firm pressure over the anterior aspect of the fracture site of the ulna in order to straighten this or to complete the fracture if it is of the greenstick variety, similar pressure should be made over the radial head. After the ulnar deformity has been corrected and the radial head slips back into place, the forearm should be supinated and the elbow should be flexed. Extension should again be tested, and, if the orbicular ligament is not interposed between the radial head and the lesser sigmoid notch of the ulna, the radial head should stay in place provided the ulnar fragments are adequately reduced. If the position of both of these remains satisfactory, the elbow should then be flexed again to an angle of eighty or ninety degrees and immobilized in anterior and posterior molded splints extending from the axilla to the metacarpophalangeal joints. Frequent roentgenographic check-ups should be made in the following two weeks to determine if the ulnar fragments are remaining in place and if the radial head is remaining in the reduced position. If either one becomes displaced, open operation should then be resorted to and internal fixation used to maintain the position of the ulnar fragments; and at the same time repair of the orbicular ligament should be carried out. Should the original reduc-

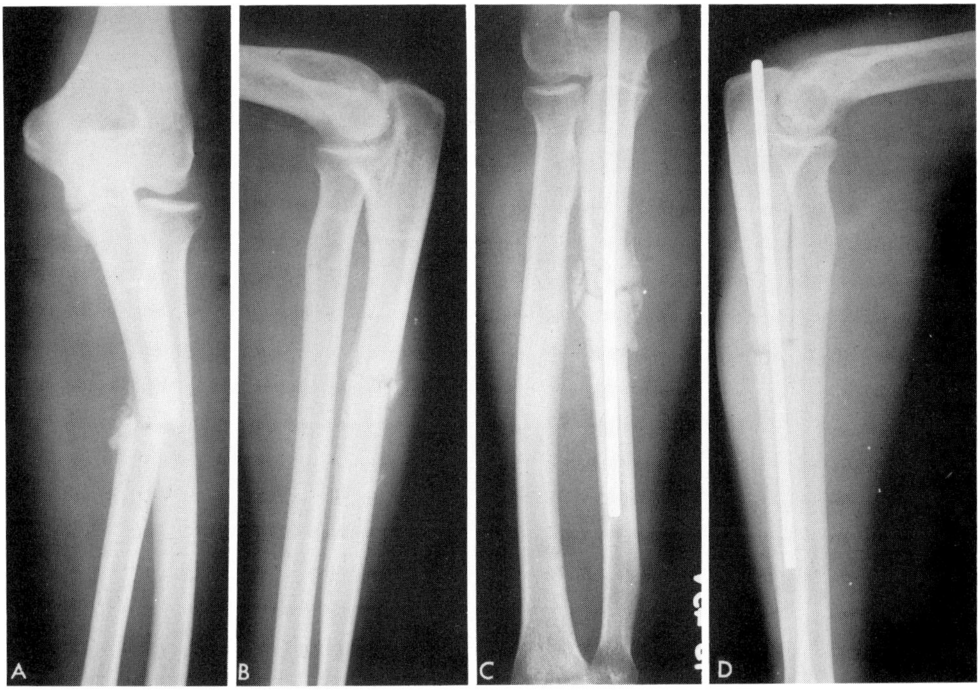

Fig. 83. Monteggia fracture with angulation of ulna persisting after two months of inadequate plaster immobilization. The patient, a 34-year-old man, sought treatment because of continued pain. Operation was performed and the ulna was straightened and fixed internally with an intramedullary rod. (A) and (B) Views two months after injury. (C) and (D) Views of same forearm two and one-half months after operation. Bony healing eventually became solid, but was slow.

tion not be completely successful from the standpoint of perfect reduction of either bone, operation should be performed. If angulation of the ulna is not completely corrected, the chances are good that the ulna will continue to angulate further, and, in an adult, it is very likely to develop non-union or malunion and with secondary loss of position of the radial head.

Open reduction, owing to the great risks of secondary loss of position following closed reduction in adults, is a much better form of treatment since it not only permits correction of the deformity, secures rigid internal fixation, and insures a much better functional result. Fixation of the ulnar fragments must be rigid, however, if early active motion is to be permitted. The orbicular ligament is repaired at the same time. Should the ulnar shaft be severely comminuted so as to preclude rigid fixation by plate and screws, it might be advisable to use intramedullary fixation by means of a Steinman pin or small calibre Kuntscher nail inserted distally through the olecranon process. Such intramedullary fixation should be done with the fracture site exposed rather than attempt to guide the pin "blindly" into the medullary canal of the distal fragment.

Exposure of the fracture site and the radial head may be made through

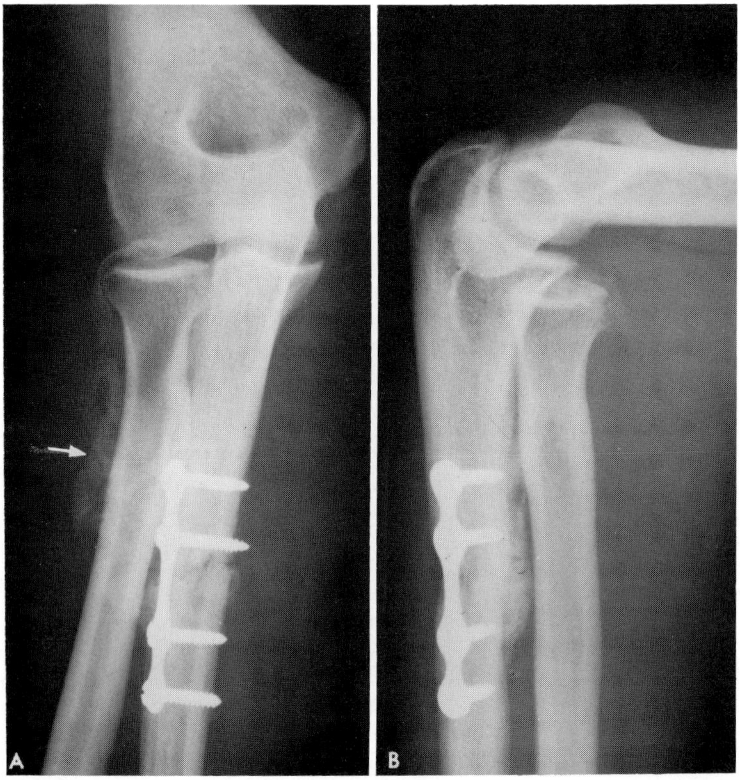

Fig. 84. Monteggia fracture in 21 year old man treated by immediate closed reduction of radial head and by open reduction of ulna with internal fixation two weeks after injury. (A) and (B) Antero-posterior and lateral roentgenograms two months after operation showing extensive calcification, i. e., myositis ossificans around the head, neck and upper shaft of the radius and between it and the ulna due to the operation having been performed as late as two weeks after injury. Note also that the radial head dislocation has recurred (or persisted) in spite of an attempt to reduce it by closed methods. This patient has marked limitation of elbow flexion and rotation. Operation to excise the radial head at a later date must be considered to improve function of the elbow.

two separate incisions, or both may be approached through a posterior incision as described by Speed and Boyd. If on exposure of the radial head it is found that the orbicular ligament is folded in behind it, this should be lifted out and sutured after replacing the radial head. If the radial head has pulled out from beneath the orbicular ligament, it may be necessary to divide the ligament before reduction of the dislocation can be obtained, following which the orbicular ligament is repaired with sutures. At open reduction it is usually advisable to correct the deformity of the ulna and to apply internal fixation first before reducing the radial head dislocation. Anterior incisions for approaching the radial head should never pass directly across the flexion crease of the elbow but should be made Z-shaped, otherwise a contracted keloidal scar will result. A posterior longitudinal incision does not tend to give a thickened scar. In the anterior approach the radial nerve and all its branches should be retracted laterally in approaching the joint in the interval between the brachioradialis and the brachialis anticus muscles so that none of the branches of the nerve will be harmed. In the posterior approach the periosteum and the attachment of the supinator muscle to the ulna must be elevated subperiosteally. This protects the dorsal interosseus nerve by displacing it forwards, since it lies between the two layers of this muscle.

After-treatment

Following successful closed reduction the elbow should be kept immobilized for six weeks in children and for at least eight weeks in adults or until there is definite evidence of bony union on roentgen examination. Function may then be restored by progressive active exercises, heat, massage and mild use. If open reduction and internal fixation has been resorted to early, protection by splint should not be necessary for longer than two weeks and elbow exercises and physiotherapy may be started as soon as the operative wound has healed.

Disability Time

The disability time for children usually is about two to three months with either closed or open treatment. For adults it will usually run to about three months for early cases if operated upon and to four to six months if treated by closed methods.

Prognosis

The prognosis is very good if the complete diagnosis is recognized and the patient is given early and adequate treatment.

Cases, however, in which the dislocation of the radial head has not been recognized and do not come in for treatment before one month or longer after injury are not apt to do well even if operated upon. Not only is the operation difficult in the late stage, but it is often impossible to correct the ulnar angulation completely and maintain correction of this. If it is not possible to repair the orbicular ligament to hold the radial head in place, it may be necessary to construct a fascial sling around the radial neck as a substitute for the orbicular ligament.

It is preferable to operate upon these cases *early* if operation is necessary and it is best to do this within the first two weeks following injury. It is better still to operate upon them within the first 48 hours. There should be no difficulty with posterior interosseus nerve palsy if it is treated adequately from the start. The nerve should recover full function.

Chapter XII

The Upper Extremity of the Radius

FRACTURES OF THE HEAD AND NECK

General Considerations

THE MAJORITY of fractures at the upper extremity (head and neck) of the radius are sustained by falls upon the outstretched hand. The force of impact is transmitted upwards along the shaft of the radius and jams the head of this bone against the articular surface of the capitellum. Not infrequently the patient may sustain a Colles fracture of the lower radius at the same time. There are of course other mechanisms causing radial head fracture, the commonest being dislocation of both bones at the elbow in which the fracture is an associated lesion, but much more serious from the standpoint of prognosis and treatment than if no dislocation were present. The reasons for this are discussed further on in this chapter.

The types of fracture of the radial head commonly seen in adults are as follows: linear fracture without appreciable displacement, sometimes called chisel fractures; fracture with displacement of one or more fragments; comminuted fractures; fracture at the junction of the head and neck with extensive displacement of the former; or this same type with angulation and impaction of the head upon the neck. In children the main types of fracture are epiphyseal injury without displacement (which diagnosis must be made on clinical rather than roentgenologic evidence); epiphyseal separation of the head either with angulation and impaction or with complete displacement from the neck. Fragmentation of the radial head in children is extremely rare. Trauma to the epiphyseal plate whether associated with displacement or not may cause subsequent growth disturbances and for this reason the surgeon should be careful in making his prognosis.

The head and neck of the radius from the anatomical standpoint are completely *intra-articular* in position. The clinical implications resulting from this peculiar anatomy are of considerable interest. First, a displaced fragment of head (aside from its mechanical derangement) may fail to unite by bony union, because of its lack of blood supply. Second, any bleeding from the fractured surface of the neck causes blood to collect within the elbow joint without possibility of escape (unless the joint capsule has been extensively torn by an associated dislocation of both bones). The hemarthrosis thus created under increased tension not only causes severe pain, but marked limitation of function even without marked displacement of a bony fragment (see under Treatment).

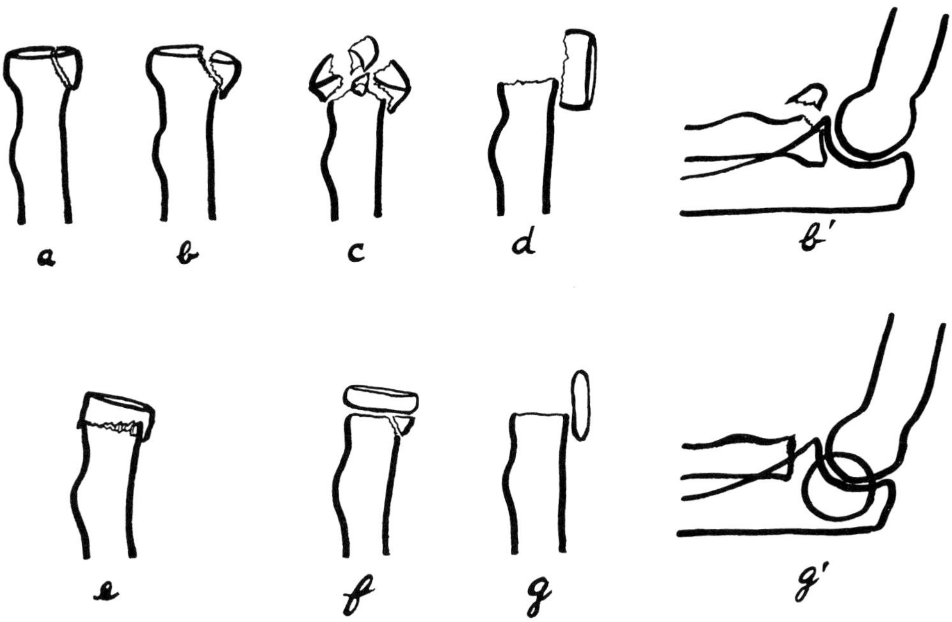

Fig. 85. Fractures of the radial head: a, b, b', c, and d are the types commonly seen in adults; e, f, g, and g' are those commonly seen in children.

Fractures of the radial head are extremely common both in adults as well as in children. Roentgenograms frequently fail to reveal many of these fractures without displacement and the injury is often considered to be merely a simple sprain. In such cases without displacement this is often to the patient's advantage, because his elbow is not subjected to prolonged splinting and instead he is allowed to exercise and use it from the beginning which is the ideal form of treatment for this type and aids in more rapid restoration of function. Accurate diagnosis of fracture in such cases often can only be made early by such clinical findings as tenderness located directly over the radial head, aggravation of pain on extremes of rotation, and by the presence of a hemarthrosis in the elbow joint. This latter condition is detected by a tense, fluctuant, tender bulge in the portion of the elbow joint capsule overlying the postero-lateral aspect of the joint. This bulge is either visible, palpable, or both and lies within a triangle bounded by the following three bony landmarks: lateral epicondyle of humerus, radial head, and tip of the olecranon process—the hemarthrosis triangle (see Fig. 91).

If the original roentgenograms immediately following injury fail to reveal evidence of a radial head fracture, this may be because (without displacement) the surfaces of the fragments fail to lie in the proper plane to become projected in profile upon the film. Should additional films be taken at the end of two or three weeks following injury, one will more frequently than not be able to discern evidence of the fracture due to rarefaction of the bone immediately adjacent to the fracture surfaces and thus be able to confirm definitely the original clinical diagnosis.

Hemarthrosis to some degree accompanies every fracture of the radial head and neck. This may be so slight as to cause very little discomfort or disability. If, on the other hand, bleeding into the joint becomes sufficient to cause increased tension, then pain becomes severe and disability great. Bleeding from a small crack without appreciable displacement will be slow and may take several hours before it creates tension and distress. A patient with such an injury frequently gives a history of a fall upon his hand followed by mild pain at the elbow in the region of the radial head. He usually pays very little attention to it at first, believing he has sustained a mild sprain. After an hour or two he notes that the elbow is becoming "stiff" and that the pain is becoming more constant as well as severe. He may even describe it as a sensation of throbbing. Sometimes he tries hot soaks or hot applications, but finds that none of these give relief. He cannot by this time flex or extend the elbow joint more than ten or fifteen degrees without increasing pain and spasm and almost certainly cannot get it into any comfortable position that will allow him to get to sleep. Such a story is characteristic of hemarthrosis in the joint. Although he has a fracture of the radial head, the patient is suffering not from the fracture itself, but from the effects of the hemarthrosis. Relief from the symptoms of hemarthrosis by aspiration (decompression) of the joint may be easily obtained, and this procedure is often indicated. Besides giving immediate relief of symptoms, it allows early active motion which in turn is most important in the restoration of function. (See Technique of Aspiration of Elbow Joint, Chapter XIII.)

Treatment

Rationale. Before treatment of any fracture of the radial head or neck is begun, one should formulate a definite rationale. This should be based on the type of fracture (whether in an adult or child), upon the general principles of fracture treatment, and upon as complete and early a restoration of function as is possible. Naturally, if no displacement is present, no reduction need be performed and no immobilization is necessary except to give comfort to the patient for possibly as long as twenty-four hours to two days. Immobilization for as long as two weeks or more may permit the formation of fibrous adhesions between the fracture site and the joint capsule which no amount of well-meant physiotherapy can relieve and restore to full and painless function. It is important that function be restored in all these fractures. The only way that this can be accomplished is by instituting on the part of the patient early active motion and exercises (within pain limits). Aspiration will relieve the bulk of the pain and thus allow the patient to carry out his exercises on his own and thus obtain recovery much more rapidly than if he had to wait until all the blood in the joint were absorbed, as well as run the risk of formation of intra-articular adhesions.

On the other hand, if a fragment of the radial head is markedly displaced or the head is badly comminuted, the same rationale must be followed, i. e., make it possible for the patient to regain his function early by exercises and use. Aspiration and exercises alone are not sufficient in such a case because of the displacement or comminution which causes an internal derangement and mechanical interference or irritation of the synovial lining of the joint. Therefore, help is needed in the form of operative removal of the entire radial head, following which the same regime of *early* active exercises within pain limits should be carried out.

There is one type of radial head fracture associated with posterior or postero-lateral dislocation of the radius and ulna upon the humerus that needs special consideration. The rationale of treatment by excision of the radial head followed by early active motion is the same as described above. However, incision for removal of the radial head and the time of removal are different than with radial head fractures not associated with dislocation of the two forearm bones upon the humerus. The reason for this is because of the pathology resulting from the dislocation. As has been stated previously, all posterior dislocations of the forearm bones are accompanied by extensive tearing of the soft parts on the medial and anterior aspects of the joint. The tissues thus torn consist of the medial collateral ligament, anterior capsule of the joint, brachialis anticus muscle and numerous small and medium sized blood vessels. Extensive hemorrhage and extravasation of blood and inflammatory cells and fluid into the torn brachialis anticus muscle causes marked swelling and tension in the anticubital region. Unless this extreme soft tissue pathology is gotten rid of by operative means, it will take an excessively long time to become absorbed and in the meantime creates an ideal "set-up" for the formation of a myositis ossificans which may progress even to the formation of complete bony ankylosis. (For treatment of this particular injury and avoidance of myositis ossificans, see Chapter XIV.)

ADULT. Conservative Treatment. 1. Fracture of Head of Radius without Displacement of Fragment (Chisel fracture).

If pain is severe and motion is markedly limited and there is definite tense hemarthrosis, the elbow joint should be aspirated under local anesthesia. Following this the joint should be immobilized in a posterior molded plaster splint and sling at an angle of 90° flexion for rest, comfort and to allow intra-articular bleeding to stop. (See Fig 25.) The splint should be discarded after twenty-four to forty-eight hours and a sling worn for one more week. Active flexion, extension, pronation and supination exercises should be started immediately upon discarding of the splint. These should be performed frequently (at least once an hour) by the patient and always within pain limits. Soaks in warm water every two or three hours are soothing, help to improve the local circulation, and hasten the disappearance of swelling. Under no circumstances should passive stretching or manipulation be employed in order to obtain a quicker return of function.

Under the regime just advocated most patients obtain full functional re-

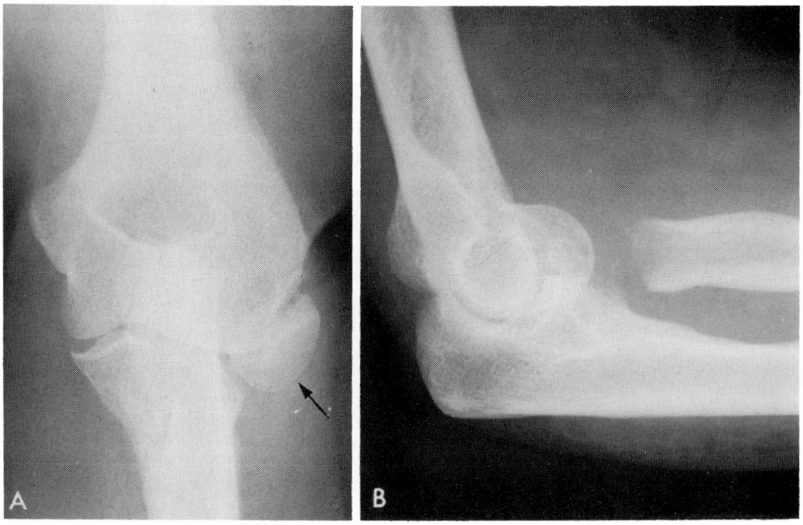

Fig. 86. Fracture of radial head. (A) Antero-posterior view showing radial head intact, but rotated and displaced in lateral direction. (B) Lateral view after operative removal of head.

covery in 10 days to two weeks for all but heavy work. Should aspiration not be done, but the treatment otherwise remain the same, it will require approximately four weeks to recover full function of the joint.

Operative Treatment. 2. Fracture of Head of Radius with Displacement of Fragment.

If the fragment broken off the radial head is displaced or tilted as much as two or three millimeters (especially if it is displaced from the anterior margin), operation should be performed and the *entire* radial head should be removed. To remove only the displaced fragment is a poor operation and allows the remaining fracture surface of the head to scratch and irritate the synovial lining within the orbicular ligament, thus causing a synovitis and possible formation of fibrous adhesions. Either of these conditions, if given a chance to occur, will result in pain on the extremes of rotation and in limited rotation.

The operation should be performed as soon as possible after injury and certainly no later than four days. The results are better if it is performed within the first 24 hours.

The incision used for removal of this type of radial head fracture is usually the postero-lateral one beginning just above the lateral epicondyle and extending distally five centimeters along the axis of the radius. The extensors carpi radialis longus and brevis are split and retracted. When the joint capsule is reached, the radial head may be identified by rotating the forearm. The capsule is then split over the lateral aspects of the radial head and capitellum, and in so doing there is an immediate escape of old blood

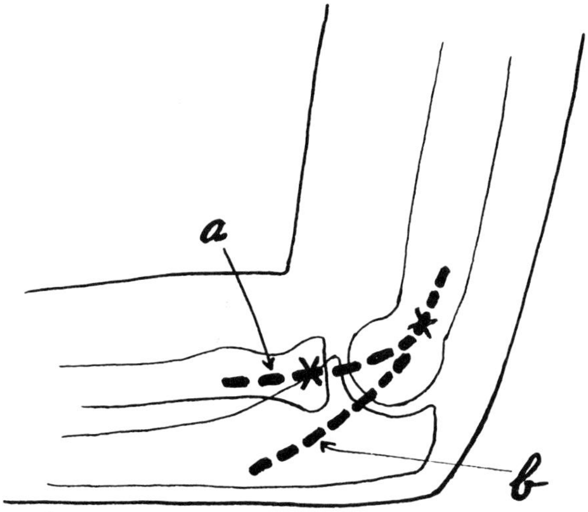

Fig. 87. (a) Lateral. (b) Postero-lateral incisions for approach to elbow joint and radial head.

from the joint cavity. The capsule should *not* be split more than 1.5 cm (5/8 inch) distal to the inferior margin of the head of the radius nor should forceful retraction be made in this area for fear of dividing or contusing the posterior interosseus nerve that courses around the radial neck approximately 2.0 cm. below its head. The old blood and clots should be sponged out of the joint. Any completely loose fragments should be lifted out. The head of the bone is then removed by a transverse cut with a thin sharp osteotome. In order to make a clean cut without any remaining spurs or jagged edges, the forearm should be rotated back and forth while using the thin chisel. If any projecting spurs remain on the end of the neck after taking these precautions, they should be bitten off with a sharp rongeur. The raw surface of the neck thus left may be touched with an electro-coagulator to "discourage" the re-formation of new bone. The important point is not so much the actual treatment of the raw bone end as is the institution of early and frequent active exercises 24 hours after operation. To put any operated case of this type in plaster and keep it immobilized for two to four weeks is to defeat completely the purpose of the operation. (Before closing the joint it is advisable to irrigate it with a forceful stream of normal saline solution to wash out any tiny bone fragments chipped off during the procedure and to rid the joint of remaining blood clots.) The wound should be closed loosely with interrupted sutures of fine silk or catgut for the capsule and likewise for the deep fascia. The skin may be closed with either a continuous or interrupted suture of silk or dermal suture.

3. Fracture of Head of Radius with Comminution or with Complete Displacement of the Intact Head from the Neck.

Treatment for fracture of radial head is identical as described under No. 2.

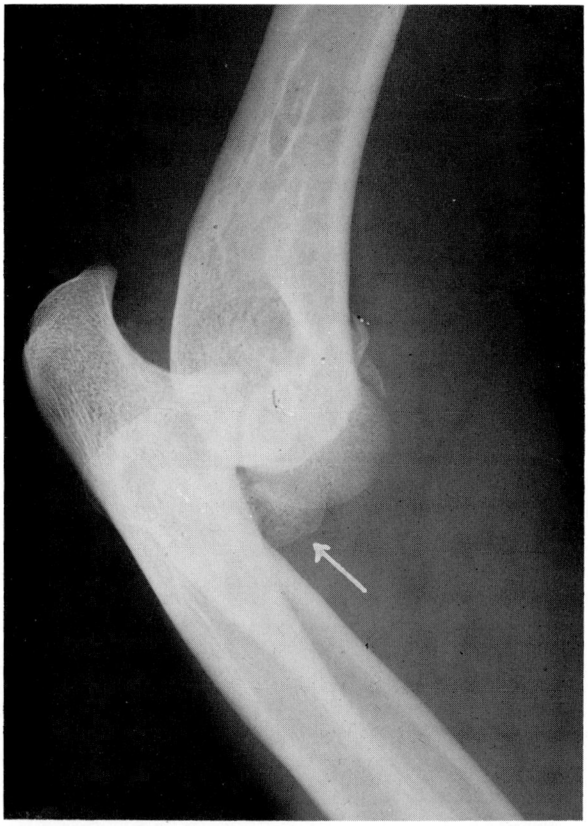

Fig. 88. Fracture of radial head associated with dislocation of elbow joint. Note displaced fragment of radial head. Extensive tearing of capsule and brachialis muscle and swelling occurs, predisposing to myositis ossificans.

4. Fracture of the Head of the Radius Associated with Dislocation of Radius and Ulna upon the Humerus; or Where the Dislocation Has Been Reduced.

In either type there is extreme swelling and induration in the front of the elbow due to the extensive tearing of the joint capsule and brachialis anticus muscle. Much hemorrhage and extravasated blood are scattered throughout the torn muscle. Unless this extensive soft part pathology is evacuated early and allowed to escape, the chances of development of myositis ossificans is about fifty percent. Therefore, these cases are best operated upon *within the first 24 hours* after injury and certainly within 48 hours. The incision should not be a lateral or postero-lateral one, but should by *necessity* be placed anteriorly in order to get rid of the extravasated blood, etc. in the antecubital fossa. When closing the wound after removal of the radial head, the capsule should be closed very loosely and *the deep fascia should not be closed at all.* This is for the purpose of allowing the escape of old blood and cellular exudate into the subcutaneous tissues, thereby getting rid of the chief factors leading to the formation of myositis ossificans.

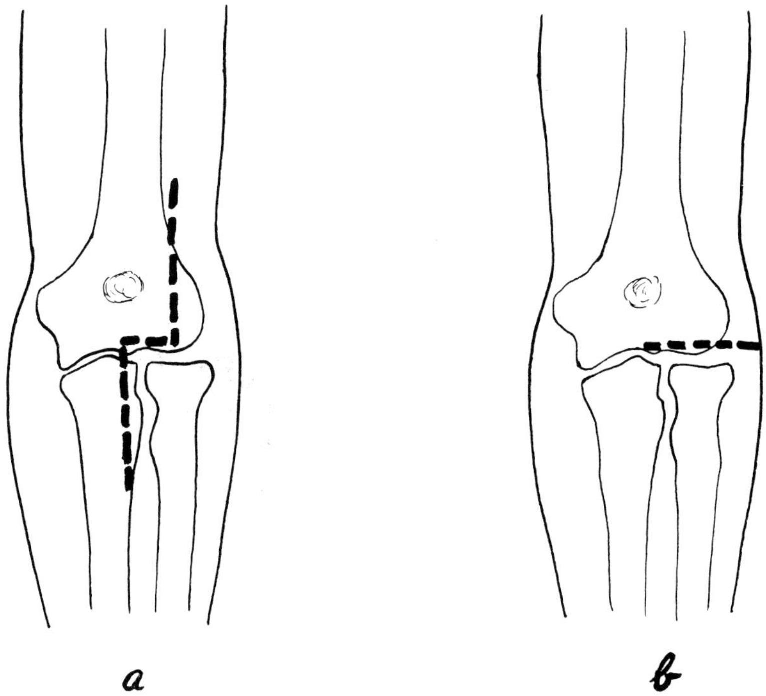

Fig. 89. Anterior skin incisions used for removal of fractured radial head accompanying dislocation of both bones at the elbow. (a) The Z-type of incision, the vertical portions of which are likely to give a thick contracted scar. (b) The straight transverse incision which will remain narrow and is cosmetically far superior to any incision that crosses the flexion crease of the elbow.

The incision used for the anterior approach may be either the Z-type or the transverse for the skin and subcutaneous tissues. The latter heals with a narrower scar and with less tendency to keloid formation.

The deep part of the incision passes between the brachio-radialis and brachialis anticus muscles. The radial recurrent vessels may have to be clamped, divided and ligated to allow for better retraction lateralward of the brachio-radialis muscle. The radial nerve must be identified and both its motor and sensory branches must be retracted *laterally*. By so doing none of the muscular branches from the main nerve will be harmed, since they all pass in a lateral direction. The joint capsule is opened longitudinally and the technique of actual removal of the radial head should then be carried out as described under No. 2. Following operation active exercises are begun within 48 hours and should be performed frequently and always within pain limits. Hot soaks or whirlpool baths may be begun as soon as the operative wound has healed. No massage or passive manipulation should be permitted at any time.

CHILDREN. Conservative Treatment. 1. Fracture (Separation) of the Radial Head Epiphysis without Displacement.

This diagnosis can only be made on clinical examination by the presence

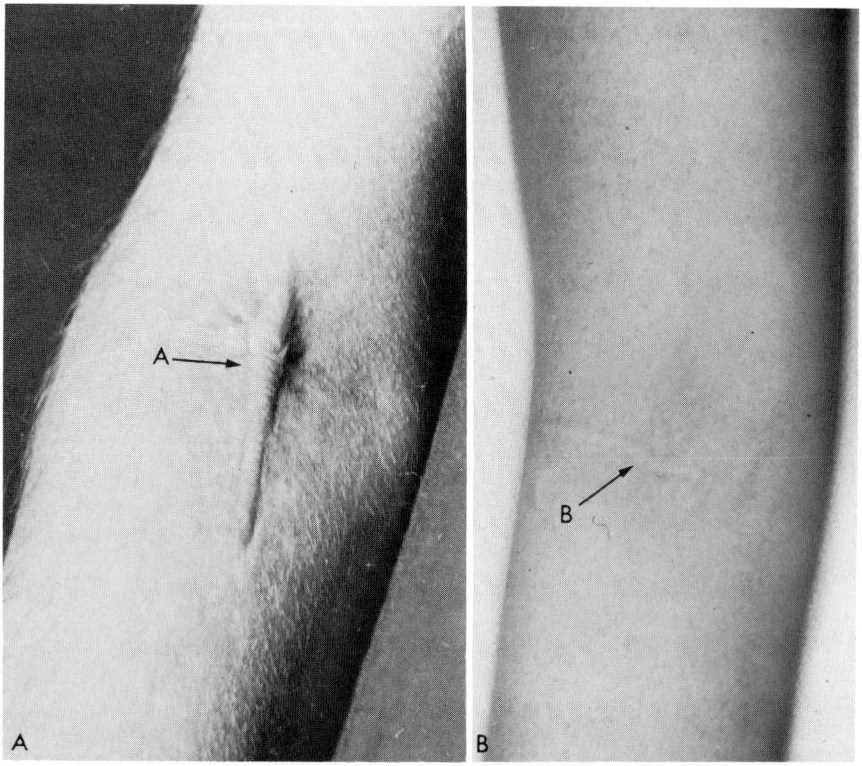

Fig. 90. Clinical photographs of operative scars in elbow region showing the difference between the vertical scar (A) crossing the flexion crease, and (B) the transverse scar lying in the flexion crease.

of tenderness over the radial head, limited motion and hemarthrosis, since roentgen examination is entirely negative. The treatment is the same as for adults with undisplaced radial head fractures, namely: aspiration of the joint if necessary to relieve pain, splint immobilization for 48 hours, then a sling and frequent active exercises for 10 days to two weeks. As soon as 50 percent of motion range is recovered without causing pain, mild active use may be permitted and encouraged. All passive motion, stretching procedures, massage, weight-carrying, hanging from trapeze or door casing to increase joint motion should be avoided as was advised against in adults, even if the child is disinclined to move the elbow.

The parents of the child should always be warned of the slight possibility of subsequent difficulty from growth disturbance.

2. Fracture (Separation) of the Radial Head Epiphysis with Partial Displacement or (Angulation with Impaction.)

This lesion in a child is usually fairly obvious clinically and can be confirmed by roentgen examination (see Fig. 85). If hemarthrosis is present, the joint should be aspirated. Following this (under general anesthesia) the displaced or angulated radial head epiphysis should be replaced as close to its anatomical position as possible. This can usually be accomplished by firm pressure with the operator's thumb over the anterior or lateral aspect of the radial head while with his other hand the patient's forearm is pronated and supinated several times. It is usually advisable to check the reduction of the fragment with the fluoroscope and to determine in what position of rotation and flexion this fragment remains in best position. The arm should then be immobilized in a posterior molded plaster splint from axilla to metacarpophalangeal joints and sling for two to three weeks followed by active exercises and mild use. One need have no fear in keeping a child's elbow joint immobilized for this period of time and this protection will aid in early union of the displaced epiphysis and offer less chance of later growth disturbance.

Open operation to reduce displacement of a radial head epiphysis *should be avoided* if it is possible to replace the head fragment in nearly normal position and axis. The reasons for avoiding open reduction are two, namely: (1) increased chance of growth disturbance; and (2) increased possibility of a synostosis (cross-union) developing between the upper ends of the radius and ulna with resulting loss of pronation and supination.

Operative Treatment. 3. Fracture (Separation) of the Radial Head Epiphysis with Complete Displacement.

This is a very rare and serious injury (see Fig. 85g). Frequently the displaced head epiphysis cannot be reduced by closed manipulation and repeated attempts to do so may cause additional damage to the epiphyseal plate. On the other hand the head must be operated upon if completely displaced and found impossible to replace by closed manipulation. One should therefore give a very guarded prognosis for the reasons stated above under No. 2. When the radial head has to be operated upon and replaced, it may be advisable to fasten it in place with a suture through the periosteum of the neck. Under no circumstances should a radial head epiphysis in a child be excised unless it be badly comminuted (a rarity in children) or unless it is found that it will not remain in contact with the neck when the forearm is pronated and supinated. Then a growth disturbance must be expected with resultant Madelung type of deformity at the wrist with loss of function.

There have been reported several cases of radial head fracture with complete displacement in children with the head of the radius turned upside down after closed reduction (180 degrees), i.e., with the fracture surface of the head facing the capitellum. These obviously require open reduction and correction of the mal-position obtained.

After operative replacement of the radial head epiphysis has been performed, plaster immobilization and subsequent treatment should be carried out as in No. 2. These operations, if they must be done, should be performed no later than 48 hours after injury.

FRACTURE (AVULSION) OF BICIPITAL TUBEROSITY OF RADIUS

(See under Rupture of Lower End of Biceps Tendon—Chapter XXII.)

Chapter XIII

Aspiration of the Elbow Joint

a. Purpose
b. Site for aspiration
c. Precautions
d. Technique

Purpose. Aspiration of the elbow joint is a procedure commonly used to relieve pain resulting from hemarthrosis. When the joint capsule remains intact, the blood which collects within it causes tension. This frequently is accompanied by severe pain which may be aggravated by attempts to move the joint actively or passively. Minor fractures in the head of the radius without displacement may be relatively painless at first, but after several hours during which time bleeding has occurred, the patient may be unable to get to sleep because of the pain. These fractures require no immobilization or splint protection, but should be treated by a regime of early active exercises in order to allow recovery of joint function. It is impossible to begin this regime of exercises satisfactorily while the patient suffers severe pain. If the joint is not aspirated, the disability time will be approximately one month. The fact that the blood remains in the joint to be absorbed offers a chance for the formation of adhesions between the articular surfaces and capsule, which in turn causes loss of joint motion or pain on extremes of motion. If, on the other hand, the same injury had been treated by early aspiraton and active motion, the disability time would be shortened to two weeks and there would be less chance of adhesion formation. Pain would likewise be less or even absent.

A second reason for aspirating a joint is for diagnostic purposes. Some cases of tuberculosis may have the diagnosis made on guinea pig inoculation of fluid removed from the joint before any positive roentgenographic evidence of the disease has appeared. If yellow fluid is recovered on aspiration and the usual bacteriological cultures and smears are negative for pathogenic bacteria, one should always request guinea pig inoculation so as not to lose valuable time in possibly establishing a positive diagnosis of early tuberculosis.

Suppurative arthritis due to staphylococcus or streptococcus, or joint infections due to pneumococcus, gonococcus, or other organisms may have a positive bacteriologic diagnosis made by smear and culture of the aspirated joint fluid.

From a therapeutic standpoint the joint may be aspirated to remove exudate, and penicillin or other antibiotics may be instilled, thus attacking

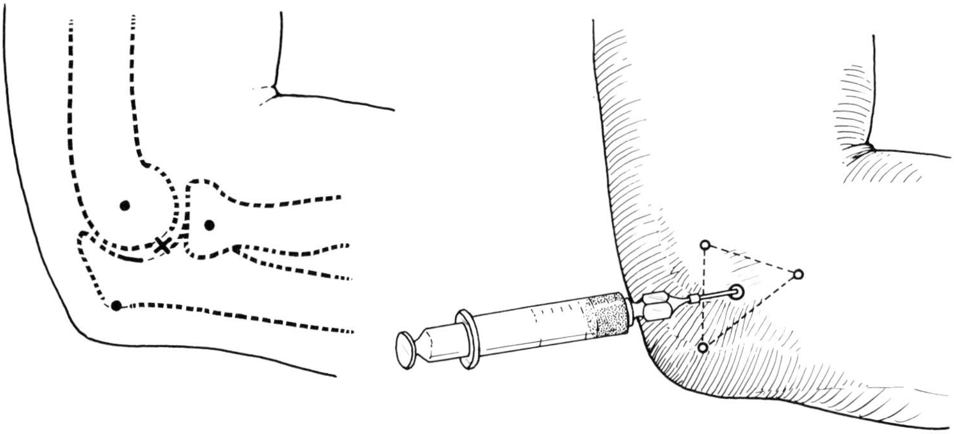

Fig. 91. The "hemarthrosis triangle" of the elbow joint formed by the lateral epicondyle of the humerus, radial head and posterior corner of the olecranon (see insert). The site (X) for insertion of the aspirating needle is equidistant from all three bony points and at the summit of the bulging capsule.

directly the infective organism and possibly making surgical drainage unnecessary. This of course depends upon the virulence of the organism and its sensitivity to the antibiotic used.

Site for Aspiration. The elbow is not a difficult joint to aspirate. The most ideal site for aspiration is at the point where the capsule bulges prominently on the postero-lateral aspect. In the center of the hemarthrosis triangle formed by the three bony prominences (all easily palpable), lateral epicondyle of humerus, radial head, and tip of olecranon is the spot where the aspiration needle should be inserted.

Precautions. Aspiration of a joint is a surgical procedure and should not be done in a haphazard manner. The skin must be shaved, then carefully cleansed with green soap, water, alcohol and ether to remove all dirt and grease before applying iodine or other skin antiseptic. With such precautions there should be very little risk of infection. The entire procedure must be carried out with careful *aseptic* technique. The surgeon should adhere as closely as possible to the principle that nothing should be introduced into the joint cavity except the aspirating needle. By thus keeping the entire procedure a "one way" affair, the risk of inadvertently introducing a few organisms into the joint cavity is kept at a minimum.

Technique of Aspiration. After careful cleansing and preparation of the skin as described above, the elbow must be rested on a sand bag, firm pillow, or pile of folded towels in a position comfortable for the patient, so that it will be steady and the patient will not wish to move it during the procedure. The joint should be partially flexed and the patient's hand and forearm may rest upon his chest and abdomen. Sterile towels should be placed beneath the prepared elbow and around its lateral aspect exposing only the immediate area for the aspiration. The triangle formed by the lateral epicondyle, head of radius, and tip of olecranon should be identified. A site equidistant from all three points is then chosen and an intradermal wheal made with one percent procaine solution. A sharp pointed scalpel should then be used to make an incision one-eighth inch long in the center of this wheal and extending through the entire thickness of the dermis. This makes it easier to insert a large caliber aspirating needle without risk of forcing skin organisms ahead of it and with minimal pain. As soon as this incision is made, the anesthetic solution should be infiltrated via a narrow intravenous needle through successive layers of subcutaneous tissue, deep fascia, anconeus muscle and joint capsule. The needle should be directed perpendicularly to the surface of the skin and will thus pass medially, slightly forward and distally into the joint cavity between the radial head, capitellum, and lateral surface of the ulna. Should bony resistance be encountered with the point of the needle, the latter must be withdrawn slightly and its direction changed until it slides easily into the joint without resistance. As soon as the needle traverses the joint capsule, blood will be forced into the syringe. This needle should then be withdrawn and a No. 17 or 18 gauge needle substituted and inserted in the same direction, infiltrating with additional anesthetic solution if necessary. The aspiration of blood should be continued until the flow ceases. Pressure applied over the front of the joint through the sterile towels may assist in obtaining an additional few cubic centimeters of blood. When no more blood is readily obtained the needle should be withdrawn and a sterile compress applied over the aspiration site.

Following aspiration it is often wise to immobilize the joint completely in a posterior molded splint for twenty-four hours. This puts the joint at rest, permits bleeding to stop, and thereby lessens the risk of recurrence of the hemarthrosis and the necessity for repeating the aspiration procedure.

The amount of blood that it is possible to remove from an elbow following trauma varies from five or six to fifteen and rarely twenty cubic centimeters. The relief thus obtained by decompression (aspiration) is often dramatic. The same may be said of immediate increase in joint motion.

Chapter XIV

Complications Following Elbow Injuries

GENERAL

EARLY COMPLICATIONS following fractures around the elbow are circulatory impairment (Volkmann's ischaemia), vessel damage, nerve paralysis, increased fragmentation of bone, compounding of the fracture, interposition of soft tissue, bleb formation, skin maceration, and loss of reduction. Severe circulatory impairment may progress to the point of actual ischaemia following reduction even if it had not been present earlier. Anatomical reduction of the fracture, splinting and elevation are the best means of over-coming an initially impaired circulation. Flexion of the elbow *without* reduction in a displaced supracondylar fracture may shut off the circulation distal to the elbow. Flexion should be used *only to maintain reduction* in such a fracture but *never* to the point that it compromises the radial pulse at the wrist. Too tight bandaging of a molded splint may tend to act as a tourniquet causing excessive swelling, bleb formation, and pain. Circular plaster casts applied to immobilize a reduced fresh elbow fracture are unsafe since subsequent swelling within a rigid circular casing tends to obstruct the veins and act as a potential cause of Volkmann's ischaemia. High elevation of the injured elbow will lessen the degree of swelling and risk of serious damage.

Loss of reduction in plaster will cause obstruction to the circulation and requires a further attempt at reduction by closed manipulation or by one of the methods of traction. Subsequent closed manipulations must be performed immediately and not be repeated over a period of several days to a week else the trauma caused by these may bring about the conditions favoring myositis ossificans. If dressings are too tight, they must be loosened. If flexion is too acute, the elbow must be partially extended. If circular casts are in use, they must be removed. If reduction is lost, treatment by Kirschner wire or Dunlop traction must be strongly considered and instituted early.

Damage to vessels or nerves may occur during treatment and is sometimes due to too great force employed in reduction. It is better that the patient be well relaxed under anesthesia and less force will thereby be necessary for the reduction. Increased fragmentation of a bone or compounding of a simple fracture by rough handling and manipulation is inexcusable.

Bleb formation is due to excessive swelling and possibly to too tight bandaging. Prevention of such swelling by a compression dressing evenly applied is the best means of avoiding it. At times bleb formation occurs in spite of all prophylactic measures used to avoid it. If they occur, they must be kept clean. Aspiration of their contents may prevent rupture and secondary infection.

Maceration of the skin is due to inadequate evaporation of perspiration between the apposed skin surfaces of the forearm and arm which come in contact with each other with the elbow in acute flexion. A few layers of surgical gauze placed cross-wise in the antecubital fold will act as a wick to permit evaporation of moisture.

Late complications following fracture in this region are Volkmann's contracture (which follows ischaemia) and myositis ossificans. Prevention of either of these complications is the only treatment of real benefit to the patient (see p. 187). If it is found that myositis ossificans is developing, all forms of treatment that may cause or increase it must be stopped immediately (see p. 185).

Late nerve complications cannot be expected, but with certain injuries we must forewarn the parents of the possibility and be on the look-out for them even years after the original injury. They may be treated as they arise (see p. 181).

Sudeck's atrophy is fortunately not common following elbow injuries. If one were to encounter such a complication, it would seem advisable to administer to the patient repeated sympathetic (stellate ganglion) nerve blocks with procaine hydrochloride and to increase active exercises and use for the entire extremity.

Causalgia, severe burning pain, usually results from incomplete injury to a peripheral nerve caused not infrequently by a gun-shot wound. The treatment is the same as for Sudeck's atrophy described above. If stellate ganglion blocks do not give permanent relief, it may be advisable to perform a stellate ganglionectomy.

VASCULAR INJURIES COMPLICATING FRACTURE AND DISLOCATION

When bone fragments are badly displaced in a fracture or the forearm bones are displaced in a dislocation at the elbow there may be serious damage to the major blood vessels. Though these will stand some stretching if not excessive they often are the site of direct contusion or laceration from the sharp anterior edge of the proximal fragment of the humeral shaft in a supracondylar or dicondylar fracture. (See Fig. 21-B, e.) The entire neurovascular bundle, enclosing the median nerve, brachial artery and brachial veins may be injured. Severe contusion of these vessels may result in thrombosis. If this occurs in the artery, gangrene of the hand may result. If it occurs in the veins, venous stasis will result and swelling may become excessive and Volkmann's contracture may occur. It is not necessary that the artery be completely lacerated before its circulation is shut off. Should it become badly scratched by a bone fragment, arterial spasm may supervene, which may also threaten the circulation to the forearm and hand. Spasm in the artery occurs more commonly than is supposed and often clears up following reduction of the fracture and release of the vessel from its contact with the lower shaft of the humerus. Should the radial pulse not return to normal within two hours following adequate reduction of the fracture or dislocation by closed manipulation, or following traction and suspension and should the hand and fingers remain pale and cool, operative exploration of the brachial artery should be resorted to immediately to determine the cause of its failure and correct it if possible.

NERVE INJURIES COMPLICATING FRACTURE AND DISLOCATION

The three main nerves (median, radial, and ulnar) at the elbow are rather frequently injured in fractures and dislocations. They are subject to direct contusion, stretching or partial laceration as a result of the initial trauma. It is very rare that one of them becomes completely severed except by gunshot injury, knife or glass cuts, or in severe open (compound) fractures such as those known as "truck-swipe" fractures. Each of these nerves has both sensory and motor function. When injured in the vicinity of the elbow the medial and ulnar nerve will lose both its sensory and motor function. The radial nerve divides about four centimeters above the elbow joint into a

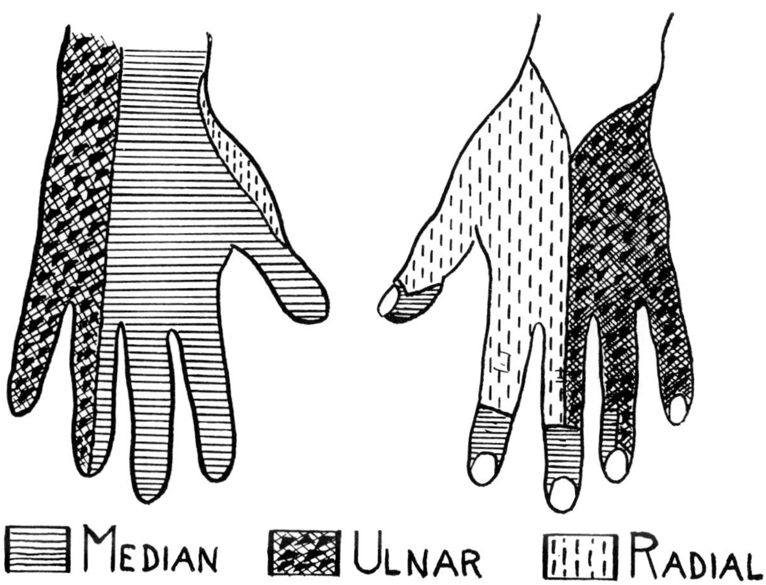

Fig. 92. Sketch showing sensory distribution of the median, ulnar, and radial nerves in the hand and fingers.

motor branch (posterior interosseous) and a sensory branch (superficial radial nerve). Either one or both of these branches may be involved in elbow injuries with respective loss of function.

With the MEDIAN NERVE paralyzed at the elbow due to local trauma the loss of motor function consists of inability to pronate the forearm, to flex the thumb or to oppose the thumb to any other finger; flexion of the wrist is weak and it tends to adduct on flexion due to the pull of the flexor carpi ulnaris muscle; flexion of all the fingers is weak. The thenar eminence is atrophied if the lesion has been present for two to three weeks or longer. The thumb as a whole is adducted towards the second metacarpal and index finger. The index and middle finger are extended at the metacarpophalangeal joints, but are slightly flexed at the proximal and distal interphalangeal joints as a result of the loss of function of the two lateral lumbrical muscles innervated by the median nerve. If the condition has been present for several months there will also be marked atrophy of the flexor muscles in the forearm and there may be atrophy of the skin and pulp on the tips of the thumb and two adjacent fingers.

Muscle Innervation by MEDIAN NERVE

Forearm

- Pronator Radii Teres
- Flexor Carpi Radialis
- Palmaris Longus
- Flexor Digitorum Sublimis
- Flexor Digitorum Profundis (Lateral one-half)
- Flexor Pollicis Longus
- Pronator Quadratus

Hand

- Abductor Pollicis Brevis
- Flexor Pollicis Brevis (Superficial head)
- Opponens Pollicis
- Lumbricales (First and Second)

The ULNAR NERVE when paralyzed at the elbow following trauma shows its loss of motor function by inability to abduct and adduct the fingers and to adduct the thumb; flexion of the wrist is weak and it may tend to abduct due to the pull of the flexor carpi radialis muscle; flexion of the fourth and fifth fingers is weak. There will be atrophy of the hypothenar eminence and of the adductor pollicis muscle belly if the lesion has been present for several weeks. The fourth and fifth fingers have their metacarpophalangeal joints extended, but their interphalangeal joints slightly flexed. There may likewise be pulp atrophy in these two fingers.

Muscle Innervation by ULNAR NERVE

Forearm

Flexor Carpi Ulnaris
Flexor Digitorum Profundus (Medial one-half)

Hand

Palmaris Brevis
Abductor Digiti Quinti
Flexor Digiti Quinti Brevis
Oppones Digiti Quinti
Lumbricales (3rd. and 4th.)
Flexor Pollicis Brevis (Deep head)
Adductor Pollicis
Interosseous (Volar and Dorsal)

As noted above, the RADIAL NERVE may have its sensory branch affected, or only its motor branch, or both. If the former, there will be loss of sensation on the dorsum of the thumb and index finger. If the motor branch (dorsal interosseous) is affected, the patient will be able to extend the wrist joint, because the extensors carpi radialis longus and brevis muscles are innervated by a separate branch from the main radial nerve which comes off at a slightly higher level than its main bifurcation. He will be unable to extend the proximal phalanges of the fingers at the metacarpophalangeal joints or the thumb, because all the extensor muscles of the fingers and thumb are innervated by the dorsal interosseous nerve. He will be able, however, to extend the middle and distal phalanges of the fingers at the two interphalangeal joints, since this function is performed by the lumbrical and interosseous muscles. If the patient lacks the ability to extend

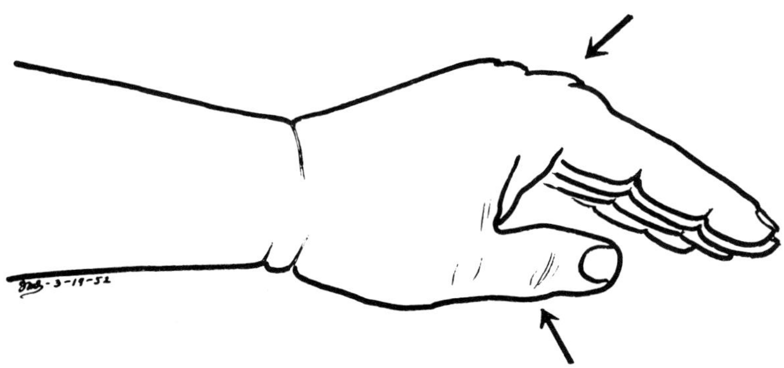

Fig. 93. Sketch showing result of paralysis of the posterior (dorsal) interosseus nerve. The patient is able to extend the hand at the wrist joint because the extensor carpi radialis longus and brevis muscles receive their innervation from branches of the main radial (musculospiral) nerve before it divides into the posterior interosseus (motor branch) and the superficial radial (sensory branch) nerves. He is *unable* to extend the fingers at the metacarpo-phalangeal joints and the thumb at its interphalangeal joint.

his wrist as well as the metacarpophalangeal joints, then the entire radial nerve (both motor and sensory) is paralyzed.

Muscle Innervation by RADIAL NERVE

Forearm

Brachio-radialis
Extensor Carpi Radialis Longus
Extensor Carpi Radialis Brevis
Extensor Digitorum Communis
Extensor Digiti Quinti Proprius
Extensor Indicis Proprius
Extensor Carpi Ulnaris
Anconeus
Abductor Pollicis Longus
Extensor Pollicis Brevis
Extensor Pollicis Longus

Hand

None

There may be late nerve complications occurring after fractures and dislocations at the elbow region. The nerve most commonly affected is the ulnar. The cause is scar tissue which forms in the region of the groove on the posterior surface of the medial epicondyle of the humerus. This, if excessive, may cause pressure on the nerve and even cause a constriction of the fibrous roof overlying the groove and may happen months after the original injury. The symptoms consist of numbness or tingling in the ring and little fingers. Objective findings are loss of or diminution of sensation to pinprick in the sensory distribution of the nerve. If the condition is allowed to progress, motor palsy or complete paralysis may supervene with all the physical signs described under nerve paralysis. Such a condition is occasionally seen after dislocations at the elbow joint.

There is still another type of late ulnar nerve neuritis which is not too uncommon following conditions that give rise to an increased carrying angle (cubitus valgus) deformity at the elbow. The commonest injury leading to this deformity is a fracture of the lateral condyle of the humerus in children which is occasionally followed by non-union of the fragment or by growth disturbance which shortens the lateral condyle and capitellum thereby increasing the carrying angle. Such a deformity puts a stretch upon the ulnar nerve by virtue of making it take a longer course to reach the forearm as it passes behind the medial epicondyle. Also, on full extension of the joint with the carrying angle increased to 25 degrees or more, the tip of the olecranon swings further medially and impinges upon or "crowds" the ulnar nerve. This constantly repeated trauma may set up a late neuritis with eventual palsy, etc. if not corrected. The long delayed onset of ulnar neuritis has been known to occur as late as thirty-three years after the original injury. Conversely, if a patient complains and shows objective signs of ulnar neuritis in the presence of a markedly increased carrying angle and no toxic cause can be found to explain its presence, further questioning is in order relative to previous elbow injury in childhood. Almost always this can be found to be present and roentgenograms will usually show evidence of deformity of the lateral condyle of the humerus characteristic of late pictures following such fractures.

Other conditions leading to increased carrying angle deformities and possible ulnar nerve neuritis are: (1) persistent anterior dislocation of the head of the radius following fracture of the upper third of the ulna (Monteggia fracture) which has either been incompletely reduced or has passed unrecognized from the beginning; and (2) the absence of the lateral condyle of the humerus when it has been necessary to excise this fragment for malunion.

The treatment of ulnar nerve neuritis is operative by transposition of the nerve to the anterior surface of the medial humeral condyle. This, of course, should always be performed if the condition appears to become progressive. If it is to be done, it should be done before atrophy becomes marked, otherwise there will be little functional recovery.

MYOSITIS OSSIFICANS

Myositis ossificans is the formation of new bone in injured muscle. It may extend to periosteum, bone, joint capsule and ligaments. It may occur following supracondylar or lateral condyle fractures of the humerus in children and more commonly after posterior dislocations at the elbow particularly when these dislocations are not promptly reduced.

The causes of myositis ossificans are few, but definite. These are: (1) repeated manipulative attempts at reduction of an elbow dislocation or fracture; (2) repeated attempts to mobilize a partially stiff elbow joint by vigorous or forceful passive stretchings (pump-handling); and (3) deep, vigorous massage. As was seen under the heading of repair of fractures the necessary factors for the formation of bony callus were hemorrhage, death of tissue, and an adequate circulation. So too, in the formation of myositis ossificans, the same factors are present. There has been hemorrhage, and damage to muscle and periosteum; the underlying bone from which the periosteum has been stripped acts as a source of calcium; granulation tissue begins to form and the reaction of the local area is acid. All attempts to stretch the joint passively to give it better motion or all attempts to reduce the dislocation or fracture repeatedly, especially late, adds insult to injury. Passive manipulation over-stretches and tears the infiltrated and no longer elastic muscles and periosteum, causes additional hemorrhage and tissue death, it increases the amount of inflammatory cell exudation and granulation tissue formation, which in turn gives an increased local hyperemia. With each attempt the additional damage to the tissues not only prolongs the period of acid pH reaction in the local tissues, but this withdraws more calcium from the underlying bone. Each attempt at manipulation or stretching or any attempt to give deep vigorous massage will obviously diffuse the calcium thus mobilized throughout the injured muscle and reparative granulation tissue. Consequently, we have an ideal "set-up" for the formation of new bone in injured muscle (usually the brachialis anticus) which is immediately adjacent to the anterior surface of the humerus and elbow joint.

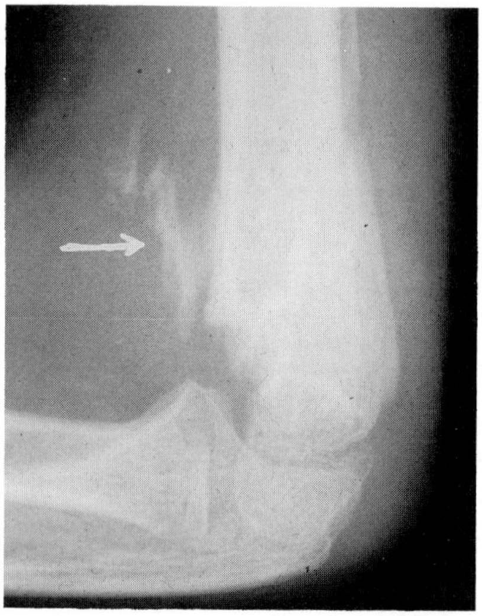

Fig. 94. Myositis ossificans (early) in brachialis anticus muscle following supracondylar fracture of humerus. This complication results from repeated attempts to improve reduction of the fracture over a period of a week to 10 days, passive stretching or manipulation to improve motion, deep massage, or a combination of these.

The onset of myositis ossificans, when it occurs in front of the elbow, is usually around the second to the third week after the initial injury. Clinically it is manifested by progressive decrease in joint motion, and by palpation of a firm lump or mass in the antecubital region which may be tender. This should lead one to suspect the condition and should suggest the necessity of further roentgenograms. The first evidence that these reveal is a faint cloudy mass of calcium density in the brachialis anticus muscle. As time goes on this becomes larger and more dense on the film. Eventually, after four to six months the new bone formation becomes stationary. It remains thus for a period of roughly three additional months after which it finally regresses and may disappear completely and spontaneously. Under no circumstances should operative removal of the ossifying area be attempted (even if it appears to cause a definite mechanical hindrance to flexion and extension) *until maximum regression has taken place.* This will be at least twelve months after the onset of the myositis ossificans formation.

The immediate treatment of early cases of myositis ossificans consists in stopping whatever factors have caused it. In other words stop all passive stretching or manipulations whether given by a physician, masseuse or over-enthusiastic parent; do not allow the child to chin himself or hang from an over-head bar or door casing with the idea of increasing his own motion by virtue of his own weight; prohibit the carrying of flat-irons, sand bags, buckets of water or school bags on the affected side. All of these procedures are notorious for causing myositis ossificans, and once the condition has started, their further use will only increase it—perhaps to a point where bony ankylosis of the joint may result.

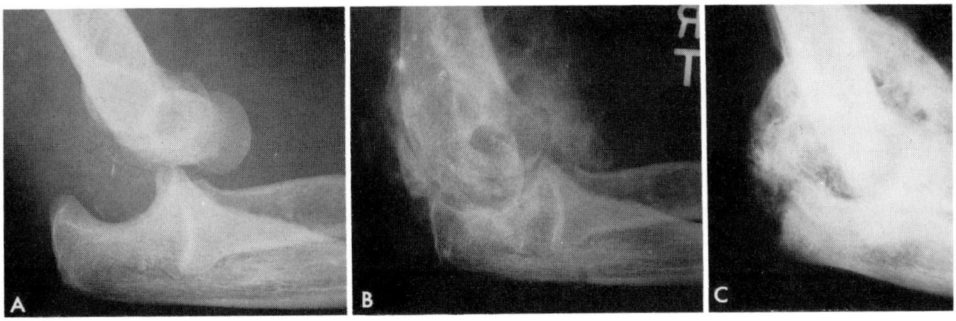

Fig. 95. Myositis ossificans (full blown). (A) Lateral view of two weeks old elbow dislocation in 50 year old patient (unreduced after two manipulative attempts, one on day of injury and the second 10 days later). Note faint calcium shadows just behind posterior aspect of lower extremity of humerus (beginning calcification). Open reduction was performed on 16th day after injury which is not the optimum time for such a procedure. (B) Same elbow five weeks after the late open reduction showing extensive myositis ossificans. (C) Lateral roentgenogram in a 30 year old man who had an arthroplasty performed for stiffness of the elbow following a dicondylar fracture of the humerus. The arthroplasty was followed by *passive* manipulation and stretching given with the mistaken purpose of improving joint motion, but succeeded only in creating extensive myositis ossificans and an ankylosed joint.

The very best positive treatment for myositis ossificans once it has commenced is to allow the child full activity. Do not try to hurry him by advising active exercises. Recovery is slow at best and the child will guard his usage of the extremity according to how it feels. In other words he will not move the joint beyond the point where it begins to hurt. Consequently, he will not cause further damage to the soft tissues, but will by virtue of this limited active use improve the circulatory status, rid the area of edema, and will restore elasticity to the muscles. This constant activity alone will restore joint motion to its full or nearly full capacity. It may take nearly a year to do this, however.

One of the most difficult problems in attempting to carry out such a regime is a disgruntled and well-meaning parent, who is unable to understand why Johnnie's elbow cannot be restored to normal in the course of a few weeks or months. Sound surgical judgment should not permit itself to be warped by the lack of understanding or the rantings of an over-emotional parent. If the parent is dissatisfied, or, if the physician is not entirely satisfied with the progress that is being made by the child, *insistence* upon consultation with an older surgeon experienced in treating fracture cases should be of mutual benefit to the parent, physician and the patient.

VOLKMANN'S ISCHAEMIC CONTRACTURE

The most dreaded complication of an elbow fracture or dislocation is Volkmann's ischaemic contracture. It is dreaded because of its ugly deformity and also because the hand and forearm are rendered practically useless.

Different degrees of the deformity and consequent loss of function are seen, but any loss from this cause is to be considered regrettable. The patient and his family can never be made to understand the complication and therefore many unjust malpractice suits have been instituted.

The usual Volkmann's ischaemia occurs most often following supracondylar fractures (extension type) of the humerus, fractures of both bones of the forearm, or after dislocations at the elbow. It may occur in cases of bleeding into deep muscle spaces in hemophilic patients following slight injury. Arterial embolism, severe soft part injury, and operation under Esmarch bandage have also been cited as antecedent causes of Volkmann's contracture.

The first decade claims the greatest and the second decade the next largest number of Volkmann's contracture, after which the lesion is rare.

Clinical Features. Within a few hours of injury there may appear the first symptoms and signs of ischaemia. These may be delayed in their appearance, however, for 24 to 48 hours. The most characteristic symptom is constant unabating pain of a burning character in the forearm, although with major nerve injury the onset may be quite painless. There may be coolness and pallor of the hand and fingers—both serious signs. On the other hand the fingers may be swollen and cyanosed. The radial pulse is almost always absent. The pain is aggravated by attempts to move the fingers actively or by passive attempts to extend the flexed fingers—also a very serious sign. The reason the child does not move the fingers early is not because of nerve involvement at this stage, but because the attempt to do so causes increased pain. After the process has continued to the point where the muscles are completely infiltrated, ischaemic, and paralysis has set in, the damage has been done and further emergency measures will be of no avail. By this time actual flexion contracture has occurred.

Deformity. The typical deformity of an established contracture is caused by shortening of the forearm muscles which have undergone necrosis and have become replaced by scar tissue. There is seen extension contracture of the metacarpophalangeal joints and flexion contracture of the interphalangeal joints. The contracture in mild cases may be limited to one or two fingers. When the wrist joint is passively extended the degree of flexion of the fingers is increased and when the wrist is flexed the degree of finger flexion is decreased.

Morbid Anatomy. Voluntary muscle when deprived of blood and thence oxygen undergoes necrosis. According to Griffiths the dead muscle mass behaves just like any other infarcted tissue. All cellular activity (infiltration) and all fibrosis occur at the periphery of the dead muscle. Interfibrillary fibrosis does not occur as after atrophy or contracture following sepsis or denervation. Fibrosis eventually proceeds from without inwards and replaces the necrotic muscle with fibrous tissue. This contracts and shortens to form the characteristic deformity of an established Volkmann's contracture.

Diagnosis. Accurate diagnosis must be made *early* if disaster is to be avoided since the only treatment of any use is prophylactic in nature. Once paralysis and contracture have occurred there is little to do but carry out measures to minimize the degree of contracture.

The following four words: PAIN, PALLOR, PULSELESSNESS, and PARALYSIS should be remembered in order to avoid them if Volkmann's ischaemic contracture is to be prevented.

Pathogenesis. It was formerly believed that Volkmann's ischaemia and contracture was due to obstruction of the venous circulation from too tight bandaging, circular plaster casts, or to too acute flexion of the elbow after reduction. Subsequent clinical observations by numerous surgeons have shown that this lesion can occur without any one of the above causes being present. Volkmann, himself, originally felt that the cause was arterial obstruction from too tight bandaging. Putti believed the contracture due to a nerve lesion and that the circulation was of secondary importance. J. B. Murphy considered the cause of the condition was venous obstruction. Jepson believed likewise. These surgeons considered that venous congestion resulting from one or more of the above causes plus tension hematoma beneath the deep fascia increased to the point where the venous pressure and surrounding soft tissue tension equalled the arterial pressure—thus bringing about an ischaemia of the entire area distal to the lesion. The ischaemia with associated anoxia thus affected the striated muscle sooner and more seriously than other tissues with fewer demands for oxygen. The muscle so affected became infiltrated with hemorrhage and underwent necrosis. Paralysis resulted. Healing took place by replacement of the dead muscle with fibrous tissue which in turn caused contracture of the wrist and fingers.

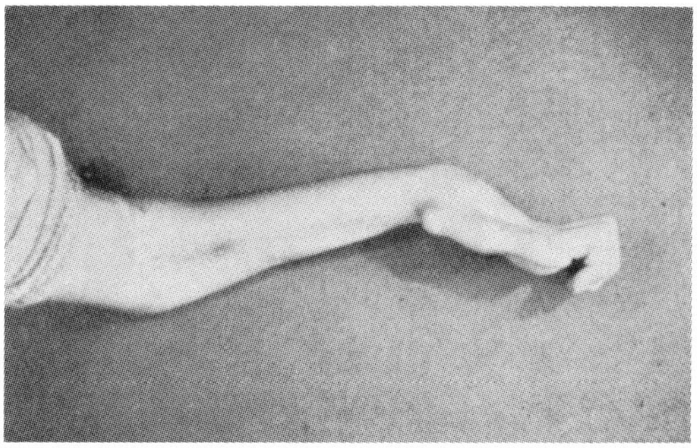

Fig. 96. Volkmann's ischaemic contracture following an unreduced supracondylar fracture. A decompression operation was performed but not early enough to prevent sloughing of all flexors. (Bunnell, S.: *Surgery of the Hand.* Lippincott, Philadelphia, 1948.)

Brooks carried out considerable experimental work by ligating the vein to the sartorius muscle in dogs and produced some contractures, but according to Griffiths these were never quite the same type as seen in a true Volkmann's contracture.

Griffiths in 1940 blamed arterial injury as the main cause of Volkmann's ischaemia. The artery becomes injured through contusions, or laceration, or gets caught on the lower end of a supracondylar fracture fragment. Reflex vasospasm constricts the artery and interferes with the pulse. If the collateral circulation is poor gangrene will result. If the collateral circulation is good nothing may happen; but if the collateral circulation is not entirely adequate, ischaemia will result and this affects muscle tissue first. The muscle undergoes necrosis and becomes infiltrated with edema and subsequently with red blood cells as in other infarcted tissues. Eventually this is replaced by scar tissue and this in turn causes the typical deformity of Volkmann's contracture.

Griffiths states that Volkmann's contracture is due to arterial injury and occlusion and to nothing else. He also states that external compression (constricting dressings, splints, or casts) is a contributing factor. Therefore, it would seem that venous congestion in his mind may continue to be a factor in this lesion.

Watson-Jones agrees whole-heartedly with Griffiths that Volkmann's contracture is due to arterial injury and occlusion. On the other hand he states that "Volkmann's contracture may be due to: (1) flexion of a swollen elbow (or swelling of an acutely flexed elbow): or (2) pressure splints or plaster on forearm fractures."

Garber states that arterial injury is not always the only factor in producing ischaemic lesions. He states that in cases of Volkmann's contracture after forearm fractures which he has studied the hands have shown cyanosis, *not* pallor, at onset of the circulatory disturbance; he therefore feels that venous obstruction may have been the primary causative factor.

Hemophilic patients sometimes develop contractures similar to Volkmann's, but certainly this is not on the basis of arterial injury. Slow bleeding takes place beneath the deep fascia and tension develops, blocking the venous circulation long before the arterial circulation is slowed and before ischaemia can develop.

In view of the two schools of thought concerning the etiology of Volkmann's contracture, it might be said that both have their merits. It is most difficult for the author to believe that of 16 out of 55 consecutive elbow fracture cases developing Volkmann's contracture as reported by Putti the cause could be solely on a basis of nerve injury according to his own belief or on a basis of arterial injury alone according to Griffiths. This is all out of proportion to the experience of other surgeons with the development of Volkmann's contracture from any cause. In over 650 consecutive supracondylar fractures treated in the past 22 years at the Presbyterian Hospital, New York City, not a single case of Volkmann's contracture has developed. Certainly, if the etiology were arterial obstruction following arterial injury, it is highly probable that several cases should have occurred in this series in spite of all precautions (see Treatment). Many of these patients entered without a palpable pulse and some with primary nerve lesions. In every instance the pulse returned after reduction or within two hours following the institution of over-head traction.

The author does not feel that either arterial or venous obstruction alone is the cause of Volkmann's ischaemia and contracture. To blame the original arterial injury as the sole cause is in his opinion extremely dangerous, because it implies that nothing can be done to prevent it. Even the strongest advocates of arterial etiology suggest such preventive measures as release of too tight bandages or splints, decrease in the angle of flexion of a reduced elbow fracture all *before* operative exploration of the brachial artery is to be undertaken as a last resort.

Treatment

If it is difficult for expert surgeons to decide what is the exact etiology of Volkmann's contracture, it is certainly too much to expect the average surgeon or physician to determine it. Therefore, one must keep in mind both possibilities and try to avoid anything in the form of treatment that might dangerously constrict either the arterial or the venous circulation.

Preventive Treatment. Prophylaxis is the most important type of treatment. It must therefore be instituted early since the characteristic ischaemic contracture can occur within six hours after injury. Absence of the radial pulse accompanying an elbow fracture or dislocation must be considered of serious import. Pallor and pain must likewise be regarded with grave suspicion.

Embarrassment of the circulation calls for the following urgent steps: (1) release of any tight bandage, splint or plaster that may be causing external constriction. (2) Decrease of the angle of acute flexion of the elbow to maintain reduction if marked swelling is present. (3) Reduction of the supracondylar fracture immediately by manipulation if it remains unreduced. (This alone often relieves the circulatory impairment completely by releasing a trapped artery.) *Do not wait* for the swelling to go down. To do so may permit the onset of ischaemia. If it is impossible to reduce the fracture when first seen and swelling is excessive and possible ischaemia threatens or is feared, some form of traction (Dunlop skin traction or Kirschner wire skeletal traction) may be started (Chapter X). (5) If, despite all these procedures and precautions, the circulation fails to return, one must not delay more than two hours before operating and exposing the brachial artery. This is done to release a trapped artery, bathe with saline solution and massage an artery in spasm, and to excise a badly contused or lacerated segment of artery. If the vessel is in spasm and this fails to relax after massage, one-fourth grain of papaverine should be injected intravenously. (6) In addition to the above five precautions, but not as a primary form of treatment, one may administer a sympathetic block of the stellate ganglion with 2 percent procaine hydrochloride.

Additional precautions which may help as a safeguard are the avoidance of circular plaster, too tight bandaging of splints, avoidance of elbow flexion following reduction of the fracture to the point where the radial pulse becomes compromised. *Never* utilize the Jones' position of acute flexion *to reduce* a supracondylar fracture. This position should only be used to maintain reduction *after* it has been obtained. Adhesive figure-of-8 dressings are likewise dangerous because they are not adaptible to swelling. Any patient

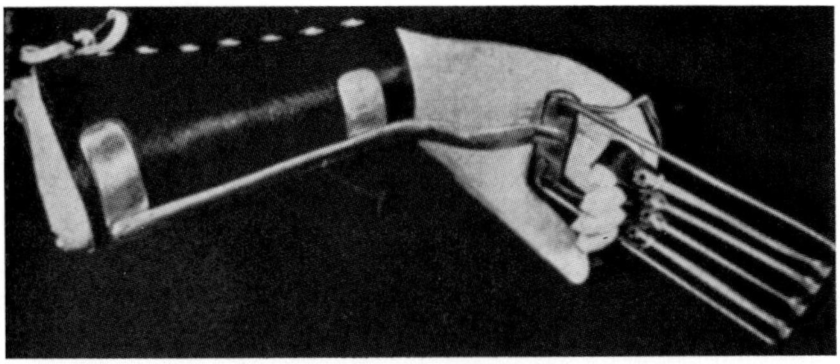

Fig. 97. Elastic traction splint used to overcome Volkmann's ischaemic contracture. (Steindler, A.: *Traumatic Deformities and Disabilities of the Upper Extremity*. Springfield, Ill., Thomas, 1946.)

with a severely swollen elbow should be kept in the hospital over-night for observation of the swelling, an hourly check on the presence and quality of the pulse. color and temperature of the hand and fingers, for high elevation of the injured part in order to assist gravity drainage of the veins and lymphatics, and for the institution of any other measures deemed necessary should the emergency arise. It is very unwise to reduce a supracondylar fracture in a child and allow him to go home with instructions to the parents to feed him aspirin or codeine if he continues to suffer pain. A "full-blown" ischaemic paralysis can occur in six hours.

Early Treatment of Contracture. Treatment of Volkmann's contracture, once it has become established, consists principally in protective splinting to prevent contractures which will otherwise be inevitable. Gentle passive stretching exercises and elastic traction, alternating between flexion and extension of the fingers should likewise be given. This treatment is difficult to carry out and must be continued for at least a year if any appreciable benefit is to be derived from it. If this regime is followed assiduously along with active exercise and use, much of the bad deformity may be overcome and some return of useful function may be regained.

Late Treatment of Contracture. On the other hand if the case appears late and contracture has already occurred, it is too late to accomplish much in the way of correcting severe deformities. Several procedures may be done and the most likely one to succeed is gradual stretching of the contracted fibrotic bellies by the use of a splint and gentle manipulation. Tendon lengthening procedures may be tried, but are frequently unsatisfactory due to the formation of the fibrous adhesions around the operative site. Transplantation of the common tendon of origin of the flexor-pronator groups of muscles from its origin at the medial epicondyle of the humerus to a point five or six centimeters distal on the ulna will help to relax the contracted muscles, but at the same time it weakens what little power remains in these muscles.

Prognosis

In an established case the prognosis depends mainly upon the severity. A Volkmann's contracture is a real tragedy. It is something to be *prevented,* not treated.

Chapter XV

Operative Treatment of Fractures

General

ALTHOUGH THE various methods of conservative and operative treatment of fractures about the elbow have been discussed at length under each type of fracture (Chapters X, XI, and XII), it would seem wise to review the advisability of open reduction for these injuries. In general the great majority of fractures anywhere may be adequately treated by conservative means and a good result expected. In the elbow region this still holds true since the commonest types of fracture are in children and often very mild in nature. On the other hand one should try to appreciate the types of fracture in which conservative treatment is useless from the beginning, or where, though properly carried out, it has failed to accomplish its purpose. Some surgeons have been criticized for advising open reductions where conservative treatment promised a good functional and anatomical end-result. Others may be similarly and justifiably criticized for advising or insisting upon the use of conservative treatment.

This brings up the advisability of recommending operative treatment as opposed to conservative treatment. It should also cause one to pause and consider that operations may be divided into two main types; those of *necessity;* and those of *choice*. Each of these has disadvantages as well as advantages. There are certain types of fracture in which very definite harm may be caused the patient by injudicious or over-enthusiastic operative surgery. The question of the use of internal fixation will be discussed further on in this chapter.

Necessary Prerequisites for Open Reduction

Operations of *necessity* may have to be performed under circumstances far from ideal and by general surgeons without extensive experience in open reductions. A serious compound fracture is such a case where the general condition of the patient or the time element precludes transporting him a long distance to a more properly equipped hospital. Under the circumstances the surgeon must treat the case according to the recognized surgical principles and employ what equipment and skill he has to the best of his ability and in the best interests and welfare of the patient. If strict adherence to principles is maintained (Chapter VI), more patients will obtain better results than if the surgeon forgets these principles (and what they will accomplish) by improvising new methods, by trying out the latest "gadget," or by compromising on thorough surgery. This truth suffered a considerable set-back at the beginning of World War II when chemotherapy was held by some to be a sure prevention of infection in compound fractures and gave "sloppy" surgeons a ray of hope in covering up their inadequate surgery. By the end of the War the magic myth about the wholesale use of chemotherapy for such prevention of infection had disappeared and the medical services of the Army and Navy began to emphasize, as authoritative civilian surgeons had done long before, that one must carry out and emphasize the adherence to strict surgical principles in treating the badly injured patient.

Operations of *choice* on the other hand are not dire emergencies. They may be performed as emergencies if the surgeon wishes, or they may be put off for a day, a week, or longer. Where such choice exists, it is logical that all operative facilities and anesthesia be as perfect as possible, and that the surgeon and his assistants be qualified and trained in the proper technique of handling fresh bone injuries not only at the operating table, but in the carrying out of the after-treatment as well. They must understand the pathology of acute injuries and appreciate the time element so necessary in handling these properly. They must also keep in mind the importance of quickly restoring the normal physiology to the injured part. They must be able to think in terms of hours and days—not merely in weeks or months.

Unnecessary risks should not be taken in operations of choice unless the risk be considered so slight as to be far out-weighed by the advantages to be gained as compared to other methods of treatment. These risks are: possible injury to nerves and vessels due to distorted pathological anatomy or injudicious or prolonged use of a tourniquet, possible loss of reduction, loss of function, infection, and the complications of anesthesia, and need not be discussed here in detail. Any procedure (open or closed) is accompanied by some risk to the patient, however slight, so we cannot say dogmatically that no risk should be taken. Again, the surgeon must consider all the factors, circumstances, and the patient's mental and economic status, and try to base his judgment as to the method of treatment to be employed on what he believes will give the patient the best possible result (both immediately and later).

Operations of Necessity

Certain fractures absolutely require open reduction. The following types come under this classification according to Kennedy: fractures with interposition of soft tissue, irreducible fractures, joint fractures, and those in which a complicating nerve injury is present. At the elbow these would include in adults such lesions as fracture of the radial head with marked displacement (with or without an accompanying elbow joint dislocation), fractures of the lateral condyle or capitellum with displacement, fracture of the medial condyle with displacement, or other irreducible fracture. In children the only fracture that regularly requires open reduction is a separation of the medial epicondyle epiphysis with displacement into the elbow joint. In general all other epiphyseal injuries at the elbow should be treated by conservative means if possible. Occasionally, it may be necessary to perform open reduction upon an irreducible radial head epiphysis, and, if such is done, the head should be replaced rather than excised as is the accepted method in adults—otherwise growth disturbance is almost certain to follow. Fracture of the lateral humeral condyle in children in which the fragment is displaced and rotated very frequently requires open reduction, since it is often impossible to replace it by closed reduction. The fracture line often passes through the condyle immediately adjacent to the epiphyseal line, but it also passes through the articular surface of the capitellum (though invisible on roentgenograms). Consequently, the fragment including the articular surface must be replaced accurately for function to be recovered even though operation may enhance the possibility of subsequent growth disturbance. A fair number of these fractures show growth disturbance at a later date even though no appreciable displacement was originally present. In an exceptionally rare instance it may be necessary to operate to bring about reduction of a supracondylar fracture of the humerus when there is an impending Volkmann's paralysis, but operation should never be performed until treatment of the fracture and impaired circulation by traction has been tried and proved a failure in restoring the radial pulse.

Operations of Choice

There are some fractures in which a satisfactory result is to be expected only by open reduction, or where, if given the best conditions, a better result may be expected than by any form of conservative therapy. This latter type must never be operated upon indiscriminately. At the elbow it would be necessary to include in the former group fractures of the olecranon with displacement, of the radial head with moderate displacement, and Monteggia fractures (fracture of ulnar shaft with dislocation of the head of the radius). Some dicondylar fractures of the humerus should be included in this group when comminution is not a factor.

Operations That Must Be Avoided

In some fractures open reduction is not only of questionable or no value, but it may be definitely harmful. Such is the case in badly comminuted fractures, because it is impossible to reassemble all the fragments anatomically without stripping their periosteal and muscular attachments so extensively that it disturbs their nutrition; also, because it is impossible to employ internal fixation in adequate mechanical form. In other words such an injudicious procedure if attempted would merely add insult to injury and certainly accomplish no useful purpose from the standpoint of the patient. Delayed open reduction in the presence of beginning myositis ossificans must never be undertaken, since it will very *definitely* increase the possibility of extra-osseous bone formation and thus cause impairment to elbow function.

Open reductions on epiphyseal separations at the elbow should be avoided if it is at all possible except in the occasional instances mentioned above.

Advantages of Open Reduction

In operations of necessity it is obvious that no other treatment is of any benefit. In operations of choice on the other hand many advantages are to be gained by open reduction as noted above, *provided* all the qualified personnel, equipment, and circumstances are present to permit carrying out such operations successfully. The advantages are more perfect reduction and maintenance of reduction by internal fixation, without the continued use of external plaster fixation. This in turn permits early active motion and exercises for the adjacent joints, thus minimizing muscular atrophy and joint stiffening, and promoting early return of the injured part to its normal physiological status. This permits early use (if the injured bone has been adequately fixed internally), promotes a more complete return of function, and cuts down disability time, which is often of extreme importance in adults. Where possible—open reduction, internal fixation, early active motion and use will make late rehabilitation unnecessary. The only rehabilitation necessary is that which the patient can carry out himself (exercises and mild use) *while* the bone is healing. No regular physiotherapy treatments are needed if this regime is adhered to conscientiously. Occasionally, the patient may need guidance in his exercises or may even need prodding, but one should avoid giving him "baking and massage" daily or three times a week and not expect him to help himself between treatments. Occupational therapy may also be employed to advantage—not as a diversional measure—but as an adjunct to exercises to help improve muscular strength and coordination as well as to improve motion range.

Disadvantages of Open Reduction

The disadvantages of open reductions of choice are evident to the surgeon who has seen a large number of fracture cases, but it is to the less experienced that these must be pointed out, hoping that he may be able to profit from the experience of others. Operative wounds still occasionally become infected in spite of careful technique and the wishful use of prophylactic antibiotic and chemotherapy. Such infection in bones and joints, the site of acute trauma, is oftentimes disastrous and may lead to amputation or ankylosis aside from prolonged disability. Inadequate internal fixation due to too much comminution or to the use of improper materials may lead to loss of position of the fragments and the necessity of employing plaster fixation, which in turn negates one of the main purposes of the open reduction (i. e., early motion and use). Some surgeons still employ wire loops, catgut or kangaroo tendon sutures for fastening shaft fractures together. No such fixation can give the desired rigidity and the extremity will require external plaster fixation. It would be better not to operate than to insult the tissues (bone and soft parts) and then not give them or the patient the advantages of rigid internal fixation. True rigid fixation can only be obtained by the use of plates or by screws and nails (including intramedullary), except for such fractures as the olecranon or medial epicondyle of the humerus. If plates are used, the fixation will be vastly improved by the additional use of a transfixion screw where possible to use it. It must also be appreciated that internal fixation is likely to be less secure in cancellous than in firm cortical bone.

Certain fractures though they should be operated upon do not require actual reduction or fixation, but must have excision of the displaced fragment (radial head or capitellum in the adult). Others may require reduction, but no internal fixation (radial head epiphysis in children).

The hasty and indiscriminate plating of fractures is to be frowned upon. However, if the surgeon believes that a fracture should be operated upon and takes the trouble to expose and reduce it, (and subjects the patient to the risks of open reduction) he should not hesitate to employ internal fixation. To omit the use of internal fixation where it is indicated because of fear of its acting as a foreign body is pure folly. Even though the wound were to become infected, the plate often acts as an excellent temporary splint (provided adequate surgical drainage has been established), preventing wide-spread infection and giving comfort to the patient meanwhile. Later when the acute infection has cleared and fracture healing is taking place, the plate may be removed.

This is no place to enter into a prolonged discussion of the types of metal best employed for internal fixation. The type of metal used (in spite of what some authors advocate) probably makes less difference than the technique of the surgeon using it. The two best metals for internal fixation are Vitallium and SMO stainless steel. These metals are strong yet cause very little tissue reaction ordinarily. However, either one of these metals will cause tissue reaction if it is improperly applied, i. e., screws put in loosely or under strain.

Open reduction with internal fixation is regaining its prestige and more and more patients are being benefitted by its usage. It behooves the fracture surgeon to know *when* to use it and *how* to use it.

Optimum Time for Open Reduction

When open reduction is to be performed for fracture or dislocation, the *optimum* time is within the first twelve to twenty-four hours following the injury. It is difficult for many surgeons accustomed to performing open reductions as late as a week or ten days after injury to understand the great importance of early immediate operation. The advantages are obvious to those who perform them regularly as emergency measures within two to six hours after injury.

What are these advantages? *First,* the entire operative procedure is more easily done. Swelling though present is soft; induration is at a minimum; inflammatory reaction and beginning organization are not present to impede reduction of the fracture; the soft tissues are still elastic which permits easier reduction of the bone fragments and makes it possible to obtain closure of the skin wound without resorting to the use of extreme tension. Much of the extravasated blood and edema fluid is permitted to leak out and, consequently, with primary closure without tension, wound healing is enhanced rather than delayed. *Second,* if internal fixation has been employed, and adequate rigidity has been obtained, the surgeon need have no fear of starting the patient upon a regime of early active exercises for keeping up motion in the joints and for continuing physiological function of the muscles and circulation. *Third,* the after-care required is less, since frequent changes of plaster are not necessary. This after-care is more in the nature of supervision and requires less physical effort. It is also unnecessary to keep the patient "coming-back" for treatments since he rehabilitates himself while the bone is healing and not afterwards.

For the patient the advantages of early open reduction are even more obvious. It assures him of satisfactory anatomical reduction early making repeated attempts at further reduction unnecessary, thereby giving him a minimum of surgical trauma. By operative removal of the products of tissue death (following the original trauma) the patient does not have to absorb these into his system and consequently has a smoother post-operative course, little or no fever, and, if he has been in shock, will respond better to the treatment for it. The circulation of the injured part will return to normal more rapidly, swelling will be less in extent and persist less long, all due to the continuance of muscular activity so important for support of the venous and lymphatic circulation. There will be less muscular atrophy and no loss of muscle elasticity. Return to weight-bearing or to active use of a non-weight-bearing joint such as the elbow (at the proper time) may be performed with less effort, fatigue and fear. The disability time is often half that of similar cases treated by plaster immobilization and the patient may return to his regular work in a similar period. This is not only a great economic saving, but is also vastly important for the patient's morale.

Skin Preparation Prior to Operation

Open reduction should never be performed without very careful preparatory cleansing of the skin. This preparation must be in the nature of mechanical cleansing rather than rely upon chemical antiseptics with their dubius bactericidal powers. Any antiseptic with sufficient strength to kill bacteria when applied to the skin will also kill epithelial cells. Skin antiseptics though theoretically excellent are prone to give the surgeon a false sense of security especially if they are of a brilliant color. One of the reasons for disastrous results in open reduction due to infections has been through the employment of iodine or other skin antiseptic applied over the operative area, but without first getting rid of the skin oils, dirt and perspiration beforehand.

Prior to operation, whether immediate or delayed, the skin must be thoroughly shaved for a wide area above and below the operative site. When operation is to be delayed, as is sometimes necessary, it is advisable to give the patient a thorough skin preparation forty-eight hours before operation and to repeat this twenty-four hours before operation. The skin should be prepared by scrubbing it thoroughly with green soap and water for a minimum of five minutes. The surgeon or nurse performing this procedure should wear sterile rubber gloves and use sterile gauze compresses. The main purpose of the soap and water scrub is to remove mechanically all surface dirt and grease. The limb is then washed free of soap by pouring sterile water over it. The entire area to be prepared is next painted with seventy percent ethyl alcohol, followed by ether, and again by alcohol. The entire prepared area is then wrapped in sterile towels and the latter bandaged carefully in place to prevent their slipping and exposing the skin. At the time of operation another similar preparation is given before the extremity is draped in sterile sheets. It has been thoroughly demonstrated through years of experience with such skin preparations that they are far more effective than a single preparation with iodine and alcohol immediately preceding operation.

In emergency operations the technique of skin preparation is identical except that the preliminary soap and water scrub should be carried out for ten minutes instead of five.

When an immediate operation is necessary and an abrasion of the skin is present in the vicinity of the operative area, it is safer to proceed with the operation early (provided the skin *and abrasion* are thoroughly cleansed as described above) than to wait two or three days at which time the abrasion may be infected. Abrasions are no more infected when treated early than are compound wounds. They are contaminated, but may be easily converted into clean wounds. Later they are more difficult to convert and may carry virulent organisms which, if introduced into the operative wound, will very probably lead to infection and perhaps disaster.

In (compound) open fractures preparation of the operative field should be carried out in similar fashion with a preliminary soap and water scrub. The compound wound is protected and kept covered with a sterile compress while the surrounding skin is thoroughly washed and scrubbed for ten minutes. Following this the skin immediately surrounding the wound is similarly cleansed. The whole field is then painted with alcohol, ether and alcohol, and the extremity is then ready for draping. No attempt should be made to scrub the wound itself, nor should any antiseptics be poured or swabbed into the wound during the preliminary preparation.

Treatment of the Wound in Open (Compound) Fractures

The primary purpose in treatment of the wound associated with a compound fracture is to convert a contaminated wound into one that is surgically clean and which will heal without infection of the bone or soft parts. The treatment of the open (compound) fracture per se is a separate problem and one of utmost importance and, although it must be dealt with at the same time, it need not be brought into the immediate discussion of the care of the wound of compounding. *All* traumatic wounds are contaminated with bacteria to a lesser or greater degree, but *none* of these wounds regardless of the extent of contamination are infected at the onset. Infection, if it supervenes, probably does not occur for a minimum period of time (eight to 12 hours) after injury. The "safe" period varies somewhat depending upon the degree of contamination impairment of the local blood supply, and the type of first-aid treatment that may have been rendered.

Certain principles of treatment are of extreme importance in the care of a compound fracture wound. The first of these is *protection of the wound* with a sterile dressing to prevent further contamination with organisms from clothing or the examiner's fingers or respiratory passages. It is wise for the examiner to wear a mask to minimize further contamination from this source. No probing of the wound with instruments (even though sterile) must be permitted in order to prevent surface contamination from being carried deeply into the wound. No antiseptics should be applied to the wound and no washing should be attempted until the patient is in the operating room where all proper facilities are available for carrying out the operative treatment of the wound and the fracture. Should bleeding be excessive, a pressure dressing may be applied over the sterile dressing or, in the case of arterial bleeding, a tourniquet may be temporarily employed. A tourniquet thus applied should be released every one or two hours for five minutes otherwise gangrene of the extremity may result. The fracture must be splinted for protection and to reduce additional soft part injury as well as for the patient's comfort. Traction, if employed, must not be for the purpose of pulling a contaminated and exposed bone end back under the skin, but purely for stabilization of the fragments. Shock treatment must be commenced early if necessary. Careful physical examination must also precede any operative procedure to rule out other serious injuries that might otherwise be over-looked in the presence of an obvious compound fracture.

The second principle to be followed is *thorough preparation of the skin*. Under general anesthesia and after shaving of the extremity, the skin must be very thoroughly scrubbed with green soap and water (while the immediate wound is kept covered with a sterile compress) for a period of ten minutes. Following this, the skin immediately surrounding the wound is similarly washed for five minutes. This is in turn followed by the application of alcohol, ether, and alcohol in this order to the entire cleansed area.

The extremity is now draped with sterile sheets, etc., as it is for a regular operation.

The third principle in the treatment of this type of wound is *conversion of the contaminated wound into a clean wound.* This may be accomplished by two means—debridement and *lavage*. Debridement must be thorough and complete except for important nerves, tendons and major blood vessels. Debridement actually consists of excision of the contaminated wound as completely as possible. Debridement must be performed layer by layer, removing all dead or devitalized tissues such as skin, subcutaneous tissue, fascia, muscle, periosteum or completely loose bone fragments if not of large size. All foreign material such as bits of clothing or dirt must likewise be removed. The purpose of debridement is to get rid of the contaminated and devitalized tissues that will not survive and which (if not removed) would undergo necrosis and furnish an ideal culture medium for bacteria. Debridement must be performed with sharp scalpels rather than by scissors since the latter cause additional damage by crushing of tissues. After debridement of each layer, lavage should be carried out with copious amounts of warm, normal physiological saline solution taking care to wash outwards from the wound with a forceful stream and not allow the fluid to run over the skin and into the wound. The lavage serves three purposes: (1) getting rid of particles of devitalized tissue and bloodclots; (2) removal of gross dirt not removed by debridement; and (3) dilution of the bacterial contamination to the point where the natural defenses of the tissues can take care of it.

The fourth principle under consideration is *complete exploration of the wound.* This is for the purpose of opening up the wound to relieve tension, and to make debridement and lavage thorough. It is also for the purpose of ridding the wound of all possible pockets that might harbor bacteria or collections of blood which would act as an excellent culture medium.

The fifth principle is *perfect hemostasis.* Without this there will result hematomata, tension in the wound, and very likely infection.

The sixth principle in treatment of a compound wound is the *avoidance* of tension. Certain compound wounds showing little or no contamination or soft part damage, if treated early (under eight hours), may be closed primarily. Under no circumstances, however, must tension be created in the closure or disaster may result. Other compound wounds are so badly contaminated and have extensive soft part damage that it is impossible even to close them partially. These are best left wide open and packed very loosely with plain, sterile, fine-mesh gauze to permit escape of serum or other exudate. It may be possible, safe and highly desirable to perform secondary closure upon some of these wounds five to six days later. If this is to be done, it must be performed in the operating room with complete aseptic technique and the skin edges may be undermined to permit closure without causing tension. Many wounds, if packed wide open and permitted to granulate and heal by second intension, will become superficially infected or even develop infection of the bone. It may therefore be desirable and advantagous to apply dermatome grafts at the original operative procedure in order to obtain closure, lessen scar tissue formation, and decrease the risk of secondary infection. Any scars resulting from such a procedure which are cosmetically poor, may be corrected at a later date by plastic surgery.

Finally, the last principle is *maintenance of support to the circulation* of the injured part. This may be accomplished by a compression dressing which furnishes even pressure to obliterate dead spaces and which will support the venous and lymphatic circulation, thus preventing stasis and swelling.

Chemotherapy in Compound Fractures

There will always be two schools of thought concerning the advisability of employing chemotherapeutic agents or other antibiotics in compound fractures as a purely *prophylactic* measure. There is no question that once infection has become established in the wound, all possible surgical, chemical and physical agents should be employed to check and eradicate the infection. These measures are absolutely necessary (see p. 203).

Too much hope was extended to surgeons in general by premature reports at the beginning of World War II on the prophylactic use of "sulfa" drugs in compound fractures. This seemed to offer a ready answer to the serious threat of infection, leading many surgeons to forget temporarily the most important of such surgical principles (i. e., thorough debridement of the wound). Before the war had terminated, it was generally agreed that "sulfa" drugs and penicillin were of little or no benefit in *preventing* infection of a compound fracture wound. This was also well shown in civilian hospitals that cooperated with the National Research Council Wound Study where control cases were used for comparison. In other words the most important treatment still remains strict adherence to the surgical principles. No corners must be cut. Debridement must not be omitted or spared in thoroughness. If antibiotics are to be used, they must be employed as an adjunct to thorough surgery and *not* as a substitute for obvious inadequate surgery. The author is opposed to the indiscriminate use of these drugs as a prophylactic measure, because it is now well known that many patients having received "sulfa" have likewise developed hepatic or renal damage. Penicillin on the other hand may do little harm to the patient, giving him an urticaria, but it may give the surgeon a false sense of security and cause him to relax the high standards of important surgical principles that have been preached for years.

There is probably no question that "sulfa" or penicillin have prevented some infection in compound wounds, but in general they do not. They may lessen the severity of the infection even if not preventing it, which is in itself of considerable advantage. The principle type of wound to receive such advantage would be the battle casualty that had to be transported a considerable distance before he could receive adequate definitive surgery. In civilian practice this great delay should not occur.

Another most important consideration in severe traumatic wounds of the extremities is their location. In general compound fractures in the lower extremity (especially in the region of the lower tibia) are prone to develop a high incidence of infection (25 to 30 percent); those in the upper extremity become infected much less often. Aside from the factors of greater tissue damage and contamination in compound fractures of the lower extremity, this extremity is noteworthy for circulatory stasis because of arteriosclerosis, varicose veins and dependency. Poor circulation plus stasis are probably the most important factors determining the difference in infection rate between comparable wounds of the upper and lower extremity.

Treatment of Established Infection

(a) Following compound fracture.

(b) Following Open Reduction and Simple Fracture.

Up to this point all discussion has been directed towards the prevention of bone infection in clean fractures coming to operation or to contaminated fractures. The surgical principles of protection, gentle handling of tissues, strict asepsis, perfect hemostasis, and avoidance of creation of tension in wound closure have been stressed as all important and must never be overlooked. We now come to the group of infections that occur as a result of poor surgery or in spite of excellent surgery.

Infection Following Open (Compound) Fractures

Increased or continued pain at the site of fracture, increased swelling not due to constrictive dressings and in spite of high elevation, persistent or increased fever, elevated pulse rate, leucocytosis, and general malaise should cause the surgeon to suspect infection at the site of the fracture. He must of course rule out the respiratory, genito-urinary and gastro-intestinal tracts as well as other associated fractures or serious injuries as being the cause of the pain, fever, etc. If any doubt exists, the compound wound must be inspected under strict aseptic precautions. Care should be taken to handle the extremity painlessly and all clamps and forceps coming in contact with adjacent skin or dressings must be sterile. If it is necessary to palpate the tissues alongside the wound, sterile rubber gloves are indicated. If the cardinal signs of infection are all present, the patient should be taken to the operating room where the wound, if closed or partially closed, can be opened widely. All pockets containing exudate should be opened completely and the wound should be irrigated with saline solution. Tubes may be placed in the depths of the wound for instillation of penicillin or other suitable antibiotic. The remainder of the wound must be loosely packed wide open with plain fine mesh gauze. The fracture fragments must be kept adequately immobilized in plaster for the patient's comfort as well as to prevent their constant motion from irritating the wound and prolonging the infection. If internal fixation with plate and screws had been performed at the original operation, there need be no hurry to remove these, for they will continue to give rigid fixation which is all to the good of the patient's comfort and local infection. Simply because metal is a foreign body, one need not fear it will increase infection. Later, when the acute infection has subsided, and if absorption has appeared in the bone around the metal, the plate and screws may be removed. By this time there has often been built up enough callus to stabilize the main fracture fragment so that no more than a molded plaster splint is required for protection.

One should be on the watch for infection due to gas forming organisms such as Clostridium Welchii. High pulse rate, foul odor and subcutaneous crepitus (the result of gas in the tissues) is characteristic of this type of infection. Immediate operation is indicated not only to open the wound completely but far enough in a proximal direction to stop the spread of clostridial infection. If wide open drainage is not sufficient, amputation may be necessary to save the patient's life. Zinc peroxide cream dressings should follow such wide open drainage or amputation in order to bring oxygen into direct contact with the tissues to kill the anerobic organisms.

Late surgical care of an infected compound fracture will consist of maintenance of wide open drainage, removal of all completely dead bone or sequestrated fragments, and obliteration of dead spaces and rigid walled cavities that mitigate against filling in by granulation tissue growth. Very often an impasse is reached and the wound does not seem to improve. Antiseptic and chemotherapeutic agents do not improve its appearance. The reason for this is that a ring of scar tissue has formed around the wound and nutrition to the skin edges becomes impaired. A chronic ulcer forms which neither gets better nor worse. Likewise with a large dead portion of bone attached to one main fragment, no blood supply is available to separate this from the live bone or to carry antibiotics to the dead bone. Unless antibiotics are made available where needed (i. e. via good circulation) they cannot be expected to accomplish their purpose of destroying bacteria. Further surgery is therefore necessary to assist wound healing. This must be in the form of excision of dead bone and excessive scar tissue. It may even be necessary to employ pedicle skin grafts to cover soft tissue defects in order to secure wound closure or preparatory to subsequent bone grafting for loss of substance.

Infection Following Open Reduction in Clean Fractures

Infection of a clean operative case is a very distressing sequel. The fact that it can still occur in modern surgery is something that should never be overlooked. It is often easier to detect than in compound wounds since the post-operative reaction ordinarily should be less severe. The same precautions should be taken in investigating the wound. If infection is thought to be present, haste is necessary in opening the wound completely, in its entirety (length and depth), and to evacuate all the exudate and permit of freer escape of further exudate. Original clean wounds are usually closed in layers. If infection supervenes, the infection may become more severe than in a compound wound where the wound was either left open or closed only loosely. It is therefore important to open all the layers down to the bone if necessary in order that no further pocketing of exudate may occur which would increase the chances of spread of infection and cause increased necrosis. Late surgical removal of excessive scar tissue or of dead bone may be called for as described above under compound fracture infections.

Chapter XVI

Operations on Soft Parts Associated with Fracture or Dislocation

THE FOLLOWING conditions though not commonly associated with fractures or dislocations in the elbow region (except in the "truck-swipe" or gun-shot type of injury) must always be kept in mind and measures taken to correct them (if possible) before serious damage or disaster occurs or before healing has progressed to the point where attempts to correct them may cause as much harm as good: —

a. Interposition of tissue—muscle, ligament, periosteum, nerve, vessels.
b. Ligament tears.
c. Nerve lacerations, contusions, impingements, transplants.
d. Vessel rupture, laceration, thrombosis, spasm.
e. Capsulotomy (?) to release caught radial head in Monteggia fracture.
f. Decompression of antecubital space.
   1. Circulatory impairment.
   2. Prevention of myositis ossificans.
g. Removal of loose bone fragment.

Muscle tissue (brachialis anticus) may become interposed between the fragments of a supracondylar (transcondylar) fracture or muscle and joint capsule between a displaced radial head fragment and the main head or neck of this bone. The necessity for operative correction in the former is rare indeed, since manual manipulation or over-head Kirschner wire traction will usually achieve sufficiently good bony contact between the fragments so that one need not fear non-union as in shaft fractures of the femur, etc.

A radial head fragment displaced anteriorly into the brachialis muscle especially if there is marked hemorrhage, swelling, and induration in the antecubital region usually means that a dislocation has occurred between the forearm bones and the humerus (though spontaneously reduced) and must be considered an extremely serious injury. It is serious because of the high rate of development of myositis ossificans unless the radial head fragment and remainder of the radial head is removed *through an anterior incision and not later than forty-eight hours* after the injury. The reason for the anterior approach is to get rid of the soft part pathology (hemorrhage, edema and tissue debris), the products of which are acid and tend to promote absorption of calcium from bone fragments or cut end of the neck of the radius, later to be laid down in the healing tissues as extra-osseous bone. Not only should the soft tissue pathology be evacuated in this fashion, but the deep fascia must be left open to permit further escape of blood, serum, etc. into the subcutaneous layer.

Ligaments may become interposed and prevent reduction. The best example of this is the orbicular (annular) ligament which often gets caught behind the radial head when it becomes anteriorly dislocated in association with high ulnar shaft (Monteggia) fractures. It may be necessary to unfold this ligament and resuture it across the radial head after reduction. If the radial head has pulled out of the orbicular ligament and caused a tear of the thinner joint capsule distal to it, allowing the ligament to become interposed between the radial head and the capitellum, it will be necessary to incise the ligament before it is possible to reduce the radial head. Repair of the ligament should then follow (Chapter XI).

Other soft tissues that occasionally become interposed between fracture fragments are: periosteum, vessels, and nerves. These may interfere with closed reduction, but can usually be managed by the same methods used to correct interposition of muscle between fragments of a supracondylar fracture. If closed reduction is possible, but the fragments continue to slip upon each other in spite of the position of acute flexion used to maintain reduction, there probably exists interposition of periosteum. Operation may be necessary to correct this. If a nerve or vessel were interposed, there should be signs of vascular or nerve lesion in addition to the mechanical difficulty in maintaining reduction. Over-head Kirschner wire traction should be tried for two to three hours to see if this will improve the circulation. If improvement does not occur at this time, operation should be performed to explore the brachial vessels, untangle them from the fragments if necessary, and to decompress the deep fascial space of the antecubital area. Early nerve lesions are due to contusion or stretching (except in severe compound injuries where laceration may occur), and do not require early operative exploration per se. They show a high rate of recovery if reduction is carried out by gentle manipulation or traction and followed by protective splints, exercises, etc. It is possible for a nerve to become drawn into the elbow joint cavity. The author has seen one case of dislocation of the radius and ulna in a posterior and lateral direction in which the medial epicondyle epiphysis had become avulsed from the medial condyle and displaced into the elbow joint. Although the dislocation had been reduced by a physician, the medial epicondyle was found to be still in the joint at the end of one month and a complete paralysis of the ulnar nerve was present. It was necessary to operate to withdraw the epicondyle fragment and attached flexor-pronator tendon from the joint, and, at operation it was found that the ulnar nerve also lay within the medial aspect of the joint cavity between the humerus and ulna, having been avulsed from its bed and carried laterally. The nerve was withdrawn from the joint and transposed.

Torn ligaments at the elbow are common especially in simple dislocations of both bones and these usually heal well after closed reduction. Under certain conditions, however, it is not only advisable, but extremely important to operate and repair a torn ligament. This should be carried out with the orbicular ligament following inability to reduce or maintain reduction in a Monteggia fracture (Chapter XI). In some fractures of the lateral condyle of the humerus with comminution in adults a lateral dislocation of the forearm bones may be present. If the broken off fragments are large and include the lateral portion of the trochlear process, the medial collateral ligament is usually completely torn. Unless this be repaired there remains no support to prevent recurrence of the lateral subluxation of the ulna if it has been necessary to excise the condylar fragments or if there has been difficulty in maintaining reduction of this fragment.

The greatest number of nerve lesions at the elbow are the result of stretching or contusion. These ordinarily require no immediate operative procedure, but should be conservatively treated by closed reduction, proper splinting, etc. In the types of fracture requiring open operation, a paralyzed nerve should be explored at the same time and its sheath injected with saline solution to assist in its recovery. If the fracture is treated conservatively, the progress of recovery of the nerve should be frequently checked. If no evidence of recovery has appeared in three to four months, the nerve should be explored and proper treatment given. If recovery begins to appear as it should at two months if proper conservative measures have been employed, no operative procedure is indicated.

In severe compound fractures at the elbow, gun-shot "side-swipe" fractures, or stab wounds with nerve injury, the nerve must be explored. It may be inadvisable to repair a lacerated nerve or a nerve defect due to loss of substance in the presence of severe injury and contamination, but the nerve ends should be identified and marked with black silk or tantulum wire sutures. This will facilitate locating their ends at a later date when reparative nerve surgery is undertaken.

Impingements upon nerves from a fascial band may be seen at open reduction. It may be found that the sheath over-lying the ulnar nerve is hemorrhagic when the elbow is explored for removal of a medial epicondyle displaced into the joint. If such be the case, one may anticipate subsequent fibrosis of its sheath with compression of the nerve. The nerve should therefore be transposed primarily rather than wait for permanent loss of function (Chapter XXI).

Interposition of a portion of capsule may occur requiring operative correction and repair. This has already been dealt with above under interposition of the annular ligament in Monteggia fractures.

Decompression of the antecubital fossa may have to be performed: (1) It may be necessary to do this for severe impairment of the circulation as a result of swelling and venous stasis in some cases of supracondylar fracture where other methods have failed, but it is rarely necessary. The deep fascia should be incised longitudinally in several areas and the enclosed hemorrhage and edema fluid allowed to escape. The skin incisions should be short and multiple (overlying the longer fascial incisions), otherwise difficulty will be encountered in closing them since they tend to spread markedly. (2) The deep fascia must be opened anteriorly in removal of a fractured radial head accompanying dislocation of the elbow and left open in order to allow for the escape of damaged muscle, hemorrhage, serum, etc. to minimize the risk of myositis ossificans.

Chapter XVII

Surgical Approaches to the Elbow Region

THERE ARE MANY approaches to the elbow joint, lower humerus, upper radius and ulna. The approach to be employed should depend upon the nature of the operation in mind so that the pathology may be fully studied, corrected as far as desirable and repair accomplished without causing unnecessary trauma to vessels, nerves, ligaments and joint surfaces. It is impossible to explore the posterior aspect of the elbow joint through an anterior incision, and vice versa. Similarly it is impossible to explore the medial aspect through an anterolateral incision. In some instances it may be best to employ two separate approaches at the same operation, but a single incision is preferable if it can be so planned that everything necessary to be done can be performed through it. A thorough knowledge of the normal anatomy of this region is absolutely essential if one is not to blunder through some of the very simple approaches. What is still more important is a thorough appreciation of this knowledge in the presence of superimposed pathology (acute trauma, hemorrhage, deformity, and scarring of the soft tissues). Approach to the elbow joint may be for the purpose of: aspiration (diagnostic or therapeutic), drainage, open reduction of fractures or dislocations (new or old), exploration and removal of loose bodies, removal of fracture fragments, resection of the joint, arthroplasty, ankylosis, capsulorrhaphy, neurolysis, exploration of blood vessels, decompression of deep fascia, excision of bursae, neoplasms, myositis ossificans or for the correction of deformities due to malunion or growth disturbance.

The skin incision for the majority of approaches to this region are usually vertical or a variation of the vertical, such as the Z-shaped, bayonet shaped, or slightly curved incision. Vertical incisions on the anterior, antero-lateral, or antero-medial aspects of the elbow region are prone to result in thick broad scars with possible contracture. For this reason numerous surgeons have attempted to avoid incisions that cut directly across the flexion crease and have employed the Z-type of skin incision with the central portion passing along the flexion crease and connecting with the vertical portions at each of its extremities. Needless to say this solves only part of the problem, the transverse portion passing along the crease leaves a thin hair-line scar, while the two vertical arms continue to give thick broad scars that are ugly in appearance even though no contracture results. Since observing these scars in many late follow-up cases the author has found it possible to perform a considerable number of explorations of the anterolateral and medial aspects of the elbow adequately through a simple transverse incision in the skin passing along the flexion crease. The skin flaps with subcutaneous tissue may be dissected upwards and downwards and retracted sufficiently to permit approach to the deeper layers via the usual anatomical planes. Removal of the head of the radius for fracture, repair of the orbicular ligament (in Monteggia fractures), and open reduction for separation of the medial epicondyle epiphysis with displacement into the elbow joint may all be performed through one of these two transverse incisions. In the latter type of case if there exists any disturbance of ulnar nerve function and possible transplantation of the nerve is contemplated at operation, a medial transverse incision will not offer adequate exposure. It will be better to employ a vertical incision that is sufficiently long to permit full exposure of the portion of the nerve to be transplanted.

One of the commonest mistakes made by younger surgeons is to make their skin incisions too short. Insufficient length of incision (in the desire to leave a shorter scar) "cramps the surgeon's style," causes unnecessary trauma to the patient because of the strong retraction required, and may lead to irreparable nerve or vessel damage through failure to visualize the anatomy adequately in the path of the exploration. Experienced surgeons employ incisions sufficiently long which will not have to be enlarged half-way through the operation. This is especially important in cases of acute injury. Marble has made the comment that "the length of a surgical incision varies in direct proportion to the age and experience of the operating surgeon."

Closed reductions of fractures and dislocations are frequently performed by general practitioners. A certain number of operations by necessity (compound (open) fractures for example) have to be performed by these same men or by "pure" orthopedists with little or no training in the surgery of acute trauma. Operations of choice on the extremities for acute trauma or deformity are more likely to be performed by general surgeons or orthopedic surgeons. Therefore, regardless of the necessity or voluntary choice of the operation, the surgeon must formulate some general plan before he proceeds. He should first think of what he is trying to accomplish by operation. This means keeping an open mind as to methods of accomplishing this purpose. Preconceived ideas rigidly adhered to for certain conditions in spite of circumstances that mitigate against their use may not only prevent the surgeon from fully discovering the important pathology, but cause him to under- or over-estimate the quality and quantity of treatment indicated. To be more specific, it is well recognized that fractures of the radial head with comminution and displacement should be operated upon and the radial head removed. On the other hand it is not fully appreciated by most surgeons that a radial head fracture associated with a posterior dislocation of both forearm bones at the elbow is a serious condition, because of the likelihood of subsequent formation of myositis ossificans in the lacerated brachialis muscle. Though most surgeons agree that the radial head should be removed in such cases, how many would perform the removal through an anterolateral incision and leave the deep fascia open to allow the escape of hemorrhage, cellular and fluid products of tissue death from the damaged brachialis anticus muscle? Also how many would perform this operation in the first twenty-four hours after injury? If the radial head (associated with elbow dislocation) is removed within the first two days after injury through an anterior incision and the fascia is left open, there is extremely little risk of myositis ossificans; if on the other hand this removal is performed through a lateral incision and the deep (brachialis) fascia is not opened and left open or the operation is performed from four days to two weeks after injury, the likelihood of development of myositis ossificans is unusually high (possibly fifty percent or greater) (Chapter XII).

The surgeon must have a plan of approach that will permit him to evaluate the pathology fully in order that he may accomplish his repair with ease to himself and without additional serious harm to the patient's already damaged tissues. There are perhaps no better principles to follow in making the choice of incision and approach than in the criteria listed by Darrach as being necessary for a good surgical approach. These are:

(1) The approach should provide comfortable access to the structures for which one is seeking.
(2) It should cause as little damage as possible.
(3) It should go between muscles rather than through them.
(4) It should not divide the blood or nerve supply of a muscle that it passes.
(5) It should permit clear visualization of important anatomical structures or "give them a wide berth."
(6) It should permit restoration of the disturbed tissues to their normal position at the end of the operation and allow them to regain normal function as early as possible.

There are in general four main approaches to the elbow joint or elbow region that can be considered safe. These are the *medial, anterolateral, lateral,* and *posterior* approaches. These will be presented and variations of each will be described in the following paragraphs. The anteromedial approach is rarely necessary and is not so safe as the anterolateral or medial approach because the brachial vessels and median nerve are in its direct path.

Medial Approach

This approach is used for exploration of the medial aspect of the elbow joint for the following reasons: removal of a loose body in the joint, the displaced tip of a fractured coronoid process, repair of the medial collateral ligament, removal from the joint and open reduction of a fractured medial epicondyle epiphysis which has become displaced into the joint, open reduction of a fracture of the medial condyle or trochlea, and neurolysis or transposition of the ulnar nerve.

The anteromedial transverse skin incision may be used for the above procedures except for neurolysis and nerve transposition where it is likely to be inadequate. For these latter two procedures a longitudinal skin incision is better.

The transverse skin incision may encounter the median basilic vein which will have to be ligated and divided to allow sufficient retraction of the skin flaps. A cutaneous branch of the median antibrachial cutaneous nerve is encountered and should be saved if possible. Nothing else of importance is met superficial to the deep fascia. The ulnar nerve lies immediately behind the medial epicondyle and should be visualized, freed and isolated by a moist tape before any deeper exploration is carried out. Should the medial epicondyle epiphysis be avulsed from its normal position and turned into the elbow joint with the attached conjoined tendon of the flexor-pronator group of muscles, the ulnar nerve may be stripped of its anterior protective covering and lie freely exposed. Hemorrhage and edema may partially mask it, but again it should be searched for and protected as described above. If it be necessary to explore the medial aspect of an intact joint, the surgeon may temporarily remove the medial epicondyle from the humerus by means of a sharp osteotome and turn it distally with its attached muscles (later to be replaced and fastened by a heavy suture, a nail or screw). A broad elevator or other flat instrument should be used to shield the ulnar nerve while osteotomizing the epicondyle or while replacing it and fastening it to the medial condylar ridge. With reasonable care no operative damage should occur to this nerve. Temporary removal of the epicondyle facilitates exposure to the medial side of the joint and permits better repair of the collateral ligament than a vertical incision through the muscles attached to it.

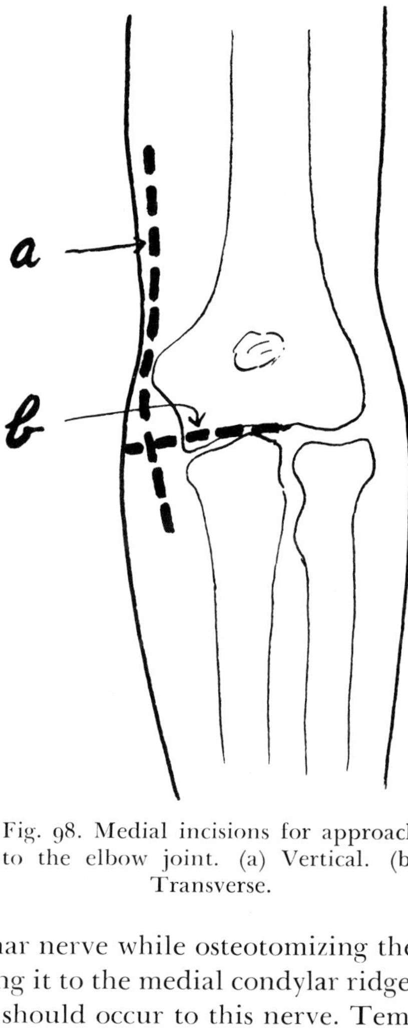

Fig. 98. Medial incisions for approach to the elbow joint. (a) Vertical. (b) Transverse.

Anterolateral Approach

This approach may be employed for removal of a fractured radial head with anterior displacement of a fragment associated with posterior dislocation of both bones, repair of the orbicular ligament in anterior dislocation of the radial head in Monteggia fractures, removal of or open reduction of a fracture of the capitellum, removal of a loose body from the anterolateral aspect of the joint, correction of osteochondritis dissecans of the capitellum, repair of a ruptured or avulsed inferior biceps tendon, and exploration of the lower portion of the radial nerve or the upper portion of its two branches (posterior interosseus and superficial radial nerves).

Incisions for the anterolateral approach are usually Z or bayonet-shaped for the skin and subcutaneous tissues, but may be transverse. (See Fig. 89.) Straight longitudinal or diagonal incisions crossing the elbow flexion crease are to be avoided for the reasons mentioned above. The Z-incision begins above the joint, passes along the medial margin of the brachioradialis muscle as far as the flexion crease, then along this for a variable distance in a lateral direction, and finally along the medial margin of the same muscle. The bayonet incision is much the same except that the two long arms are in a more vertical direction.

The transverse incision beginning at the biceps tendon passes along the elbow flexion crease lateralward almost to the epicondyle. This requires dissection of skin flaps upwards and downwards in order to obtain sufficient room to open the deep fascia longitudinally and approach the joint in the interval between the brachioradialis and brachialis anticus muscle. Any of these incisions may encounter the cephalic vein or a branch of it, and the lateral antebrachial cutaneous nerve (sensory continuation of the musculocutaneous nerve). The vein will very likely require ligation and division, but the sensory nerve should be preserved and retracted lateralwards out of the field of exposure. The transverse incision will give a much less conspicuous scar and should be used if it is felt that the operative procedure contemplated can be carried out through it.

The deep anterolateral approach is carried out by incising the deep fascia binding the brachioradialis to the biceps and brachialis muscles. The interval between the brachialis and brachioradialis is deepened just above the joint in order to visualize the radial nerve and its division. Since all the muscular branches from this nerve pass in a lateral direction, the nerve along with the brachioradialis muscle should be retracted lateralwards. The incision is then deepened through the outer fibers of the brachialis anticus muscle until the anterior joint capsule is encountered. By rotating the forearm back and forth passively it is easy to distinguish the capitellum from the radial head even through the capsular structures. The capsule may then be opened in a vertical direction directly over the radial head without fear of damaging any important structures. Incision of the capsule distal to the radial head must *not* extend more than 1 to 1.5 centimeters along the radial neck in order to avoid injuring the posterior interosseus nerve that winds laterally and posteriorly around the neck between the two layers of the supinator muscle. In order to make it possible to retract the brachioradialis muscle more easily distal to the joint line it will be necessary to ligate and divide the radial recurrent vessels (artery and vein) where these cross the intermuscular space directly. A good exposure of the anterolateral aspect of the joint may thus be obtained and when the operation is completed, the normal structures practically fall together. If the deep fascia is to be left open for drainage, the only sutures employed are for the subcutaneous tissue and skin. If the deep fascia requires closure, two or three sutures only are needed for approximation.

The bicipital tuberosity of the radius may be explored through this approach and if it is desired to pass a suture through it, this can be accomplished by making two drill holes at right angles to each other (by rotating the radius deep in the incision while the surrounding soft parts are retracted).

Lateral Approach

This approach is a good one and may be used for a number of purposes, such as: excision of the radial head for fresh fracture or old deformity, open reduction of separation of the radial head epiphysis where closed methods have been unsuccessful, open reduction of lateral condyle fracture, removal of displaced fragment of capitellum, exploration of the radio-humeral bursa or excision of calcium deposit in the extensor tendon attachment to the lateral epicondyle (epicondylitis), and resection type of arthroplasty of the elbow joint (Haas). It is also used for aspiration of the joint.

The incision for the straight lateral approach is a longitudinal one beginning along the supracondylar ridge and passing downward and slightly forward over the capitellum and radial head and neck. If either open reduction of the lateral condyle or resection arthroplasty of the elbow is to be performed, the lateral incision must be started about 6 centimeters proximal to the lateral epicondyle of the humerus. Some surgeons prefer to make the

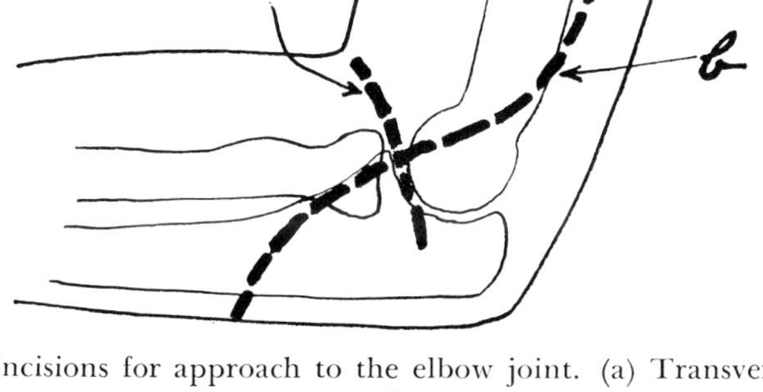

Fig. 99. Lateral incisions for approach to the elbow joint. (a) Transverse. (b) J-incision (Kocher).

incision somewhat more of a posterolateral one when removing the head of the radius. There is also a variation of this which passes obliquely along the anterior margin of the anconeus muscle and exposes the radial head from behind. None of these skin incisions encounter anatomical structures of any importance.

The deep approach exposes the lateral condylar ridge or epicondyle of the humerus, the extensor tendons taking their origin from the lateral epicondyle, and the deep fascia over-lying these. These muscles may be split longitudinally between the bellies of the extensor carpi radialis longus and the extensor digitorum communis. Directly beneath lies the joint capsule and the orbicular ligament surrounding the radial head. The head may be defined by rotating the forearm. A longitudinal incision from the capitellum to 1 centimeter below the radial head will expose the radio-humeral joint and not cause damage to the posterior interosseus nerve. This incision with retraction will furnish adequate exposure for excision of the radial head. If more exposure of the lower humerus is needed, this may be obtained by elevation of the periosteum by a sharp elevator after incising the periosteum along the supracondylar ridge. If the approach is made along the anterior margin of the anconeus muscle, it is deepened to the posterolateral aspect of the radio-humeral joint between this muscle and the extensor carpi ulnaris. This same approach may also be used for draining the elbow joint in case of suppurative arthritis.

Aspiration of the elbow joint is most easily accomplished by insertion of the aspirating needle at a point equidistant from the lateral epicondyle, radial head, and tip of the olecranon on the posterolateral aspect of the joint.

Posterior Approach

This approach may vary considerably, depending upon the purpose for which it is used. A commonly described approach is that called the posterior midline approach, but frequently this need not have the skin incision or the deep approach made directly in the midline. It is often better to approach the lower humerus, elbow joint or upper ulna slightly to the lateral or medial side of the midline.

For the lower humerus a posterior approach is valuable in the following types of operations: open reduction of fracture of the medial condyle, dicondylar fractures, and for corrective osteotomy of the lower humerus for cubitus varus deformity. For operations upon a medial condyle or dicondylar fracture an approach to the humerus on either or both sides of the triceps tendon may be adequate and simpler than in splitting the triceps. Any approach on the medial aspect must isolate the ulnar nerve and retract it out of danger before the operative procedure upon the bone is started. For corrective osteotomy on the humerus a posterior midline incision is probably the best. Old, unreduced dislocations of the elbow are also best openly reduced through this approach. Either the technique of Campbell or of Van-Gorder may be utilized for this (see below).

For exploration of the posterior compartment of the elbow joint or a MacAusland type of elbow arthroplasty (via the trans-olecranon route) a posterior U-shaped incision is made from the lateral to the medial epicondyle of the humerus curving distally to cross the ulna about one inch below the tip of the olecranon. The skin incision is carried down to the deep fascia and the proximal flap is retracted. The periosteum is split and elevated from the upper ulna and the olecranon is divided transversely at the middle of the greater sigmoid notch (2 centimeters below the tip of the olecranon) by a thin sharp osteotome. The triceps expansion and deep fascia are incised on either side, care being taken to identify the ulnar nerve and retract it out of danger by tape moistened with saline solution. The joint capsule and periosteum when divided at the level of the osteotomy will permit retraction of the olecranon in a proximal direction. A good exposure of the posterior compartment of the joint is thus obtained and the distal surfaces of the trochlea and capitellum may also be easily visualized. If their anterior surfaces need be examined, the operator may expose these by flexing the ulna further upon the humerus and by gently prying the ulna forward by means of a smooth flat elevator inserted into the joint cavity. Fibrous adhesions, degenerated articular cartilage, or loose bodies may thus be removed. It is also possible to excise the radial head through this same exposure should it be found to be enlarged, irregular in shape and causing mechanical interfer-

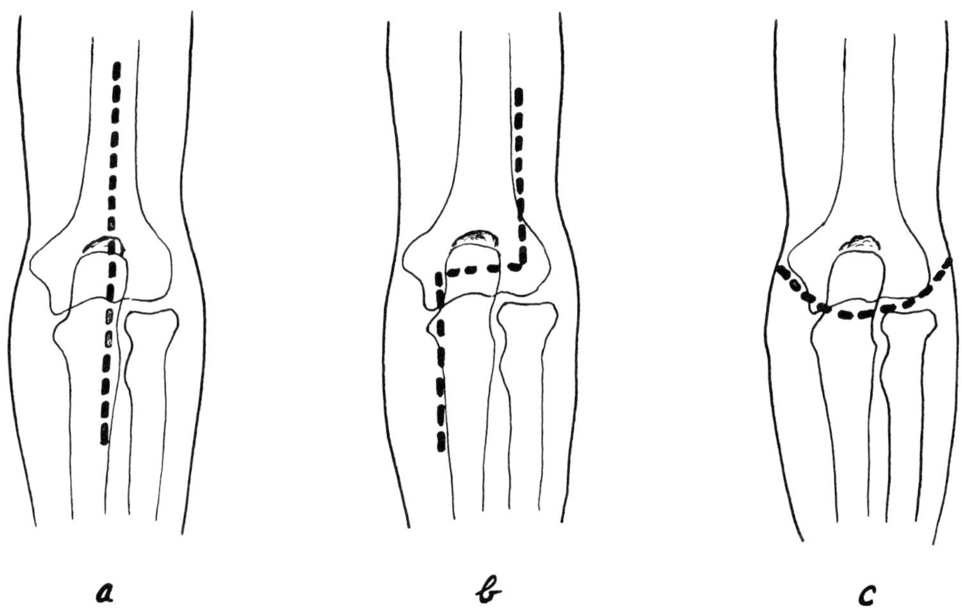

Fig. 100. Posterior skin incisions for elbow region. (a) Langenbeck's. (b) Ollier's. (c) MacAusland's.

ence in the joint. If arthroplasty is to be performed, it is possible to reshape the articular surfaces of the ulna and humerus and cover the latter with a layer of fascia lata. When the operative procedure upon the joint is completed, the olecranon should be replaced and repaired by means of a heavy wire loop (No. 22 gauge) passed through the insertion of the triceps tendon and through a drill-hole in the distal ulnar shaft. If the operator prefers, he may fasten the olecranon to the ulnar shaft by a long screw passed downwards into the medullary cavity. The ulnar nerve is allowed to drop back into its normal position and the deep fascia and periosteum are then repaired with interrupted sutures of fine silk. The skin and subcutaneous tissue may be closed according to the operator's preference. No drain should be placed in the wound. A posterior molded splint should be applied for protection, but may be removed as early as the surgeon desires for starting active elbow exercises.

For excision of an enlarged and chronically thickened olecranon bursa the best incision is a straight transverse one passing directly over the posterior aspect of the bursal swelling. This incision with retraction of its flaps gives good exposure and permits complete excision of the bursa. The resulting scar is narrow and scarcely visible.

A posterior longitudinal incision beginning just lateral to and at the level of the tip of the olecranon passing downwards seven centimeters and then curving gently medialwards across the upper ulnar shaft is an excellent approach for repair of a fracture of the olecranon with separation. This permits full visualization of the fracture site by retraction of the medial skin flap. The repair may then be carried out by one of the methods described under operative repair of this injury.

The posterior approach to the upper ulnar shaft and radial head as described by Speed and Boyd is an excellent one for use in the open reduction of Monteggia fractures. It permits internal fixation of the ulnar fragments, reduction of the dislocated radial head, and repair of the torn orbicular ligament. No other single approach will give access to and make possible the repair of both the fracture and dislocation. The incision for this approach begins one inch above and lateral to the tip of the olecranon, passes distally and medially to reach the posterior crest of the ulna approximately one inch below it, then along the crest of the ulna as far distally as is necessary to expose the fracture site thoroughly and give adequate room for repair. (If necessary, the incision may be extended the entire length of the ulna, the posterior crest of which can be readily palpated beneath the skin and subcutaneous tissue.) After the fracture site is well exposed by elevation of the periosteum and muscles from the ulna, the radio-humeral joint is then exposed by further subperiosteal dissection of the supinator muscle from its origin along the supinator crest on the lateral side of the ulna. By keeping the periosteal elevator beneath (deep) to the attachment of this muscle no damage can occur to the posterior interosseus nerve which lies between the superficial and deep layers of this thin muscle. The radio-humeral joint is then exposed and the orbicular ligament may be repaired with silk after reduction of the anteriorly dislocated radial head. Following reduction of the ulnar fragments, it is usually advisable to employ internal fixation by means of a plate and screws to prevent subsequent angulation of the ulna and redislocation of the radial head. Closure of the periosteum and deep fascia with interrupted fine silk sutures allows the muscular structures to fall back into their normal positions. None of these elevated muscles have been actually damaged or had their blood or nerve supply interfered with. Consequently, it is possible to start exercises at an early date if rigid repair of the fracture has been obtained.

The posterior midline approach of Campbell begins five inches above the olecranon and is carried downwards passing just lateral to it. The incision passes directly through the center of the triceps tendon, splitting it and the muscle beneath it. The ulnar nerve must be seen and protected on the medial aspect. Splitting of the triceps muscle in the proximal end of this incision must be done with blunt instruments to avoid cutting the radial nerve which crosses the lower third of the humerus just beneath this muscle. The split muscle may then be retracted to either side to permit full exposure of the lower posterior surface of the humerus and elbow joint. It may thus be used for repair of dicondylar fractures, corrective osteotomy, and reduction of late, unreduced elbow joint dislocations. Following completion of the operation the muscle is permitted to fall together and the deep fascia and tendon margins are approximated with interrupted silk sutures.

The posterior approach of VanGorder is used for the same purposes. The

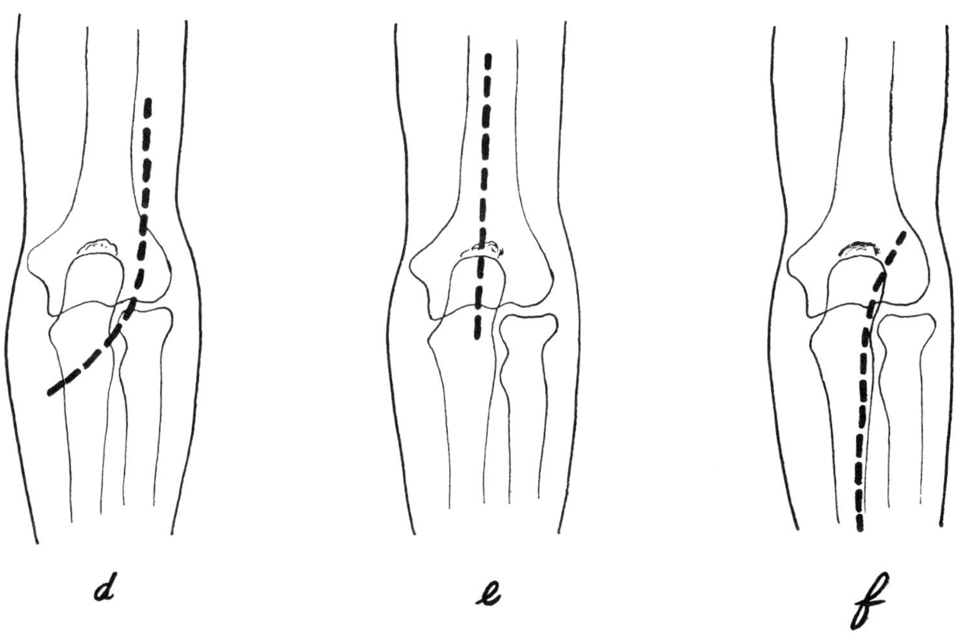

Fig. 101. Posterior skin incisions for elbow region. (d) Kocher's (posterior J). (e) Campbell's or Van Gorder's. (f) Speed and Boyd's.

skin incision is similar, but the approach through the triceps is by dissection of a tongue of triceps tendon downwards. The tip of this tongue of tendon begins approximately four inches proximal to the olecranon, and, as it is dissected distally it is also incised more deeply, so that its tip is thin and its base thick where the latter is attached to the olecranon. The entire tongue is retracted downwards, and the muscle belly beneath is split longitudinally by blunt and sharp dissection and retracted to either side. Again, the ulnar and radial nerves must be avoided. Closure is carried out by interrupted sutures of silk for the muscle to approximate the two halves. The tongue of tendon is replaced and likewise sutured along its margins to the deep fascia. If for any reason the elbow has been held in extension and the triceps is contracted, this tongue of tendon may be advanced distalwards up to one inch before re-suturing it to permit better flexion of the joint. This would seem preferable to performing a Z-shaped tenotomy on the tendon as advocated by some writers.

Chapter XVIII

Early Treatment Aids Following Injury

MEASURES TO lessen swelling and pain, to overcome venous stasis, to rid the injured extremity of exudation and to assist in carrying away the products of tissue damage, secondary inflammation and to lower the local tissue pH are described under the treatment of specific injuries. It seems advisable, however, to repeat these for the benefit of students and younger surgeons, who perhaps have not become completely familiar with them. Such measures consist of: (1) elevation of the injured part (by pillows or by suspension); (2) low intensity heat; (3) whirlpool baths; (4) compression dressings (cotton and muslin, elastic bandages); (5) gentle massage; (6) positive and negative pressure boot; (7) wet dressings; (8) active exercises, such as for finger flexors and extensors without moving injured bones; (9) sympathetic nerve blocks, and (10) periarterial sympathectomy.

Elevation, heat and active exercises can always be obtained. Light sedative massage is less readily available. Deep or heavy massage is definitely contraindicated in the elbow region since it is prone to cause additional trouble in the form of myositis ossificans.

Gravity assistance (elevation), supportive dressings, low intensity heat, and frequent early active exercises will invariably accomplish more in the reduction of swelling, in the restoration or maintenance of joint function following a fracture than will months of treatment by long or short wave diathermy, whirlpool baths, etc. applied daily or three times a week.

Sympathetic nerve blocks have been found extremely useful in hastening the disappearance of post-traumatic swelling, pain due to vascular spasm, and in assisting the initiation of early active exercises by relief of pain and muscle spasm. The employment of such blocks should be resorted to more often. For the upper extremity the sympathetic nerve block of choice is that of the stellate ganglion.

All of the above measures must be employed *early* if they are to assist in overcoming venous stasis (and its accompanying swelling and pain).

The intravenous use of procaine hydrochloride (1000 cc. of 0.1% solution in normal saline) has been advocated by Ritter *et al.* as a means of improving joint motion where pain and muscle spasm has been a factor in delaying it. Extreme caution must be employed in using this drug intravenously.

Chapter XIX

Dislocations at the Elbow Joint

GENERAL CONSIDERATIONS

THE ELBOW joint ranks second only to the shoulder in frequency of dislocation. Children and adults are about equally affected and each may show characteristic associated lesions of the bone or soft parts, such as epiphyseal separations, fractures, and lesion of nerves. It is hardly necessary to say that for dislocation to occur at the elbow or any other major joint extensive rupture and tearing of at least one of the collateral ligaments and capsule must take place. The degree of original soft tissue damage accompanying the dislocation is due in part to the direction of the displaced radius and ulna, but, still more important, it is in *direct proportion to the actual amount of displacement* of these bones upon the lower extremity of the humerus. The brachialis anticus muscle is often extensvely torn as it is stretched over the articular surface of the humerus by the posteriorly displaced ulna, a fact well to remember because of the subsequent hemorrhage within its belly which is one of the factors predisposing to the formation of myositis ossificans, an all too frequent complication following elbow dislocations. Nerve lesions may occur from stretching or contusion, or later may result from pinching by scar tissue formed during the process of healing. The ulnar nerve is most commonly affected as a result of dislocation, but the radial and median nerves may become involved. The ulnar nerve, explored because of paralysis, has been found lying within the elbow joint, where it had been displaced at the time of dislocation. The brachial artery may be torn. Fractures of the coronoid or olecranon processes, radial head, lateral condyle or capitellum of the humerus may accompany dislocations. In the rare anterior type of dislocation of the ulna and radius upon the humerus without fracture the triceps tendon is often completely torn. Any separation of the upper extremities of the ulna and radius from each other (whether one or both is dislocated upon the humerus) must be accompanied by tearing of the orbicular ligament or capsule and by some tearing of the oblique ligament and interosseous membrane.

MECHANISM OF INJURY

The exact mechanism of a particular elbow dislocation frequently cannot be determined. Many of the older textbooks stressed the mechanism in great detail and emphasized it at the expense of the existing pathology and treat-

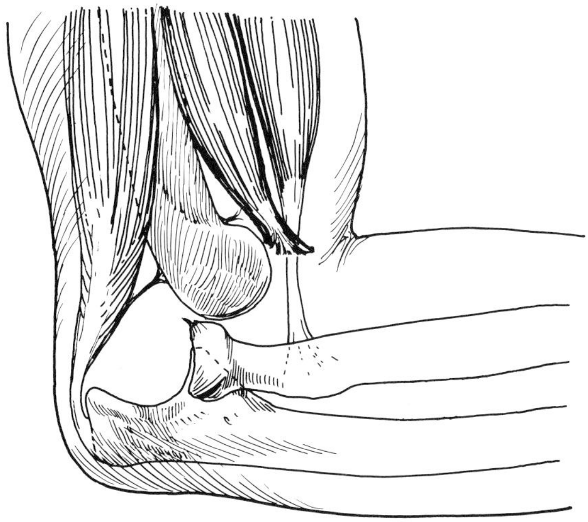

Fig. 102. Sketch of posterior dislocation at elbow joint showing how this occurs at the expense of tearing of the anterior capsule of the joint and the brachialis anticus muscle.

ment indicated. One reason for stressing the exact mechanism of dislocation has often been given (as it was said) that exact reversal of the mechanism was the best and easiest method of bringing about reduction. The futility of such reasoning would seem to be first, that the patient himself can but rarely give a truly accurate description of how the injury occurred (whether he landed on his outstretched hand first and his elbow second, or vice versa) and second, the position of the dislocated bones when the patient presents himself for treatment may be considerably altered from what they were immediately following the injury. It would seem more logical to formulate a plan of reduction following careful physical and roentgen examination and based on the existing displacement (and other pathology) than upon straight routine methods or upon an attempt at reversal of the original and questionable mechanism of the injury.

DIAGNOSIS

The diagnosis of the common posterior or posterolateral type of dislocation of the radius and ulna upon the humerus is usually not difficult on clinical examination. In children it must be differentiated from supracondylar fractures of the humerus. Roentgen examination should be made *before* any reduction is attempted if clinical examination suggests an unusual type of dislocation or if an associated fracture of a humeral condyle or olecranon is suspected. Should the injury occur on the athletic field and the team surgeon be immediately available and make a diagnosis of simple dislocation, he may dispense with immediate roentgen examination and go ahead with reduction at once by straight traction upon the forearm and with gentle manipulation. *Such cutting of corners by lay friends or "first-aiders" is to*

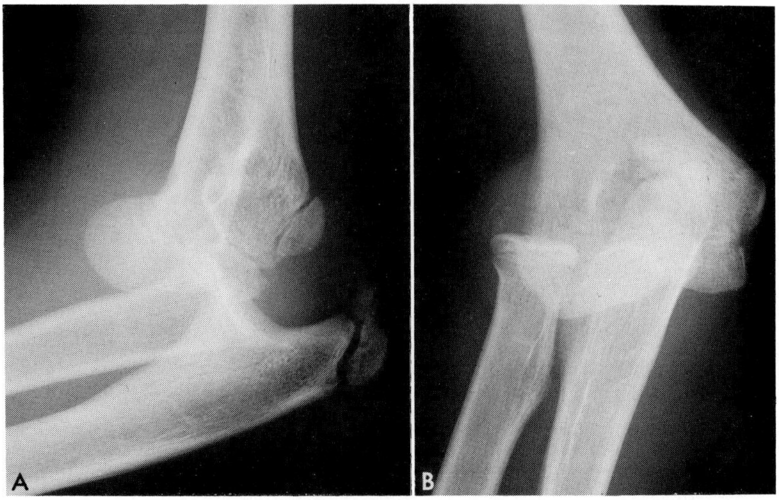

Fig. 103. Postero-lateral dislocation at elbow joint in an eleven year old boy. (A) Lateral view. (B) Antero-posterior view. Note the various epiphyseal ossification centers.

be frowned upon, since they are in no position to make an accurate or complete diagnosis and any attempts by them to render hasty definitive treatment may cause additional injury and complicate the situation for the surgeon. This can be accomplished without the necessity of general anesthesia if performed within the first 10-15 minutes after injury and may save the patient considerable pain later when muscle spasm would have become severe. It may also prevent subsequent nerve and circulatory damage. Following such a reduction the elbow should be put at rest in a sling and the patient sent for roentgen examination to rule out any possible fractures that might require additional treatment or otherwise alter the course of the treatment of the dislocation.

The clinical diagnosis of dislocation can be made on the basis of disturbed relationship of the three points making up the bony triangle at the elbow. The same may be said for differentiating a supracondylar fracture. In the common posterior dislocation the elbow appears elongated, the displaced olecranon giving the appearance of an exaggerated "heel," and the forearm is shortened. The triceps tendon is taut, stands out like a bow-string, and on profile its posterior margin is slightly concave rather than convex as compared to the normal elbow. Due to this bow-string effect of the tendon the skin and subcutaneous tissues on either side are "sucked in" and their contour is concave from side to side rather than convex. The cup-shaped proximal surface of the radial head may be visible and readily palpable beneath the subcutaneous tissue, especially if there is some lateral displacement accompanying the posterior. The anterior surface of the elbow reveals a prominent lower end of the humerus and there may be considerable induration of the soft tissues here as well.

In fresh elbow dislocations of the above type it is often possible to make the diagnosis simply on visual inspection unless the patient be very obese. After several hours have passed and considerable hemorrhage and swelling have occurred in the soft tissues surrounding the elbow joint, it may be very difficult to make the diagnosis. It is possible, however, by carefully milking away the edema fluid over-lying the bony prominences to palpate these painlessly and thereby determine whether their relationship to each other and to the axis of the humerus are normal or abnormal. If the dislocation is unfortunately of several days duration, induration and swelling will have progressed to such an extreme state that little more than a presumption of the diagnosis can be made by clinical examination and it is impossible to rule out associated fractures.

Roentgen examination of the injured elbow (except as noted above on the athletic field) should be made prior to attempts at reduction. There should be two views taken (anteroposterior and lateral) or as close to these as possible. Owing to distortion and rotation it may be advisable to take additional oblique views in one or more planes. In children it is often imperative to obtain films of the normal elbow in order not to overlook a displaced medial epicondyle epiphysis and mistake it for one of the ossification centers of the trochlea.

No diagnosis of elbow injury is complete (even with adequate roentgenograms) and no reduction should be attempted until a careful check is made to determine the motor and sensory function of the ulna, radial and median nerves and the presence and quality of the radial pulse. Any compromise of these important soft tissue structures makes it imperative to perform reduc-

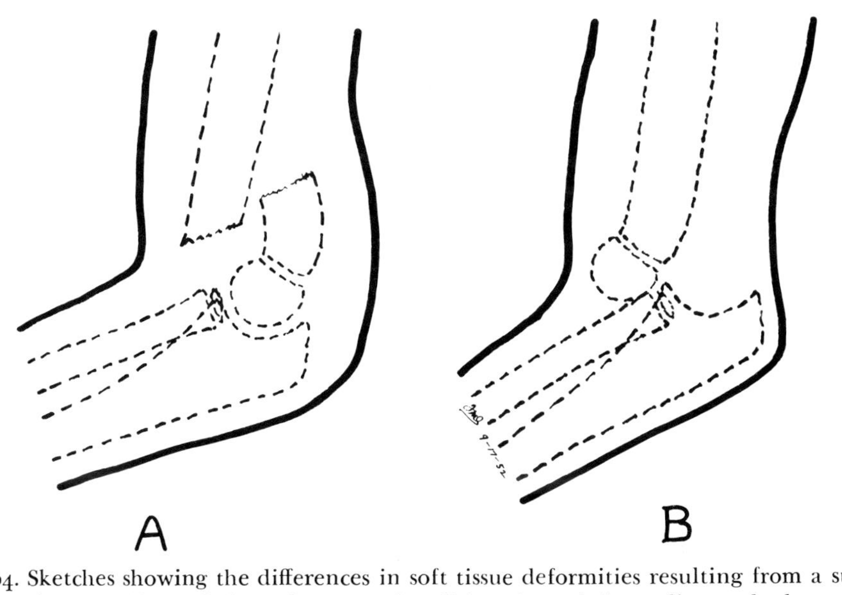

Fig. 104. Sketches showing the differences in soft tissue deformities resulting from a supracondylar fracture (A) and that of a posterior dislocation of the radius and ulna at the elbow joint (B). Compare with Figs. 22 and 23.

tion without unnecessary delay and to do so with extreme gentleness. To discover a paralysis following reduction when it was definitely known not to exist beforehand indicates either possible roughness of the manipulative reduction or the necessity for operative exploration of the nerve with possible transposition of it. Late discovery of paralysis when the pre-reduction function of the nerve was unknown would be most embarrassing and very difficult to explain to the patient or his parents.

Although open (compound, contaminated) dislocations at the elbow joint occur, they are extremely rare as such without associated serious bone injury as seen in "truck-swipe" fractures. The compounding wound in an elbow dislocation is likely to be in one of two places, (1) at the antecubital flexion crease, (2) on the medial aspect overlying the lower margin of the trochlea, where the skin has burst open from the extensive stretching, or over the olecranon from a direct blow. A small split in the skin in any of these areas from which oozes old blood in the presence of dislocation must be considered as a contaminated wound and treated as such until operation demonstrates no connection with the joint cavity.

TYPES OF DISLOCATION AT THE ELBOW JOINT

(According to direction of displacement of the forearm bones upon the humerus)

Dislocation of Radius and Ulna at the Elbow

Posterior
Lateral
Medial
Anterior

Unreduced (Old) Dislocations at the Elbow

Divergent Dislocation of Radius and Ulna at the Elbow

Anteroposterior
Medial-lateral

Dislocation of Radius Alone at the Elbow

Posterior
Lateral
Forward (without fracture)

Dislocation of Radius at the Elbow with Ulnar Fracture

Posterior, Lateral, Forward } (Monteggia Fracture)

Dislocation of Ulna Alone at the Elbow

Posterior
Anterior

Subluxation of Head of Radius in Children ("Pulled Elbow")

Congenital Dislocation of Head of Radius

Delayed Dislocation of Head of Radius Following Injury

TREATMENT OF SPECIFIC DISLOCATIONS AT THE ELBOW

Dislocation of Radius and Ulna at the Elbow

Posterior Dislocation

This is a common injury. Alone or with slight to moderate lateral displacement of the forearm bones it makes up by far the greatest majority of all elbow dislocations. The diagnosis as described above is usually fairly obvious. Tearing of the collateral ligaments and anterior capsule always accompanies the bony displacement. The brachialis anticus muscle is often extensively torn and there usually is some stripping of the periosteum and triceps muscle away from the posterior aspect of the lower humerus. Bleeding and swelling vary according to the amount of damage and length of duration after injury. Symptoms likewise vary, but considerable pain is usual.

Associated Lesions. Soft Parts. Damage to the ulnar, radial and median nerves resulting in loss of motor or sensory function or both; stretching or tearing of the brachial artery. Nerve lesions are very much more common than vascular injuries in this type of dislocation.

Bones. Fracture of the coronoid process of the ulna, fracture of the head of the radius, separation of the epiphysis of the medial epicondyle of the humerus in children (often with the avulsed fragment displaced into the joint cavity), and fracture of the capitellum or lateral condyle of the humerus.

Treatment. Reduction of the dislocation can be accomplished usually by closed methods. Occasionally open reduction must be resorted to because of inability to reduce it closed without resorting to too forceful manipulation, or because of some other associated nerve lesion or complicating fracture. General anesthesia is certainly advisable if the dislocation is more than one hour old in order to alleviate pain and especially to obtain complete muscular relaxation, without which it may be necessary to use considerable force in the reduction which in turn predisposes to additional joint and soft part injury.

Closed Reduction. There are several methods of obtaining this. (1) By direct traction on the forearm in a distal direction while maintaining counter-traction upon the humerus. Should there be present considerable lateral displacement of the ulna and radius, this should first be overcome by pushing them medially before attempting to reduce the posterior displacement. Following this, while traction and counter-traction are continued, the forearm should be *slightly* hyperextended to permit the coronoid process to slide forward beneath the trochlea. When the forearm bones are felt or seen to come forward, then they should be flexed at the elbow joint. If reduction is complete, the joint can be fully flexed with ease. If flexion is not easy and is checked at ninety degrees, reduction has not been obtained and must be done over again. If too much hyperextension is employed in this manoeuvre, increased damage may be caused to the already partly torn brachialis anticus muscle. (2) Reduction by traction on the forearm bones while the elbow is held flexed over the operator's knee. This method offers the same objection as in (1). (3) Reduction by thumb pressure pushing forward and distally upon the radial head and olecranon while using the fingers of each hand for counter-pressure upon the front of the condyles of the humerus. (4) Reduction by traction on the wrist plus flexion. In this method the operator's elbow on the same side as the hand giving the traction is used as a fulcrum against the front of the patient's humerus.

The first method described is probably the best and safest in the long run. It should be remembered that simple posterior or posterolateral dislocations at the elbow can be reduced without appreciable difficulty when done under general anesthesia. If good muscular relaxation has been obtained and if two or three gentle attempts at reduction by one or more of the above methods has failed, there must be some reason for the failure. It is probably due to intrinsic pathology such as tendon, muscle or nerve causing a definite block to replacement. Consequently, instead of using increased force or multiple repeated attempts at reduction, the intelligent surgeon will cease further manipulative trauma and resort to open reduction. At the operation

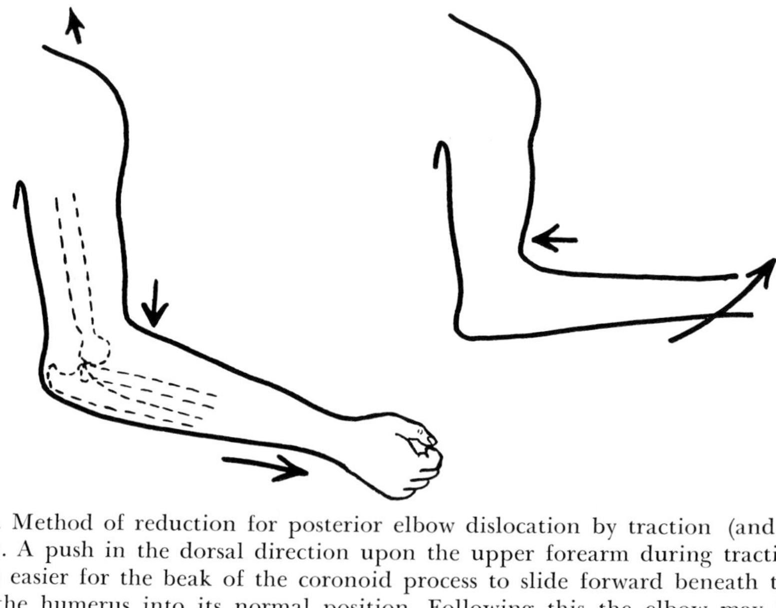

Fig. 105. Method of reduction for posterior elbow dislocation by traction (and counter-traction). A push in the dorsal direction upon the upper forearm during traction often makes it easier for the beak of the coronoid process to slide forward beneath the lower end of the humerus into its normal position. Following this the elbow may be easily flexed. If flexion is difficult, reduction is incomplete.

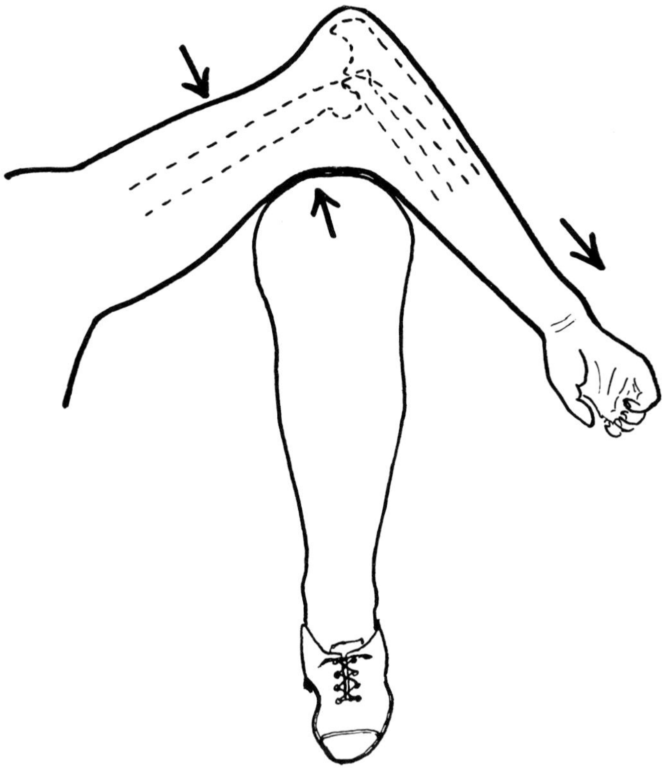

Fig. 106. Method of reduction for posterior elbow dislocation using traction and counter-traction over the operator's knee as a fulcrum (after Cotton).

the cause will be found for failure of closed manipulation and can usually be easily corrected with benefit to the patient.

Open Reduction. Resort to operative reduction for elbow dislocations is usually a matter of necessity rather than choice. It is necessary when (1) closed reduction has been unsuccessful; (2) the medial epicondyle epiphysis has become displaced into the elbow joint; (3) there is a fracture of the radial head with displacement; (4) there is a displaced fracture of the capitellar process or lateral condyle of the humerus; (5) there is ulnar nerve or other nerve damage; (6) in compound dislocation at the elbow without associated fracture. Since publication of the first edition of this book the author had seen and treated two patients with compound posterior dislocations of the radius and ulna unassociated with fracture of the radius, ulna or humerus. The lower extremity of the humerus projected through the skin, lying on the distal skin flap in the antecubital area. Needless to say, both collateral ligaments were completely torn and in one of these patients the neuro-vascular bundle (median nerve, brachial artery and veins) lay lateral to the distal end of the humerus. Treatment consisted of thorough debridement, irrigation of the wound, reduction of the dislocation, repair of the medial collateral ligament with one silk suture, and loose closure of the wound. The latter healed per primam in each case and the elbow was protected with a posterior plaster splint for two weeks. The functional results were excellent in both patients. (For specific treatment of these associated lesions the reader should consult the chapter pertaining to each.)

Post-reduction Roentgen Examination. As soon as possible following reduction another roentgen examination should be made of the splinted elbow in both planes. To allow the patient home and postpone this examination might lead to medico-legal difficulties. A fluoroscopic check-up though seemingly satisfactory at the moment is worthless as evidence in the court room. A post-reduction roentgenogram is necessary to demonstrate that reduction has been obtained. It is also advisable to have it for additional reasons: (1) reduction may not be quite complete or redislocation may have occurred; (2) a clear-cut outline of a bone fragment or articular surface may now show up within the joint that was obscured by distortion on the original films; and (3) additional fracture lines may have opened up in a condyle or radial head which may require further care or watching.

After-treatment. Treatment following reduction of a simple dislocation should be directed towards prevention of recurrence, temporary rest, re-

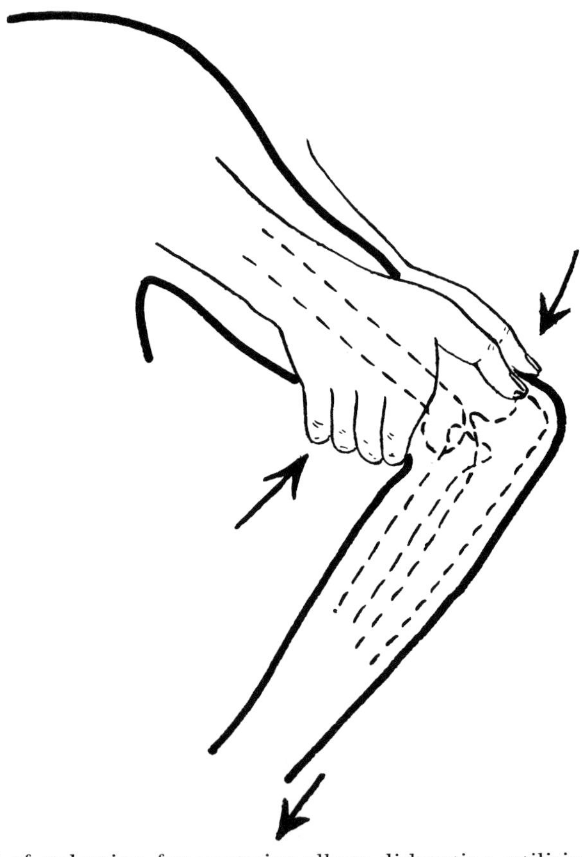

Fig. 107. Method of reduction for posterior elbow dislocation utilizing thumb pressure on olecranon while an assistant applies traction in the axis of the forearm bones.

establishment of normal circulation to the injured soft parts surrounding the joint, and to early recovery of joint motion and function. The configuration of the joint surfaces are such that recurrence of the dislocation is not prone to occur unless considerable extension of the forearm bones upon the humerus is permitted too early. Therefore, the elbow should be immobilized in a posterior molded plaster-of-Paris splint (extending from the axilla to the metacarpophalangeal joints) with the elbow at an angle of approximately seventy or eighty degrees. This splint should be supplemented with a sling. The splint should be worn for rest and protection for a week to ten days to permit the beginning of good ligamentous healing. Within two to three days following injury it is wise to allow the patient to remove the splint four or five times a day to practice active exercises for five-minute periods. He should be cautioned not to try to extend the elbow more than to an angle of 130 degrees for the first two weeks.

When the splint has been discarded after one week the sling should be continued for another 10 days or so, during which time the patient should practice his exercises hourly (always within pain limits). With the institution of active exercises the patient may be assisted with such physiotherapeutic measures as heat (thermolite, hot soaks, whirlpool baths, and very gentle massage). *Massage is contra-indicated following severe elbow injuries in children.* Under no circumstances should passive motions, such as manipulation, stretchings, weight-carrying, or encouraging the patient to hang from a door casing or trapeze be allowed. This form of brutal treatment is still too often advocated by some old-school physicians in the belief that it will help the patient regain joint motion. It accomplishes just the opposite and is one of the prime factors in the causation of myositis ossificans which may even lead to solid bony ankylosis of the elbow joint. Heat and gentle active exercises frequently carried out are stressed in the after-treatment of these injuries, because they do not cause pain or additional tearing of the swollen and non-elastic soft parts. They help to improve the local circulation, thereby assisting soft tissue healing; and also by improving the return of venous and lymphatic circulation especially, they help get rid of other products of tissue death and inflammation and thus permit an increase in joint motion and prevent articular adhesions and peri-articular capsular thickening. As motion and strength increase in the elbow joint mild active use should be permitted and encouraged.

Fractures of the coronoid process associated with dislocation require slightly more protection and care than when not present. Following reduction the elbow should be immobilized as described above but in more acute flexion (i. e. at an angle of 50 to 60 degrees), if swelling does not prohibit, and the patient should not be permitted to extend the joint beyond 100 degrees for three to four weeks. The splint should be worn for approximately the same length of time, but may be removed for application of heat and the institution of active exercises as noted above. It is good practice to prevent these patients from attempting extension of the elbow to beyond 150 degrees for at least six weeks. This will permit firmer healing of the fractured coronoid and thus diminish the chances of subsequent recurrent dislocations.

Disability Time. Uncomplicated elbow dislocations can usually return to sedentary or other light work in from two to three weeks and to heavy work in five to six weeks. If complicated by a coronoid process fracture, the above times must be roughly doubled. With other associated fractures one should consult the chapters on these specific injuries.

Complications. These may be divided into two types, early and late. Associated soft part and bony lesions are not truly complications and should not be discussed here as such.

Excessive swelling and bleb formation due to it may give considerable trouble. Prevention is the best form of treatment. The surgeon must see to it that there are no tight or constrictive turns of bandage holding the splint in place that tend to cut into the skin beneath which occurs increased swelling. Elevation of the reduced and splinted elbow on two or three pillows will overcome stagnation of the return circulation increased by dependency. Ice bags may be used to assist the prevention of excessive swelling within the first twenty-four hours. Should bleb formation occur, aspiration of the blebs under aseptic technique by means of a hypodermic needle is advisable. This should be followed by a soft pressure dressing and elevation. Bleb formation should not be used as an excuse to delay active exercises for more than a day or two at most.

Volkmann's ischaemia and paralysis may occur early after an elbow dislocation, but is not nearly so apt to as following a supracondylar fracture (Chapter XXI).

Late complications consist mainly of delayed ulnar nerve palsy and myositis ossificans. The former may occur because of excess scar tissue formation surrounding the groove along which the nerve passes behind the medial epicondyle of the humerus. The scar tissue as it later becomes dense and contracts tends to choke the nerve. The first symptoms are usually hypoesthesia or tingling in the sensory distribution of this nerve in the hand and fingers. Should the condition become progressive, operative lysis or transposition of the nerve is advisable and should be done before there occurs any atrophy of the intrinsic muscles of the hand. If performed after the motor component of the nerve becomes involves, little hope can be looked for from operative therapy.

Myositis ossificans has been mentioned before as an all too frequent complication following dislocations at the elbow. It should be otherwise. It can be minimized if the surgeon or practitioner treating the case will use common sense judgment and overcome his zeal to hasten recovery by "brawn rather than by brain." Heavy massage and forceful passive manipulations of the joint during its recovery period are the main causes of the complication. (See description and discussion of this condition under Chapter XXI.) The third most frequent cause of myositis ossificans following dislocation is a resort to often repeated attempts at closed reduction over a period of several days or a week when the original attempts were unsuccessful. Such repeated attempts not only become increasingly more difficult, but increasingly more harmful and practically "guarantee" an ensuing myositis ossificans. As mentioned under reduction of dislocations, if difficulty is encountered and reduction is unsuccessful after two or three immediate attempts under anesthesia, there must be a good reason for it—and this is best discovered and corrected by open reduction rather than by further attempts to force and insult the joint with later trials at closed reduction.

Treatment of Myositis Ossificans. Once the condition is suspected and its presence proved by roentgen examination a very definite regime should be carried out. (See Chapter XIV.)

Prognosis Following Dislocation at the Elbow. The prognosis for simple and uncomplicated elbow dislocations is usually excellent if reduction is obtained early and the above described after-treatment is carried out. About the worst that can be expected is a mild impairment (ten to fifteen degrees) of extension, which is as a rule no real handicap to the patient. It is not unusual to note some evidence of calcification in the healed collateral ligaments on late follow-up roentgenograms.

Where there has been a coronoid or radial head fracture associated with the dislocation, the prognosis should be somewhat guarded because of a tendency towards development of myositis ossificans in spite of the best and gentlest treatment.

Lateral Dislocation

This type of dislocation *alone* is very uncommon, though a certain amount of lateral displacement of the forearm bones is frequently seen in posterior dislocations. In pure lateral dislocations the coronoid process of the ulna remains distal to the lower articular level of the humerus. Damage to the soft tissues is usually very great.

There are said to be three types:

(1) Complete lateral dislocation *without* pronation in which the forearm is displaced outwards and proximally, but in supination.

(2) Complete lateral dislocation *with* pronation and rotation of both radius and ulna so that both lie in a vertical plane.

(3) Incomplete. In this type the radius is completely dislocated from the humerus, but the ulnar sigmoid is still in contact with the lateral aspect of the articular surface of the humerus.

Diagnosis. The dislocated elbow appears broader and is more flexed than in posterior dislocations. The lower inner margin of the trochlea is prominent beneath the skin. Roentgen examination is important to rule out associated fractures or to determine displacements of bony fragments.

Associated Lesions. These are commonly fracture of medial epicondyle epiphysis, lateral epicondyle, and radial head. Nerves and vessels are not especially prone to damage in this type of dislocation.

Reduction. This is usually easily accomplished under general anesthesia by pushing the two forearm bones medially and rotating them at the same time if necessary while counter-pressure is made over the medial aspect of the lower humerus. Although some hyperextension may be necessary in the manoeuvre, one should avoid changing the pure lateral dislocation into a posterior one.

If any great difficulty is encountered in closed reduction, one should not try to force it, but should resort to open reduction. The author once operated upon such a case and even at operation difficulty was encountered in the reduction until it was discovered that the capitellum had ruptured through the lateral aspect of the brachialis muscle and a portion of this muscle was caught in a groove (due to avulsion of a bone fragment) behind it. Once this was released, reduction was readily obtained.

After-treatment. (Same as in posterior dislocation.) Get a post-reduction roentgenogram.

Prognosis. Usually good unless there has been some complicating fracture. Associated fractures should be treated as such. The disability time is apt to be longer than with posterior dislocations owing to extensive soft tissue stripping.

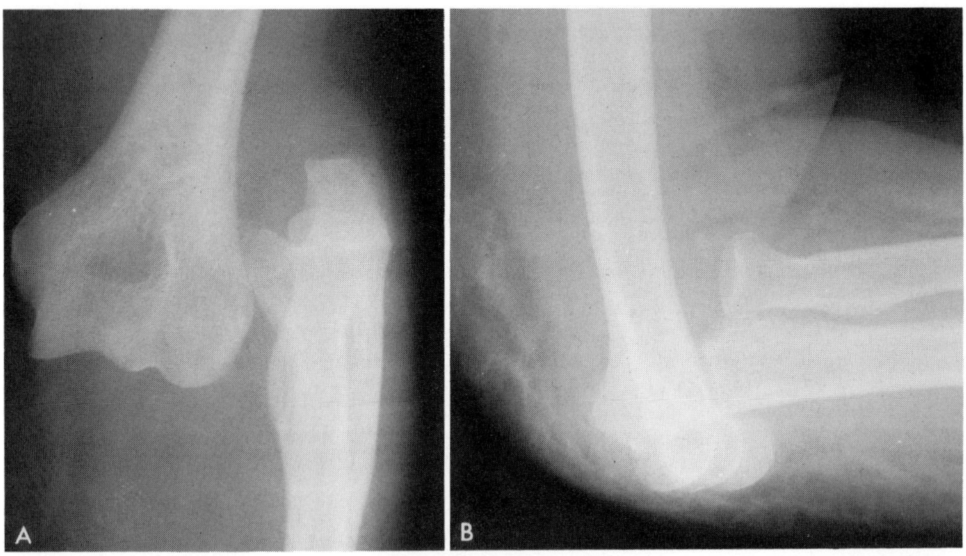

Fig. 108. Lateral dislocation at the elbow joint. (A) Antero-posterior roentgenogram. (B) Lateral roentgenogram. Note the wide displacement made possible only by extensive tearing, stripping and stretching of the adjacent soft tissue structures.

Medial Dislocation

These are rare lesions and in their pure form are usually incomplete. They are really subluxations rather than dislocations. Both the ulna and radius are shifted medially. The sigmoid fossa of the ulna may be in contact with the medial epicondyle of the humerus and the radius in contact with the trochlear surface.

Diagnosis. The olecranon is shifted medially and its fossa in the humerus is empty. The forearm deviates inwards from the main axis of the humerus.

Reduction. Under general anesthesia reduce by traction in partial extension and with direct pressure on the upper ulna in a lateral direction.

After-treatment. (Same as in posterior dislocation.) Get a post-reduction roentgenogram.

Prognosis. In general this is good because the soft part injury has been minimal.

Anterior (Forward) Dislocation

This is a very rare and unusual lesion. Though authentic cases have been reported in the literature accompanied by adequate roentgenograms, the majority reported ante-dated the discovery of roentgen rays and the diagnosis was based on clinical or operative findings, some of which showed associated compound fractures. It is also possible that anterior displacement of the radius and ulna without fracture of the olecranon may at times represent the end-point of what originally was a pure lateral dislocation. An olecranon fracture allowing forward displacement of the radius and distal ulna should not be classified as a pure forward dislocation of both bones.

Soft part damage is usually extensive in forward dislocations and not infrequently it is necessary that the triceps tendon be completely ruptured to allow it. In addition there is usually a complete tear in both collateral ligaments and of the anterior and posterior capsule of the joint. There may also be extensive stripping of the muscular attachments to the humeral condyles. The mechanism of the dislocation is said to take place by a direct fall upon the hyperflexed elbow.

Diagnosis. The elbow may be held in a position of flexion or of extension with the olecranon in front of the humerus. The forearm appears elongated. Roentgen examination is necessary to rule out fractures and to establish the diagnosis.

Reduction. Under general anesthesia the joint must first be flexed (if not already in flexion). Traction is then made on the flexed forearm and countertraction upon the humerus in order to distract the bones. Direct pressure in a posterior direction is then made upon the olecranon.

If closed reduction is unsuccessful, operation should be performed. It may be necessary to repair the triceps tendon even in the event closed reduction is possible. Take a post-reduction roentgenogram.

After-treatment. (Same as in posterior dislocation.) This injury, however, should be treated somewhat more conservatively and the elbow should be splinted for three to four weeks.

Prognosis. This depends upon the amount of muscle and possible nerve damage. One should be careful about myositis ossificans.

Unreduced (Old) Dislocations at the Elbow

In spite of modern advances in diagnosis, roentgenography, and surgical treatment an occasional case of an old, unreduced elbow dislocation is still seen. This may be the fault of the patient or of his parents in not seeking medical care. All too frequently, however, the physician in charge of the case from the beginning has failed to obtain reduction even after several attempts at manipulation over a period of a week or more, the patient finally giving up in disgust and going to another doctor or directly to a hospital. Such cases should no longer occur. The inability to reduce the dislocation may have been through no fault of the physician and perhaps was of a particular type requiring operative reduction (see under fresh elbow dislocations), but the obligation is his to get the patient to a specialist or other competent surgeon within reasonable time where reduction can be accomplished by one means or another.

Eliason has stated that "an elbow dislocation grows old early and is usually impossible to reduce by any closed treatment after ten days to two weeks." The reason for this is due to the extreme swelling and circulatory stagnation, exudation, organization of the extravasated blood, and to fibrous adhesions in and around all the joint surfaces and adjacent structures. This presents a perfect "medium" for the development of myositis ossificans since further manipulation of these inelastic tissues causes additional tearing and hemorrhage.

In order to simplify subsequent statements on the treatment of this condition it will be necessary here to omit discussion of nerve injuries and other fractures and to limit the treatment to simple unreduced and otherwise uncomplicated dislocations at the elbow. Such associated lesions and their treatment may be found under their proper sections.

Treatment. The question immediately arises as to what form of treatment can be used or is advisable to follow should such a case present itself. There are four main procedures that may be followed: (1) Traction and manipulation; (2) "sham reduction"; (3) arthrotomy and open reduction; and (4) arthroplasty.

If the dislocation is of less than two weeks duration an attempt at closed reduction should be tried. This should be performed with the patient well relaxed under general anesthesia. The traction should be applied to the forearm in the direction of its axis while counter-traction and backward pressure is applied to the humerus. At least five minutes of traction is kept up (and ten is better) following which the elbow should be gently flexed as described under fresh cases. A second attempt may be tried if the first is not successful. Should reduction be obtained, the elbow must be immobilized in a posterior molded plaster-of-Paris splint and sling for three to four weeks. The after-treatment is then much the same as in fresh injuries. The return of function is often very prolonged (three to four months) and there frequently follows permanent limitation of motion owing to scarring of the peri-articular structures and to intra-articular adhesions.

Over-head traction and suspension through the means of a Kirschner wire inserted through the olecranon may be tried for twenty-four hours before actual manipulation under anesthesia. This not only gives prolonged steady skeletal traction, but, owing to the elevation of the injured elbow, allows some of the soft tissue swelling to subside. (See section on Kirschner wire traction, Chapter X.)

If traction and manipulation fails to reduce these old dislocations or if the duration of the dislocation is three to four weeks or longer, one or more types of operative procedure may be performed. Before definitely deciding to operate the surgeon should obtain fresh anteroposterior and lateral roentgenograms. This is *exceedingly important,* because, should the films show beginning evidence of myositis ossificans in the soft tissues surrounding the bones and joint no operation should be performed at this time—(i. e., during the period of progressive bone formation)—otherwise new bone formation will be likely to increase rapidly and very probably even to the stage of bony ankylosis. If soft tissue ossification has already begun, no operative procedure should be attempted for at least nine months to a year or until the extra-osseous bone formation is well along in the regressive stage. What then can be done? It may be better then to treat the elbow temporarily by the "sham reduction" method of Hugh Owen Thomas. This is not a reduction procedure at all, but merely flexion of the dislocated elbow to slightly less than a 90 degree angle and maintaining it in this position by a collar and cuff for three weeks. Following this, the patient is encouraged to exercise and use the elbow in order to regain what motion he can at the false joint. If little function is regained and disability remains considerable, an arthroplasty may later be carried out, but certainly not until after soft tissue ossification has ceased and is regressing.

If reduction of the old dislocation has been impossible by closed methods and if there is no evidence of beginning myositis ossificans, it is usually advisable to perform arthrotomy and open reduction. This is more valuable in children than adults because the former respond better to after-treatment. In adults with very old unreduced dislocations the procedure of arthroplasty is often a better one.

The Technique of Open Reduction for Old Elbow Dislocations

(As described by Willis C. Campbell)

"An incision is made over the posterolateral aspect of the arm, beginning in the midline four inches over the olecranon process and extending down to just above the tip of the olecranon, thence slightly outward over the external condyle of the humerus, head of radius, and continuing two inches on the forearm. The flaps are elevated and retracted, exposing the tendon of the triceps muscle and posterior surface of the elbow joint.

"The tendinous aponeurosis of the triceps is dissected out at its proximal end and turned down as a tongue-like flap, remaining attached to the olecranon. A midline incision is then made through the fibers of the triceps muscle down to the humerus, extending from three inches up on the shaft to the reflection of the joint capsule around the articular surfaces. All muscular attachments over the lower end of the humerus, anteriorly and posteriorly are stripped free, together with the periosteum. The attachments of the joint capsule around the condyles of the humerus are then separated close to the bone. If dissection is carried close to the bone the ulnar nerve rarely comes into view, but may be located and detached from its bed along the groove in the internal epicondyle, and retracted out of danger. Often from stripping up of the periosteum at the time of the original injury there results considerable callus formation over the posterior surface of the humerus around the olecranon fossa; this callus with the scar tissue in the olecranon fossa must be thoroughly removed.

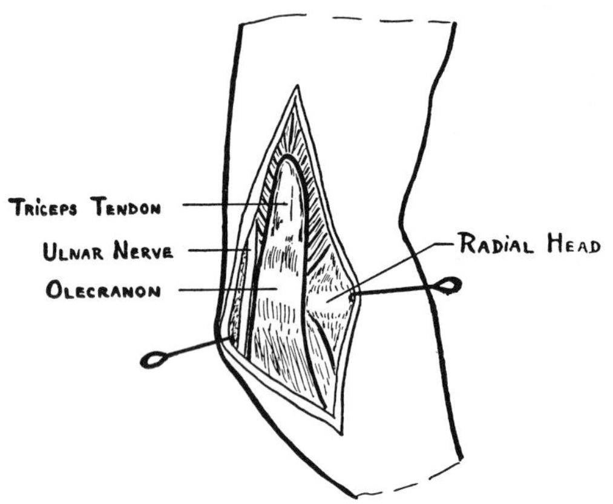

Fig. 109. *(Left)* Old unreduced posterior dislocation of the elbow. Late open reduction. Exposure of aponeurosis of triceps and isolation of ulnar nerve (after Campbell). (Bancroft and Marble: *Surgery of the Motor Skeletal System.* 2nd Ed., Chap. 32, Lippincott, Phila., 1951.) (See also Figs. 110, 111, 112.)

"Having completely freed the lower end of the humerus and exposed the capitellum and head of the radius, the forearm is twisted with gentle pressure over the capitellum, causing the head of the radius to glide forward into its normal position. If this is not readily accomplished, the soft tissues should be dissected more widely, to obviate the necessity for the use of force and consequent danger of injury to the articular surfaces. After the radius is reduced, the coronoid process may be slipped forward over the trochlea and reduction completed. The joint is then carried through the full range of motion. The periosteum and muscles are closed along the posterior surface of the humerus, and the fascia is sutured over the head of the radius. The aponeurosis of the triceps muscle is sutured into its normal position or at a slightly lower level."

After-treatment. Following operative reduction of these late cases the elbow should be immobilized at a right angle in a posterior molded splint and kept elevated on pillows for eight to ten days. The operative wound should heal by this time and the sutures may be removed. The splint should then be removed three to four times daily for heat (thermolite and hot soaks), gentle massage, and active elbow exercises within pain limits. After three weeks the splint should be worn only at night, while a sling is sufficient during the daytime. After six weeks the splint is no longer necessary at night, but should be used until this time to prevent or minimize contracture formation. The patient should be encouraged and frequently guided in his active elbow exercises to make certain he is doing them properly and often enough. Occasionally, he may do them too strenuously or for too long a time at each exercise period, thus causing himself pain and delaying his progress. If necessary, he may have to be held back slightly. The exercises should be continued for at least six months and he should be given progressively more to do in order that he may regain maximum function and strength.

Prognosis. The prognosis for old elbow dislocations is never really good, especially if they have required operative replacement. About the best that can be expected from a functional standpoint is a return of fifty percent of the normal motion range. This, however, if painless and in a strong arm may give the patient very little handicap. In others very little increase in motion is gained, but they show a definite improvement in the anatomy and in recovery of strength and use. The prognosis is naturally very much better in children than in adults.

These are serious injuries when left unreduced. No time should be lost, if closed reduction has been unsuccessful, before the patient is brought in for open reduction. The best treatment is prophylactic, i. e., *never allow an elbow dislocation to go unreduced for longer than twelve to twenty-four hours.* Early operation is far less radical treatment than (1) further delay in reduction; and (2) the necessity for later operation; and (3) offers much less risk of serious additional complications or sequelae.

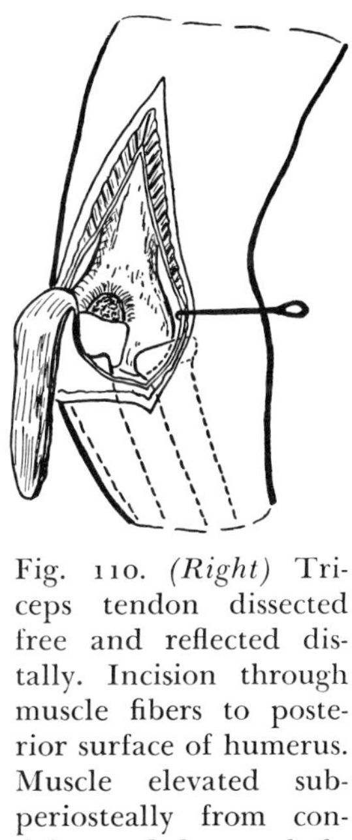

Fig. 110. *(Right)* Triceps tendon dissected free and reflected distally. Incision through muscle fibers to posterior surface of humerus. Muscle elevated subperiosteally from condyles and lower shaft, completely isolating this portion of bone (after Campbell). (Courtesy, Bancroft and Marble.) (See also Figs. 109, 111, 112.)

Arthroplasty at the Elbow Joint (See Chapter XXIV)

Divergent Dislocation of the Radius and Ulna at the Elbow

Divergent dislocation at the elbow is an extremely rare lesion. Two types have been described: the *anteroposterior,* where the ulna is displaced behind and the radius in front of the humerus; and the *transverse,* where the ulna lies to the medial and the radius to the lateral side of the humerus. The latter type is so rare as to be considered a curiosity. The exact mechanism of the injury is unknown. For either type to occur there must of necessity have been extreme violence accompanied by extensive damage not only to the collateral ligaments, but to the orbicular and oblique ligaments and even to the interosseous membrane. Clinical examination reveals marked thickening of the elbow region in the anteroposterior or lateral diameters depending upon which type is present. Along with this there is complete distortion of the bony triangle landmarks. Marked swelling occurs early.

Treatment. Reduction should be carried out under anesthesia by applying slow steady traction to the extended forearm, plus hyperextension if necessary in the manipulation, reducing the ulna first as in common forms of posterior dislocation of both bones. The radius is reduced secondarily by application of pressure over the anterior aspect of its head while the elbow is still in extension. If reduction is thus affected, the forearm should be flexed to an angle of 70 or 80 degrees while pressure is held applied to the radial head. Immobilization in this position should be carried out by means of a posterior molded splint and sling. If closed reduction has been unsuccessful, open reduction should be undertaken and special attention paid to repair of the medial collateral and orbicular ligaments. It is possible that the ulna can be reduced and stay reduced, but that the radial head may continue to redislocate anteriorly (as in some cases following reduction of a Monteggia fracture) due to an interposed orbicular ligament. Early open reduction in such cases with correction of the pathology and repair of the ligament are advisable. Closed reduction of both radius and ulna are as a rule easily obtained.

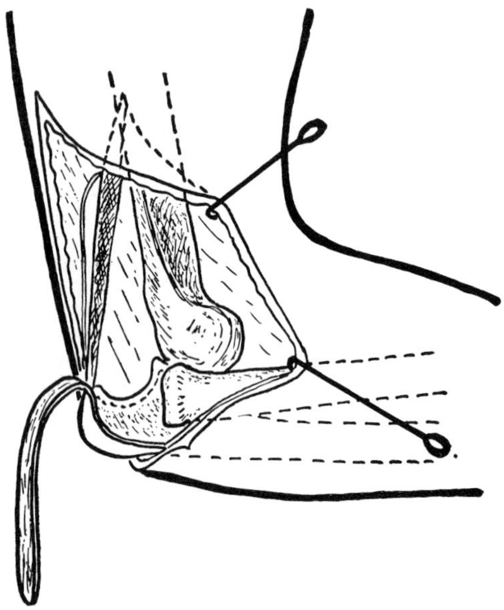

Fig. 111. *(Left)* Lateral view showing extreme limits of mobilization sometimes necessary to make reduction possible in old unreduced dislocations of the elbow (after Campbell). (Courtesy, Bancroft and Marble.) (See also Figs. 109, 110, 112.)

After-treatment. The splint should be worn for three weeks after closed or open reduction and at night for an additional two weeks owing to the extensive ligamentous or other soft part damage. The elbow should be kept well elevated to prevent extreme swelling and the pulse at the wrist and color and temperature of the hand and fingers watched carefully. No circular layers of bandage should be permitted to cut into the skin or to cause bleb formation. After three to four days the splint should be removed four times daily for the application of heat (hot soaks or thermolite), gentle massage, and mild active exercises within pain limits. It is important to start this type of physiotherapy *early* to assist in reducing swelling, to improve the local circulation, and in regaining function. This must be kept up for two to three weeks, following which exercises and mild active use are then stressed more than heat and massage. No passive manipulations or stretchings should be resorted to at any time owing to the degree of soft part damage and the great risk of increasing this with resultant pain, increased swelling, and muscular spasm.

Prognosis. Owing to the extensive ligamentous damage the prognosis must be guarded. There is a tendency for redislocation, especially of the radius. There is apt to result considerable fibrosis in the healed capsular structures with some limitation of flexion or extension or both. There is also some likelihood of development of myositis ossificans. The disability time is usually prolonged, i. e., to three or four months.

Dislocation of the Radius Alone at the Elbow

This is an extremely rare lesion when isolated. The majority of dislocations of the upper end of the radius occur in conjunction with an ulnar dislocation, a fracture of the upper third of the shaft of the ulna (Monteggia fracture), or with a fracture of the radial head. Congenital dislocations of the radius will be discussed in a later section of this chapter.

Traumatic dislocation of the radius alone at the elbow may be of any one of three types: posterior, lateral, or anterior.

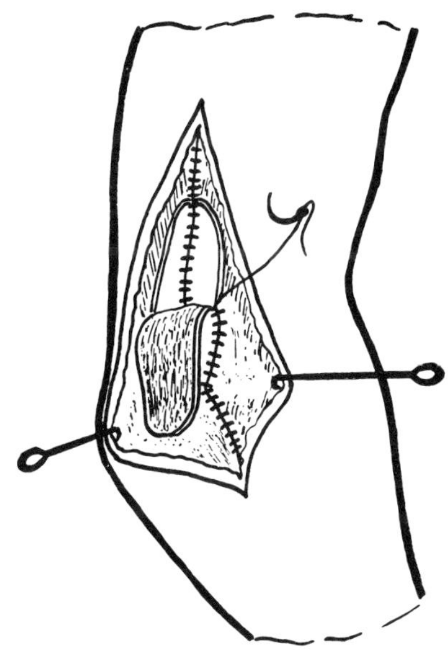

Fig. 112. *(Right)* Triceps muscle resutured following open reduction of an old unreduced elbow dislocation. The triceps aponeurosis is being resutured in its normal position (after Campbell). (Bancroft and Marble.) (See also Figs. 109, 110, 111.)

Posterior Type

This type must be accompanied by a tear in the orbicular ligament and posterior aspect of the lateral collateral ligament. There is an absence of the radial head at its normal site on palpation and instead the radial head can be readily felt posteriorly. Sometimes the superior hollowed articular surface can be palpated. The carrying angle at the elbow may be increased, but it is difficult to determine this unless the patient presents himself with the elbow held almost fully extended. Flexion and extension may be limited and supination is usually considerably limited. Associated fractures must be ruled out by roentgenograms.

Treatment. Under general anesthesia traction should be applied to the forearm and the latter adducted upon the humerus to widen the space between the humerus and radial head. Direct pressure should be made in a forward direction on the radius. Reduction is usually easy, but there is some tendency to recurrence unless the elbow is held flexed at a right angle or less in a posterior molded splint. The splint should be worn as a protection for three to four weeks except for physiotherapy and exercises as described under recent dislocations of both radius and ulna.

If the dislocation of the radial head is of long standing and causes disability, operative removal would be the treatment of choice.

Lateral Type

The orbicular and oblique ligaments must be torn in part at least to allow this type of dislocation to take place. The radial head is palpably more prominent laterally than normal. There may be slight lateral instability of the forearm upon the humerus.

Treatment. Closed reduction can usually be accomplished without difficulty using traction and forearm adduction on the humerus and by pushing in a medial direction upon the head of the radius. Following reduction splinting and after-treatment are the same as with the posterior variety. There is less tendency for recurrence and consequently the splint need not be worn for longer than two weeks. The prognosis is good when no associated fractures are present.

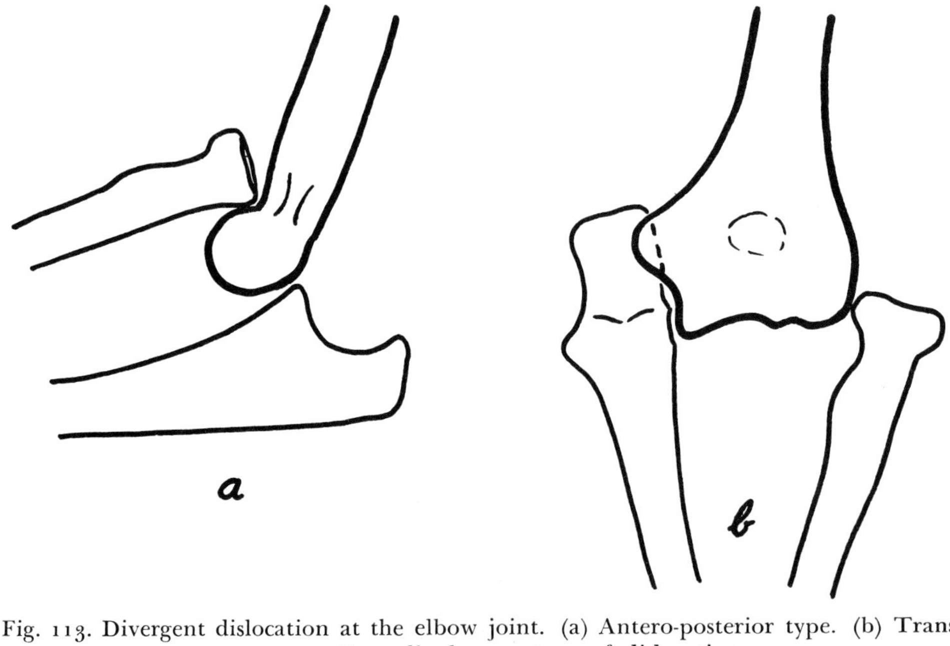

Fig. 113. Divergent dislocation at the elbow joint. (a) Antero-posterior type. (b) Transverse type. Exceedingly rare type of dislocation.

Anterior Type (without Fracture)

This is the commonest of the isolated dislocations of the radial head, but it still remains a rare lesion. One must make certain that no fracture exists in the shaft of the ulna (even as far distal as the lower third) or in the olecranon by roentgenogram before making the diagnosis of a pure anterior radial head dislocation. Monteggia fractures on the other hand are not too uncommon (Chapter XI).

The mechanism of dislocation of the radial head anteriorly without an ulnar fracture is not well understood, but the biceps tendon may be instrumental in causing it. The orbicular ligament probably becomes torn or at least badly stretched. Also, as sometimes occurs in Monteggia fractures, the radial head dislocates not by tearing across the orbicular ligament, but by pulling out through a tear in the anterior capsule just distal to this ligament. In such case it may be impossible to reduce or keep the head reduced. The radial head dislocation at times may be only partial. Flexion of the elbow is usually limited as a result of impingement of the dislocated radial head against the front of the humerus. The displaced radial head can be palpated anterior to its normal position.

Treatment. Pressure with the thumb is made in a posterior direction upon the radial head while the forearm is extended and slightly adducted. Reduction is usually easy under general anesthesia and is maintained by flexion to an angle of 80 or 90 degrees. If the orbicular ligament is not displaced or folded in behind the radial head, the latter should stay in place when the elbow is again extended to 120 or 130 degrees. It must then be splinted in flexion to protect it from recurrence and to keep the biceps tendon relaxed. The after-treatment is essentially the same as with the other types. Frequent check should be made clinically and by roentgenogram to make certain the

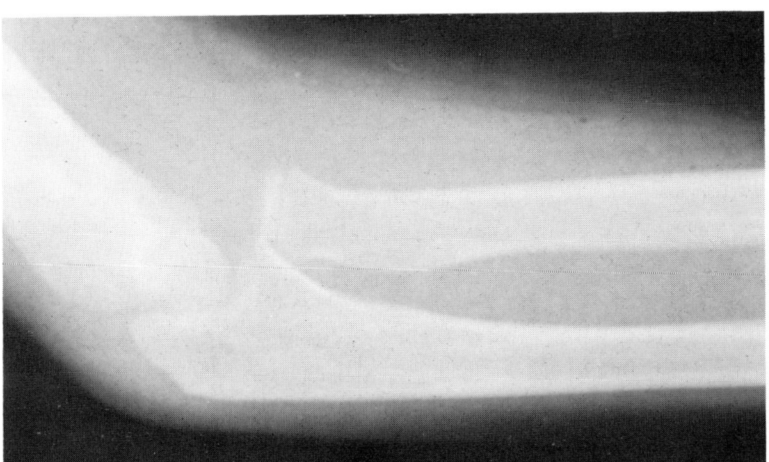

Fig. 114. Anterior dislocation of head of radius *without* associated fracture of shaft of ulna in eight year old girl. A rare injury. Closed reduction sufficed.

radial head remains in contact with the capitellum. If it tends to redislocate or if the original dislocation has been unsuccessful, open operation and repair of the orbicular ligament should be done *without delay*. (See Monteggia fractures for methods of repair, Chapter XI.) Marked delay in repairing this ligament makes the procedure not only difficult, but not infrequently results in an unsatisfactory repair which predisposes to subluxation and impaired function.

Prognosis. This is usually excellent if the dislocation of the radial head does not recur or remain unrecognized. In the majority of cases it tends to stay in place. If it does redislocate and operative reduction and repair of the ligament is performed early, the prognosis should still be excellent.

In cases of long-standing anterior dislocation of the radial head with pain on flexion and disability it is possible to improve the condition by operative means. One method may be late open reduction and construction of a new orbicular ligament from fascia after the method of Speed and Boyd. This method is satisfactory provided the head of the radius has not become enlarged and misshapen by overgrowth as sometimes occurs after being dislocated in children over a period of several years. Otherwise simple excision of the radial head followed by early and frequent active exercises and mild use would be a more satisfactory form of treatment. This is less likely to give pain or restricted motion and offers a much shorter disability time.

Dislocation of the Radius at the Elbow with Ulnar Fracture

This particular combination of fracture of the ulna in which an associated dislocation of the radial head is present is identical to and is commonly known as "Monteggia's Fracture," who originally described it in 1814 (Chapter XI).

Dislocation of the Ulna Alone at the Elbow

This is not a common injury. The dislocation of the ulna alone may take place in a forward or backward direction (the latter being more common) while the radial head maintains contact with the capitellum and acts as a pivot point. In either lesion the medial collateral ligament is ruptured.

In the *backward* type the coronoid process catches on the lower articular surface of the humerus or even slips behind the olecranon fossa. The patient holds the elbow in practically full extension. The axis of the forearm is adducted upon the humerus giving the elbow a reverse (cubitus varus) type of carrying angle and the olecranon is prominent. Reduction can usually be accomplished by hyperextension of the elbow and at the same time swinging the forearm into abduction.

In the *forward* type the beak of the olecranon catches distal to or in front of the articular surface of the humerus. The carrying angle is thus increased. Reduction is carried out by mild traction while slightly increasing the carrying angle. Direct pressure in a posterior direction is then made over the front of the upper ulna, while the forearm is gently adducted and pronated. The ulnar nerve may be stretched in this original injury and may possibly require further treatment.

The after-treatment of either type is similar to that of the usual posterior dislocation of the radius and ulna, but does not require the protective splinting for longer than one week. The prognosis is usually excellent and there is no tendency towards recurrence.

Subluxation of the Head of the Radius in Children
(The "Pulled Elbow")

This is a very common injury in young children usually occurring between the ages of two and six years. The lesion has often been called Malgaigne's luxation, who was the first to describe it, but it should not be confused with a Monteggia fracture. The mechanism of the injury is a sudden pull, jerk, or lift on the child's wrist or hand by a playmate or by a tired and annoyed parent (or nursemaid), who is trying to hurry the youngster across the street or up the steps. Sometimes while holding his parent's hand the child stumbles and the parent in an attempt to protect him from the fall pulls up quickly on his hand and wrist. Whatever the exact method or motivation, the child's arm is more or less relaxed and he is not set for the sudden jerk.

The pathology is not definitely understood, but probably one of two things occurs: (1) the radial head is pulled distally and jammed into the orbicular ligament which grips it tightly; or (2) a small fold of synovial tissue or thin part of the capsule is "sucked" into the interval between the radial head and capitellum and temporarily caught.

The main symptoms are pain and refusal to use not only the elbow, but frequently the entire arm. The child holds the elbow partly flexed with the forearm pronated. The history of a jerk on the arm is invaluable and saves the examiner needless time and the necessity of examining for clavicular, humerus, and wrist injuries in a crying and unruly youngster. Flexion and extension at the elbow are usually not limited, but supination is very definitely limited. There is no characteristic palpable deformity or tenderness. Roentgen examination is of no value except to rule out other bony injury which the physical signs have already done.

Treatment. Anesthesia is unnecessary. The lower humerus should be grasped firmly to prevent its rotation. Mild traction should then be applied to the forearm with the other hand. The latter should be pronated and followed by slow steady supination. Sometimes pushing proximally upon the radius while turning it into full supination is said to help. Very often a palpable click or snap can be felt in the region of the radial head as it becomes reduced. The forearm should again be tested in pronation and supination to make certain that the latter motion has been definitely regained. The elbow should then be moderately flexed and rested in a sling. No splint is necessary. The child within a few hours will usually begin to use the arm spontaneously. The purpose of the sling is more for the benefit of the remorseful parent than for the child.

The prognosis is excellent. Even in untreated cases these probably reduce themselves when the child later gets to sleep and becomes completely relaxed.

Congenital Dislocation of the Head of the Radius

This is a rather rare deformity and one that is not picked up until usually later in life. It may result from chondrodystrophy and not actually develop to the stage of actual dislocation until after quite a period of unequal growth of the radius and ulna. It is not infrequently bi-lateral. There are three types of this dislocation: anterior, posterior, and lateral—depending upon the direction of displacement of the radial head. There is usually loss of elbow joint motion in the anterior and posterior types, but rarely in the lateral type. In the anterior type there is limitation in flexion; and in the posterior type it is extension that is limited. In any type the radial head is apt to be misshapen and the entire radius is longer than normal. As a result of over-growth of the radius in length it impinges upon the humerus in flexion or extension, thus causing limitation of either one of these motions.

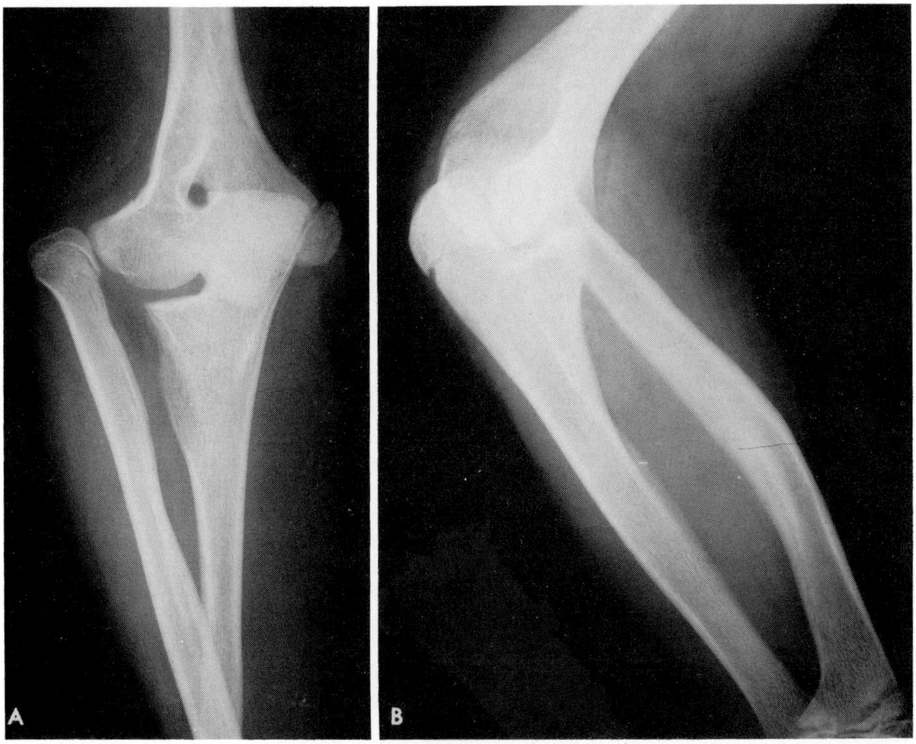

Fig. 115. Congenital dislocation at elbow joint which had been present since birth in twelve year old boy with dyschondroplasia. (A) Antero-posterior, and (B) lateral roentgenograms.

Treatment. If motion is limited so as to interfere with use and cause disability, it is advisable to operate and resect the over-grown radial head and possibly a portion of the neck. This can be done through a lateral or posterolateral incision, care being taken to avoid injuring the posterior interosseous nerve. Following operative removal exercises and use should be started within 24 to 48 hours. No splint need be worn at any time following operation. Functional recovery to the pre-operative status should be regained in three weeks, but it may take several months before marked improvement is noted in the motion that was limited before operation.

Delayed Dislocation of the Head of the Radius Following Injury

Following injury to the ulna without primary subluxation or dislocation of the radial head at the elbow, a late dislocation of the latter may develop.

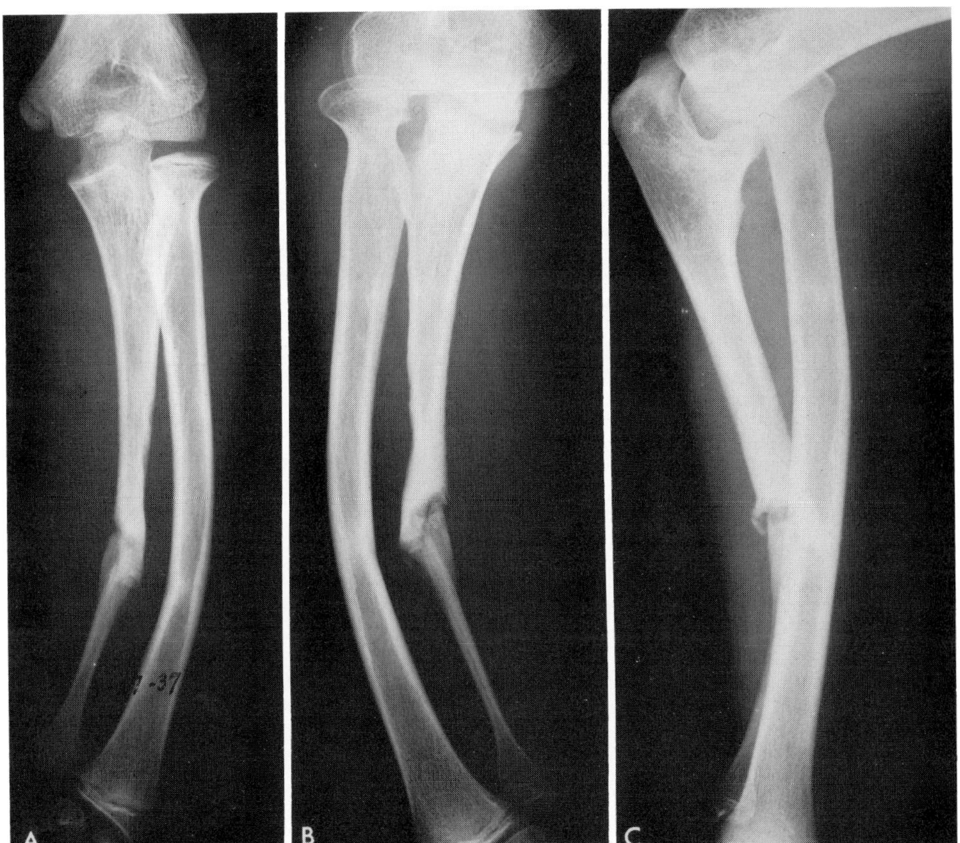

Fig. 116. Delayed dislocation of head of radius following non-union of ulnar shaft fracture. (A) Antero-posterior view of elbow and forearm taken at age of 14 years. This boy had fractured this same bone at age of 12. At 14 he re-fractured it, but no dislocation of the radius occurred. There is seen non-union of the ulna, but the radial head is in normal relation to the capitellum. Two and one-half years later at age of 16 the non-union of the ulna has persisted, the radius has over-grown, become more curved, and its head has become spontaneously dislocated from its articulation with the capitellum as seen in (B). The lateral view (C), at age 16 years, shows that this forearm is going in to a "delayed" Monteggia type deformity.

The injury to the ulna may be through or adjacent to the lower epiphyseal plate so affecting it that its subsequent growth is retarded, while that of the radius remains normal. This will give a marked disproportion to the lengths of the two bones. The first tendency towards deformity would be increased ulnar deviation of the hand. As this becomes magnified and with increased physical activity there would result a strain on the orbicular ligament at the superior radio-ulnar joint. Eventually this ligament may tear or stretch sufficiently to allow the over-grown radius to lose contact with the humerus and upper ulna.

Another mechanism by which this can happen is following a fracture of the ulnar shaft with resultant non-union of the fracture and marked angulation in a growing child. The author has seen such a case in which roentgenograms two years after injury revealed non-union of the ulna, but no dislocation of the radial head. When the patient was first brought to him for treatment, it was then four years after the original injury. At this time the radial head was found to be completely dislocated in an anterior direction at the elbow. The shaft was elongated and markedly bowed.

Treatment. The dislocated radial head should be excised if it limits motion. Other deformities or non-unions should be operated upon and treated according to their requirements. It is best to perform these procedures in separate stages rather than try to do too much at any one operation.

Chapter XX

Rehabilitation

THE DESIRE TO GET WELL

IT BECOMES obvious after several years of clinical work that there exists a marked difference in individual patients in their ability to respond successfully to treatment. This varies with the patient's individual make-up as well as with his age. The greatest single factor from this standpoint is the desire to get well. It is strongest among children. A child with a fracture ordinarily pays little attention to it once pain has ceased to be a factor. It is common to see children particpating in sports while wearing plaster casts or splints. With some adults it is only with great difficulty that one can persuade them to perform a similar feat. The child's reaction is more like that of an animal. If a particular act or exercise tends to cause pain, he refuses to use the affected extremity. An adult on the other hand is hesitant about using the extremity not because of actual pain, but because of the fear of pain or of harming himself. However admirable or otherwise these traits may be in the particular patient, they must be taken into consideration when planning his treatment. Some children must be held back and protected against over-enthusiasm or lack of caution; some adults must be constantly encouraged or forced to do things in spite of their fears.

THE DESIRE TO RETURN TO WORK

The desire to return to work is closely tied up with the desire to get well. With children (especially very young children) their main desires following injury are to get rid of the pain and to get back to their regular play. In the case of adults there are two types as regards work after injury. One is anxious to get well so that he may return to his work. This in general is the more intelligent type of individual, who has "no axe to grind," who abhors sitting around doing nothing, and is fully aware of his family responsibilities. The other type is the individual, who thinks he can collect damages as a result of his accident or who, as a compensation case, feels that he may draw his weekly compensation as long as he has a few symptoms and thinks or is persuaded that he must not work. Many of these latter are perhaps unable to carry on with their regular (heavy) occupation when they first return to work owing to prolonged inactivity and weak muscles. It is a mistake to expect them to do so; yet it is a mistake all too commonly practised both by insurance carriers and employers. An intelligent employer and insurance company will allow a man to return at first to light work if necessary at his regular salary rather than keep him off work and pay him compensation. This benefits the patient as well as the employer, insurance company and the general public.

THE ROLE OF PHYSICAL THERAPY

For hastening recovery of function following trauma, physical therapy may be of very real assistance. The author wishes to stress that for physical therapy to be of marked benefit, it must be administered *early* while it is still possible to rid the injured tissues of hemorrhage, edema fluid, cellular exudate, and products of tissue death before actual fibrosis has set in. Every possible means should be employed, such as low intensity heat, gentle massage, elevation, active exercises (even in splints) not only to get rid of soft part pathology early, but to assist the extremity in returning to its normal physiologic status as soon as possible. Reduction of a fracture followed by complete plaster immobilization without elevation, exercises or other early aids to circulation will cause muscular atrophy, circulatory stasis, and periarticular thickening, which may require many months before the patient can rehabilitate himself to a useful status.

The author feels very strongly that diathermy (regular or short wave) or other modalities are of little use to the patient at any time following a fracture. The only person who can safely increase his joint motion is the patient himself. The patient, if he begins early, may in many instances *retain* his function by exercises and never require late rehabilitation. A well trained physiotherapist who understands the value of early active exercise is invaluable at this stage in supervising and instructing patients in the proper types of exercise to be performed. In other words, the patient must never wait until the bone has healed before he starts in to limber up his joints; he must begin this immediately and thus will never lose his motion except very temporarily for a week or two at the beginning. The injured bone in the meantime has its healing qualities improved by the maintenance of a relatively normal circulation.

OCCUPATIONAL THERAPY

Often more valuable than physical therapy is occupational therapy for the simple reason that it does not rely upon artificial means and the gullibility of the patient to help him regain his strength and joint motion. Many patients will faithfully accept diathermy treatments three times a week in the hope that "it will make them well." The remainder of the week, they may do absolutely nothing to help themselves. There is therefore little wonder that convalescence and rehabilitation for many rather trivial traumatic lesions requires six months to one year. Occupational therapy on the other hand helps the patient by making him help himself. The patient, if compelled to follow this program, will increase joint motion by using the joints;

by actually doing things his strength will be increased by use. He will practice occupational therapy two, three or more times every day, not merely three times a week.

PSYCHO-THERAPY

Psycho-therapy is of extreme importance following all traumatic injuries. The most important time when this should be employed is at the beginning of treatment to explain to the patient that by following orders carefully his chances of obtaining a good functioning extremity are excellent. This will stimulate him to carry out exercises as ordered by his surgeon; it will also make him amenable to the suggestion of mild active use and help him perhaps in devising his own exercises that may be of additional assistance. The patient should be encouraged to use the extremity for eating, dressing, and, as soon as possible, to use it for carrying out simple duties around the household. It may be advisable to suggest ahead of time that at the next visit a splint may either be shortened or removed altogether if the patient in the meantime has improved sufficiently with his exercises to permit discarding of such splint.

Some particularly timid individuals must of necessity be encouraged to perform exercises or to increase the amount of work they can do with the extremity as it begins to recover from the trauma. Other patients must be constantly reminded of their improvement, otherwise they may fear that by doing too much they may be causing themselves harm. Such persons must not only be reminded, but they must be urged to continue exercises in order to increase function. The more intelligent patients will accept suggestions; the less intelligent or those apt to be somewhat stubborn or pig-headed may decide that the surgeon does not know quite all he is "preaching" and will refuse to accept his suggestions. Many of these individuals must be "bull-dozed" into carrying out the exercises as prescribed. Some must be practically threatened before they will carry them out. Others may be jollied into doing the same thing. An occasional individual may be too enthusiastic in performing his exercises and must be held back or slowed up in order that he will not actually do himself harm.

Very often, as has been mentioned elsewhere, it may become necessary during the course of treatment to stop all active forms of treatment and put the patient on a follow-up regime, i.e., not seeing him for a period of three or four months. This is because he has been made over-conscious of his condition by too frequent trips to the physician or by too frequent treatments having been given. This in addition tends to make him feel that the injury has not only been serious, but that the recovery is slow and requires prolonged and frequent treatment visits. For this reason (so he thinks) he must not do too much for fear of possibly causing himself harm. When the patient has reached a status quo as far as functional recovery is concerned, it is often best to stop his treatments completely and not see him for a period of several months. In the meantime he should be advised that he may perform all active motions and acts he wishes and not to protect the extremity in any way. By doing thus, many of these individuals forget the importance of the treatment they have been getting and will help themselves to recover function without thinking of the injured extremity.

An interesting observation in checking elbow flexion is that, with the patient's arm at his side, he will thus flex it to roughly 60 to 65 degrees, but when asked to put his hand on the back of his head and then use the fingers to crawl down the back of his neck, he will almost invariably flex this same elbow to 50 or 45 degrees, thus gaining 10 to 15 degrees of flexion when he is not *consciously* looking at his elbow. The author has found this to be true in many instances over a period of at least 30 to 35 years.

THE AUTONOMIC NERVOUS SYSTEM

The role played by the autonomic nervous system in the recovery of function and in the persistence of pain following trauma has only recently been partially understood. Pain and edema of an extremity often persist and may be greatly benefited either by drugs that affect the autonomic nervous system or by the injection of procaine hydrochloride into the ganglia to block the sympathetic nerve impulses. In the upper extremity sympathetic nerve block is accomplished by injection of the stellate ganglion. This not only aids in over-coming venous spasm, permitting edema fluid to be absorbed, but it also over-comes the pain which apparently has been partly due to venous spasm.

TECHNIQUE OF STELLATE GANGLION NERVE BLOCK

The technique of such a block is comparatively easy. Asepsis must be employed. The transverse process of the sixth cervical vertebra is identified by the operator's finger while the patient is either in the sitting or in the semi-recumbent position with the head turned toward the opposite side. The sternocleidomastoid muscle and neurovascular bundle is either displaced laterally and the trachea medially, or the muscle and neurovascular bundle is displaced medially until the finger reaches the base of this transverse process. A number 22 or 24 gauge needle four to five centimeters in length is inserted and directed in anteroposterior direction directly toward the base of the transverse process of the sixth cervical vertebra. The point of the needle is held in contact with bone and the soft tissues are allowed to recoil. The syringe is then removed from the needle to make certain that no bleeding takes place which might indicate that the point of the needle were in the vertebral artery; or, if the fluid in the needle disappears, indicating that the inner end of the needle were in the pleural space, the fluid being sucked in on inspiration; or, if clear fluid escaped from the hub of the needle that the point were within the subarachnoid space and naturally should be removed. Five cubic centimeters of a one percent solution of procaine hydrochloride is then instilled at this site. The needle is then withdrawn approximately two to three millimeters until it becomes disengaged from the prevertebral fascia and at this point an additional 15 cubic centimeters of the solution is instilled.

If the injection is successful, there should be a rapid congestion of the conjunctiva of the eye and within 15 to 20 minutes there should be progressive miosis, ptosis and enophthalmus on the side injected, giving a typical Horner's syndrome. The hand and forearm should become warm due to vasodilatation.

It should be kept in mind, however, that in spite of sympathetic ganglion blocks all other means of improving the circulation should be carried out, such as by elevation of the extremity, reduction of the fracture or dislocation, avoidance of circular bandages and of too acute flexion, if the lesion is at the elbow, so that the flexed swollen tissues will not in themselves cause further obstruction to the circulation. By all means *avoid* circular plaster casts. These hide swelling and make it difficult to relieve the effects of such swelling.

Chapter XXI

The Treatment of Late Deformities and Disabilities Resulting from Fracture or Dislocation

MALUNION

HUMERUS. Occasionally it is advantageous to remove the anterior projecting portion of the shaft in a *malunited supracondylar fracture.* Whether this operative procedure is advisable or not will depend upon the degree of limitation in elbow flexion and upon the amount of disability resulting from the deformity. A twenty to thirty degree loss of full elbow flexion (as compared to the normal elbow) is rarely much of a handicap to the patient; a loss of forty to fifty degrees of flexion may give a serious disability. Before any operative correction is attempted, the surgeon must be very certain that the block to flexion is the result of the bony deformity and not due to periarticular fibrosis, capsular contracture, or to intra-articular obstruction (bony irregularity or fibrous adhesions). It may be necessary only to remove the projecting spur of the lower shaft if the general axis of the condylar extremity is good (see Fig. 37). On the other hand, if the lower fragment is angulated posteriorly in addition to being displaced in a posterior direction, it would be advisable to perform osteotomy and to correct the position and axis. Such a procedure can often be carried out with the use of internal fixation to greater advantage than by relying upon plaster splints solely for external immobilization. If internal fixation is applied adequately, the corrected position can be maintained and active joint motion may be continued during the healing process. It is always wise to wait at least one year after injury before making a decision to employ operative correction in such cases.

Malunited fractures of the *lateral condyle of the humerus or capitellum* of long standing require operative removal *if the misplaced fragment definitely interferes with joint function.* Late correction of the malunited fragment, even if reduced and held by some form of internal fixation, rarely results in an appreciable improvement in function. Removal of such a fragment offers far greater chance of increased and painless function in the elbow joint, but perfect results should not be expected.

Dicondylar fractures with malunion are rarely amenable to operative correction and in general should not have this attempted. Arthroplasty of the elbow if carried out properly would seem to offer a better prognosis for recovery of function if the malunion of the condyles has resulted in marked restriction of motion (Chapter XXIV).

The *medial epicondyle* may occasionally heal with malunion as noted on roentgenograms, but such examination is not sufficient indication for operative correction. It is far better to avoid operation in these cases *unless* definite ulnar nerve disturbance has appeared and shows signs of progressing. If such be the case, transposition of the ulnar nerve is indicated. Malunion of the epicondyle fragment per se should cause no loss of joint function or of muscle strength. The chance of ulnar nerve disturbance following such malunion is extremely slight. (One patient only in 122 cases of simple separation of the medial epicondyle treated at The Presbyterian Hospital, New York City, developed ulnar nerve symptoms and signs.) It is the author's belief that operative correction for malunion of the medial epicondyle would cause a marked increase in nerve disturbance, necessitating subsequent nerve transposition.

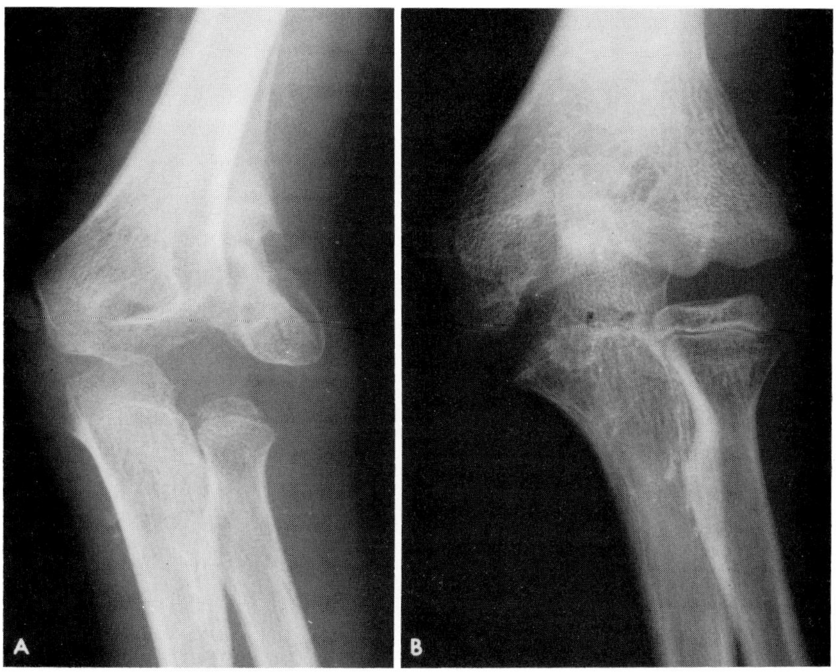

Fig. 117. Malunion following fracture of lateral condyle of humerus in nine year old boy. Several unsuccessful attempts had been made to reduce the displaced fragment prior to our examination three months after injury. (A) Antero-posterior view of elbow showing the displaced fragment in malposition and the subperiosteal callus along the lateral condylar ridge and shaft of the humerus. (B) Same elbow four years after operative removal of the fragment. Motion range was greatly improved by the operation and the carrying angle of the elbow was only slightly increased. No ulnar nerve signs had developed after six years.

Ulna. The *coronoid process* may unite in mal-position, and become so enlarged that bony block to flexion may result. If such be the case and real disability ensue, it would be justified to operate and remove the offending projection.

The *olecranon process* may show malunion and irregularity causing limitation of elbow extension (see Fig. 71). If this be present and disability be great, operative removal of the olecranon is probably the only operative procedure indicated. Following removal of the olecranon, the triceps tendon and aponeurosis should be carefully sutured to the periosteum of the upper shaft, otherwise elbow extension will remain weak as well as limited.

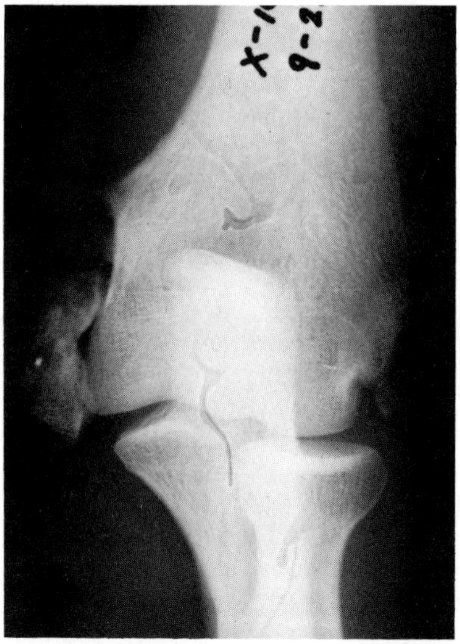

Fig. 118. Enlarged and displaced medial epicondyle of humerus five years after injury when it was avulsed from its normal position. In spite of its displacement, overgrowth, irregularity, and fibrous union, elbow function was complete and no ulnar nerve disturbance had resulted (same patient as in Fig. 39).

Malunion of the *upper shaft of the ulna* following Monteggia fracture gives an unsightly deformity. The angulation of the ulna with apex pointing towards the radius may also interfere with pronation or supination of the forearm. One should not hasten to correct such a deformity no matter how unsightly, because it is extremely difficult to do, often recurs even when internal fixation has been employed, and fibrous union of the fragments may result. It is usually necessary to excise the permanently dislocated radial head which was a part of the original deformity and has recurred if the healing of the ulna has resulted in malunion and angulation. If correction of the late deformity is considered essential, excision of the radial head should be performed as the first procedure. Subsequently, osteotomy of the ulna may be performed, the angulation straightened and the fragments fixed rigidly by a plate of adequate length plus a transfixion screw. This is an ideal site for internal fixation of the ulna by means of an intramedullary nail of the Kuntscher type.

Radius. At the elbow malunion following a *fracture of the head of the radius* may cause marked limitation of pronation and supination and, as well, pain on the extremes of these motions. If this loss of function persists for longer than six months, excision of the radial head is definitely indicated. Such operative excision should be followed by a regime of active exercises started within twenty-four hours. The prognosis for late excisions of the radial head is rarely so good as for early operation.

Following fracture of the radial head epiphysis or neck of this bone in children with tilting of the fragment left uncorrected a malunion often results giving rise to an eccentric head which impinges upon the capitellum or lesser sigmoid notch of the ulna in rotation. This causes restricted rotation and pain. Excision of such a misshapen head should be delayed until the child has attained his full growth and the epiphyseal cartilage in this area has closed, otherwise growth disturbance may follow with shortening of the radius at the wrist.

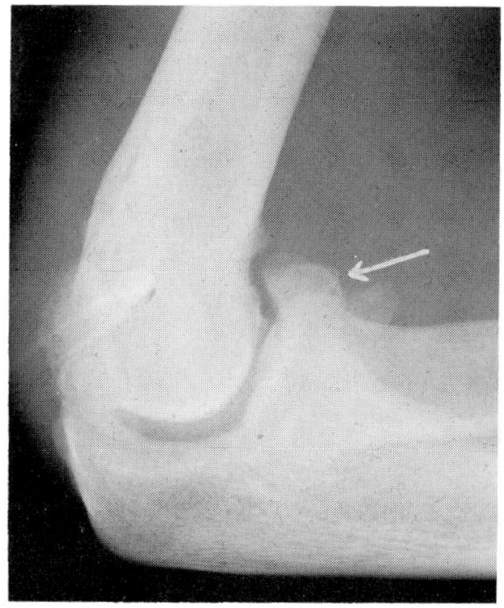

Fig. 119. Enlarged coronoid process following injury in childhood (probably elbow dislocation with fracture of the coronoid) which caused a flexion block at the elbow. Operative excision of an enlarged coronoid is sometimes indicated to improve elbow flexion.

If the entire radial head epiphysis has been displaced completely so that its axis forms a right angle with the shaft axis and the injury is of two or more weeks duration, it will be best to postpone operation for at least eight weeks. This is especially true if one or more manipulative attempts have been made to reduce the fragment previously. Operative interference within the first month would offer a high probability of development of synostosis. The child should be permitted mild active use and exercises within pain limits in order to regain as much elbow motion as possible. When this becomes stationary and all inflammatory swelling and tenderness have disappeared (usually about eight to ten weeks), operation may be performed and should consist of removal of the entire radial head. Although it is inadvisable to excise the radial head in a child in a fresh case, it must be excised in late cases. Any attempt to replace the head would be too risky from the standpoint of formation of a synostosis if not from the standpoint of mechanical impossibility. Growth disturbance will almost certainly result from the loss of this growth center and the ulna will overgrow the radius at the wrist causing a Madelung type of deformity. This should be very carefully explained to the child's parents. However, growth disturbance is far less serious than synostosis between the upper radius and ulna. The Madelung deformity may later be corrected by excision of the ulnar head at the wrist. The growth disturbance may progress for two to three years and then become stationary, so there should be no haste in performing ulnar head resection. If it is done too early, it may have to be repeated.

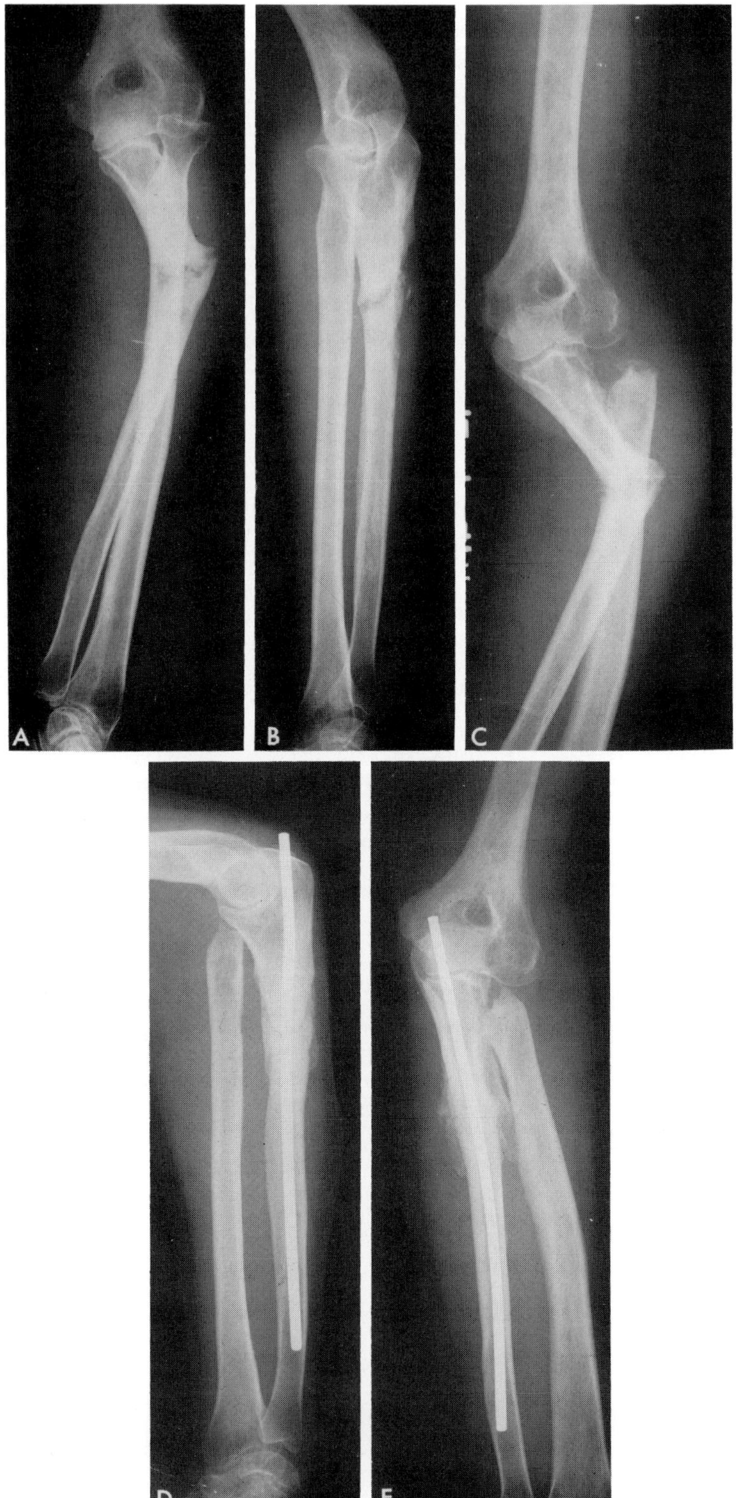
A
B
C
D
E

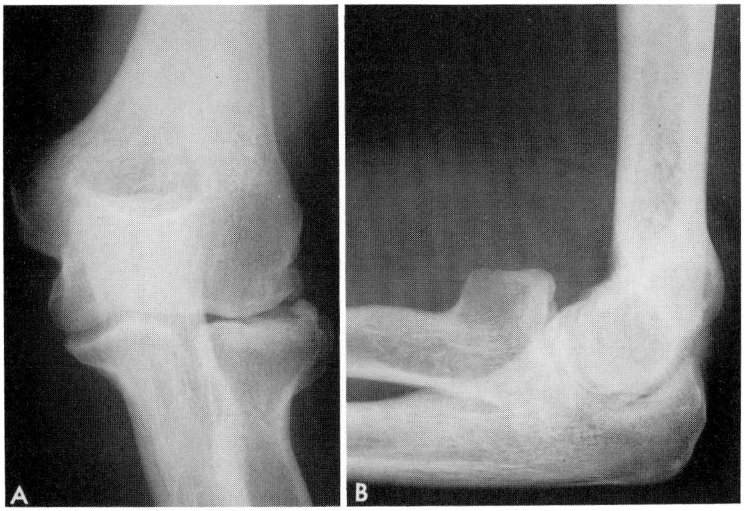

Fig. 121. Malunion following fracture of head of radius. (A) Antero-posterior view. (B) Lateral view. Operative excision of the radial head and one small loose body relieved patient's pain and improved motion range.

NON-UNION

Non-union following fracture in the region of the elbow is a rare condition except for several isolated fractures such as medial epicondyle epiphyseal separations and the rather rare lateral condyle fractures in children.

Humerus. Supracondylar and dicondylar fractures almost never result in non-union. Should one see such a case, however, the treatment would depend entirely upon the severity of the symptoms and upon the patient's disability. If the patient is having pain, it might be advisable to operate, remove scar tissue from between the ununited fragment and the shaft, and then fasten the fragments together with a plate and screws or with nails. If pain is not the predominating factor and loss of joint motion is great, it might be wise to operate, correct the position of the ununited fragments as in a case of malunion if it is felt strongly that improvement in position will increase function without resulting in subsequent pain.

←

Fig. 120. Non-union and deformity following Monteggia fracture of ulnar shaft and dislocation of radial head. This patient had been openly reduced and plated, but infection ensued, requiring drainage and eventual removal of the plate and screws. (A) and (B), antero-posterior and lateral views 11 months after injury and just prior to operative excision of the head of the radius as the first stage in reconstructing the forearm and elbow. (C) shows increase in angulation of the ulna 6 weeks after operative removal of the radial head. (D) and (E), views taken 4 months after correction of ulnar non-union and angulation with intramedullary fixation and iliac bone grafts. Fracture is solidly healed. The rod was removed at 10 months and elbow motion including rotation was greatly improved.

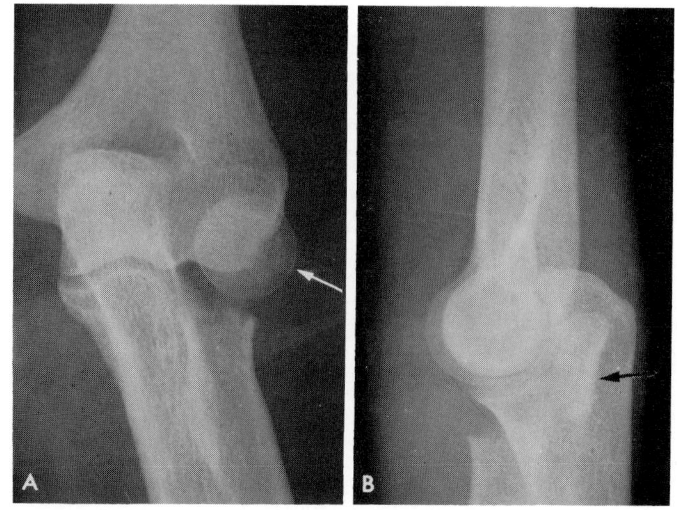

Fig. 122. Fracture of radial head in adult with complete displacement of the intact head fragment. (A) Antero-posterior view; note rotation of head 90 degrees. (B) Lateral view.

The medial epicondyle epiphysis when separated frequently fails to unite by bony union to the medial condyle. This rarely leads to any disturbance in function of the joint or even in the ulnar nerve. If ulnar nerve disturbance were found to accompany such a non-union the best form of treatment would be not to attack the ununited medial epicondyle, but to proceed with transposition of the ulnar nerve to the anterior aspect of the medial condyle (p. 263).

The lateral condyle of the humerus in children occasionally fails to unite following a fracture; if failure of union occurs, it usually results in an irregularly shaped condyle which may cause decrease in joint motion along with an increase in the carrying angle due to under-development. The fragment may seem to cause pain or loss of function by virtue of its non-union and should probably be operated upon and excised. It usually cannot be replaced accurately at such a late date. If, however, excision were to result in complete instability of the elbow laterally, some fixation of the fragments would be better than removal.

Ulna. The tip of the coronoid process when fractured within the joint cavity may fail to unite. This may result in a loose body within the joint which may interfere with flexion and extension. If it should act thus, operative removal would be definitely indicated.

The olecranon is perhaps more often seen to result in non-union when it has been treated conservatively with the elbow fixed in extension. It actually is healed by fibrous tissue, but this gives a weak extension apparatus and sometimes pain. Its displacement may also interfere with full extension of the elbow joint. Often the condition may be improved by operation, removal of the olecranon fragment and re-attachment of the triceps tendon and its expansions to the periosteum of the upper ulna. This would seem to be a far better form of treatment in late ununited olecranon fractures than to attempt to obtain bony union after excising the scar tissue.

Radius. Radial head fractures on rare occasions have been known to show failure of bony union when completely displaced to the outer side. There is only one treatment indicated for such displacement and non-union and this is total excision of the radial head.

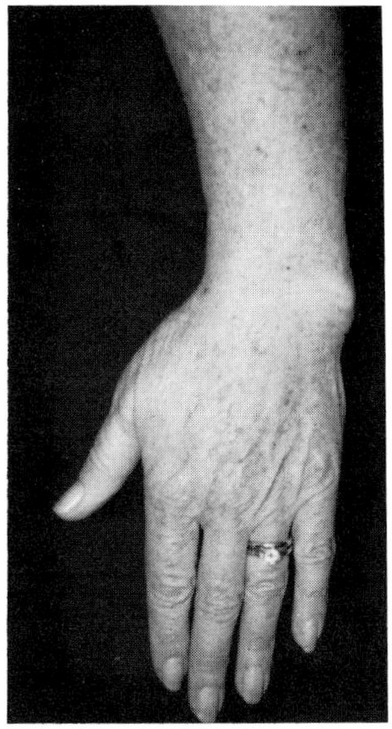

Fig. 123. Photo showing Madelung type of deformity at the wrist. Note lateral deviation of hand and prominent ulnar head. This is usually the result of shortening of the radius due to growth retardation or premature closure of the distal epiphysis of the radius. It may also occur as a result of operative removal of the radial head at the elbow in a child.

CUBITUS VARUS (GUN-STOCK) DEFORMITY

A cubitus varus deformity at the elbow not infrequently follows supracondylar fracture of the humerus, either the result of faulty reduction (incomplete correction of rotary deformity) or because of growth disturbance. This may become severe and although it does not interfere with function of the elbow joint, it is an unsightly deformity. The parents of the child may wish something done to correct it. The surgeon should be hesitant about correcting minor gun-stock deformities but, if the reversal of the carrying angle is twenty degrees or more, it might be beneficial to perform such correction. For the operative technique of such correction see the chapter on supracondylar fractures (Chapter X).

CUBITUS VALGUS DEFORMITY

Cubitus valgus deformity, or increased carrying angle at the elbow, usually follows epiphyseal growth disturbance or a fracture of the lateral condyle of the humerus in children. It rarely causes loss in joint motion, but the one thing that must be watched for with an increase in the carrying angle is a late ulnar nerve neuritis. This is due to stretching of the nerve which is made to traverse a longer course around the medial aspect of the elbow to reach the upper forearm. If ulnar nerve disturbance becomes evident and continues to progress, the nerve should be transposed anteriorly (see below). This should be done before any of the motor function of the nerve is lost. Once intrinsic muscle atrophy in the hand occurs, this cannot be expected to recover by transposition of the nerve.

LATE ULNAR NERVE NEURITIS

(Treatment by Transposition of Nerve)

Late ulnar nerve palsy in contrast to primary palsy usually follows a fracture of the lateral condyle of the humerus in children with resultant non-union, mal-union, or growth disturbance (retardation) which in turn causes a marked increase in the carrying angle (cubitus valgus) of the elbow. The nerve is thus stretched as it passes behind the medial epicondyle of the humerus as described above. A perineuritis develops and the sheath surrounding the nerve becomes thickened. Symptoms and signs rarely develop sooner than ten years following the original injury and may take twenty to thirty years before they become evident. Clinical signs develop slowly and are manifested by an ache or pain in the region of the elbow brought on by motion. Numbness and tingling subsequently appear in the fourth and fifth fingers. Should the condition become progressive, motor signs will appear in the hand in the form of weakness and subsequently intrinsic muscle atrophy.

If the condition is allowed to persist, complete ulnar nerve palsy may develop. Thickening and tenderness may be evident clinically over the ulnar nerve as it passes behind the medial epicondyle. An increased carrying angle is noted and roentgen examination will reveal an old malformed or displaced humeral condyle.

Treatment. Once the condition has been determined to be progressive,

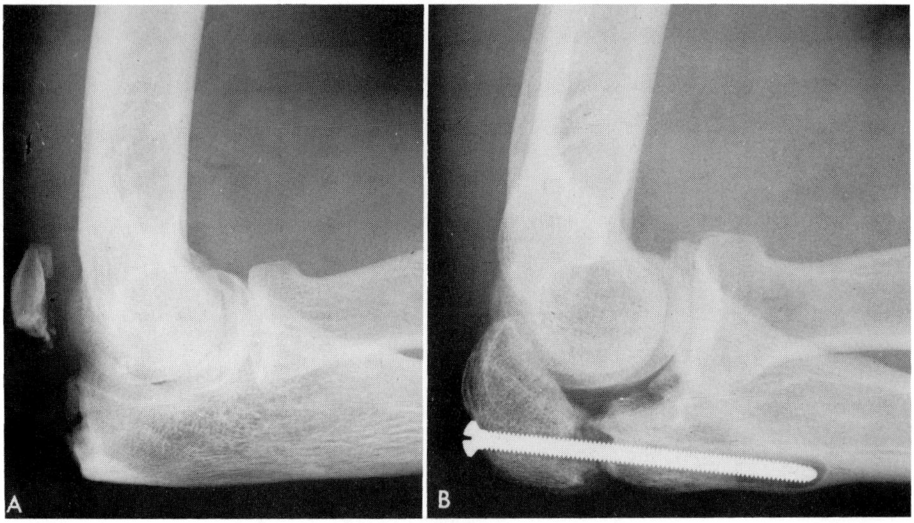

Fig. 124. Non-union following fracture of olecranon. (A) Non-union of 10 years duration in a closed fracture. (B) Non-union one year and six months following an open (compound) fracture which was debrided and fixed with a single long screw. Function and strength in both cases were good.

conservative treatment has little to offer the patient. Such forms of operative therapy as freeing of the nerve or deepening of the epicondylar groove as recommended by Broca in 1899 are totally inadequate. Correction of the cubitus valgus deformity by supracondylar osteotomy as advocated by Mouchet to relax the nerve is not only very radical, but carries with it considerable risk.

The simplest and best treatment is that of *transposition* of the ulnar nerve so that it lies in front of the medial condyle and not behind it.

Technique of Transposition. A medial longitudinal incision ten centimeters long is made with its center just behind the medial epicondyle. This is carried down to the deep fascia. The nerve is identified as it passes behind the medial epicondyle and is then freed upwards and downwards for a generous distance. A fine branch to the elbow joint may have to be sacrificed, but muscular branches to the flexor carpi ulnaris muscle should be saved as the main nerve is freed from its entrance between the superficial and deep bellies of this muscle. The nerve trunk is then swung forward making certain that no kinking or constriction of it occurs as it crosses the intermuscular septum. A small groove is then made longitudinally in the flexor-pronator group of muscles and the nerve is laid in this and the fascia sutured loosely over it.

Care must be taken to bring about perfect hemostasis since numerous small blood vessels accompanying the nerve are encountered in the groove. Following operation the elbow should be kept at rest in a sling at a right angle for approximately two to three weeks.

The prognosis is good if the nerve is transposed before motor signs develop; but, if transposition is not carried out until after motor signs have developed, recovery from intrinsic muscle atrophy and weakness in the hand and fingers can hardly be expected.

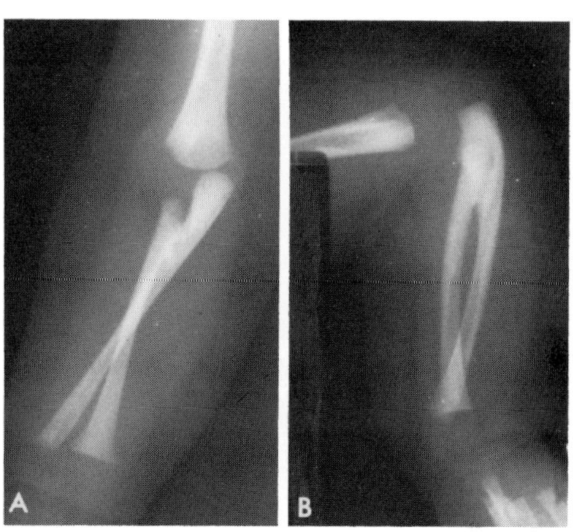

Fig. 124-A. (A) and (B) antero-posterior and lateral views of elbow and forearm in a newborn baby with a congenital synostosis of the upper radius and ulna. The forearm is fixed in complete pronation and it was impossible to supinate it at all. The hand, fingers, elbow and shoulder motions were otherwise completely normal as well as those of all the other joints in the body.

GROWTH DISTURBANCE

Growth disturbance following injury is usually the result of impairment of the blood supply to the epiphyseal cartilage. This may cause slowing up of the growth; occasionally, it may cause stimulation of growth. Depending upon which happens, various deformities may ensue and it may be necessary at a later date to perform operative correction of these.

Humerus. It has already been mentioned that the humerus may show a varus or valgus deformity. The type of treatment indicated for either one has already been described.

Ulna. The olecranon occasionally overgrows when injury has been inflicted upon its epiphysis and increases its length to such an extent that it may interfere with full elbow extension. If such be the case, excision of the excess length of the olecranon is indicated and the triceps tendon and expansions must be sutured firmly to the periosteum and through a drill hole in the upper ulna (see Fig. 71).

Radius. Growth disturbances in the head of the radius usually result in an enlarged and irregularly shaped radial head. Often the radial head may become eccentric rather than circular in shape and this may cause considerable interference with its rotary motion. If such be the case, the radial head should be excised.

FLEXION BLOCK

Due to persistent anterior displacement of the lower end of the shaft of the humerus following a supracondylar fracture, there may be interference with flexion at the elbow. This condition has been taken up already under the discussion of mal-union and the treatment is the same (see Fig. 37).

MYOSITIS OSSIFICANS

Myositis ossificans within the brachialis anticus muscle may follow elbow dislocation or supracondylar fracture of the humerus. It is more likely to occur if the elbow has been manipulated forcefully on one or more occasions and almost certainly will occur if the injury has been followed with treatment consisting of passive motion, stretching or heavy massage. This condition is not one of excess callus formation. In the early stages of myositis ossificans the treatment should be to stop all forms of treatment that may have been causing it. No attempt should be made to excise the bony mass in the brachialis anticus muscle for at least nine months to one year after the onset of the condition. The reason for this postponement is that ossification increases for an indefinite time, then becomes stationary for a period of months and eventually regresses. If operation is performed during the period of increasing calcification or during its stationary period, the trauma of the operation will very likely cause the calcification to reappear and in greater quantity than was originally seen. This will be disastrous for the function of the joint.

Late operative treatment for myositis ossificans may be unnecessary since, by watchful waiting, many of these patients within one to one and a half years after its onset may show complete or almost complete resorption of the bone in the brachialis anticus muscle. This may regress to such an extent that it no longer causes interference with function or gives any symptoms. If such be the case, operation is obviously not indicated. If a large mass of bone remains in the muscle and it appears obvious that this mass of bone interferes with elbow joint flexion or extension, operation may be performed after one year for its removal (Chapter XIV).

EXCESS CALLUS FORMATION

(Exclusive of Myositis Ossificans)

Excess callus formation in the region of the elbow is not at all the same thing as myositis ossificans. Excess callus occurs beneath the stripped up periosteum, beneath the muscle, is adjacent to the bone, and not separated from the bone by a normal clear zone on roentgen examination. The main treatment for such a condition, if noted on roentgenograms, is to leave the condition alone and to curtail the patient's activities. No operation is indicated except possibly very late if some of this callus becomes excessive in amount and is in a position where it may interfere with joint flexion. It is usually advisable to allow the child to grow out of the condition if he will.

PERIARTICULAR FIBROSIS AND CAPSULAR CONTRACTURE

Periarticular fibrosis and capsular contracture are usually due to extensive hemorrhage around the elbow joint with marked infiltration of cells into the capsule and the addition of fibroblasts which thicken the capsular structures and make these less elastic as well as to cause the capsule to become adherent in part to the articular cartilage. If attempts have been made during treatment to stretch the joint, this may have been the cause for the increased amount of fibrous thickening. As a late result, however, if it is reasonably certain that there is no bony block to flexion and extension and that the limited motion is due to thickening and fibrosis of the capsule, it may be possible to improve joint motion by performing surgical release of the entire anterior capsule as advocated by Wilson. This consists of a lateral incision exposing the anterior aspect of the humerus immediately above the elbow joint and detaching the entire capsule from the front of the bone well over to its medial side. Extension is then carried out and the capsule is stripped downwards. There is some hazard to this operation, however, in that occasionally extension of the elbow may stretch the median or radial nerve and cause a temporary paralysis. This must be carefully guarded against.

SYNOSTOSIS

Much has been said in the chapters on treatment of elbow fractures to suggest some of the causes of synostosis occurring between the upper radius and ulna and what may be done to avoid the occurrence of such a condition. The main single, but not the only, cause following a fracture is an operative attempt to replace a displaced radial head epiphysis. Synostosis is a distressing disability in which treatment is difficult and discouraging. Usually the condition is long-standing, and atrophy of the muscles that perform the normal rotary motion at the elbow joint—the supinator muscles and the pronator teres and pronator quadratus muscles—results. Following surgical correction of a synostosis it is difficult, if not impossible, to get the patient to perform rotary motions owing to atrophy and prolonged disuse of these essential muscles. As a result, the synostosis usually recurs since there remains a large raw surface on each bone across which new bony callus may form. There is probably no condition which is more difficult to correct successfully.

Congenital synostosis between the radius and ulna may be unilateral or bilateral. No immediate operative treatment is indicated in the new-born. The child should be watched for several years and may adapt to the disability remarkably well. If the patient is greatly handicapped at eight to ten years of age, operation could be undertaken with the forearm subsequently held in mid-rotation in case it "re-freezes."

The *treatment* of a synostosis consists of excision of the radial head and the bony bridge attaching this to the ulna. Hemostasis must be perfect and it is advisable to insert between the raw surfaces of these two bones some form of material which will prevent or "discourage" the re-union of the two bones by bony callus. Tantulum foil might be used or a vitallium or stainless steel cap may be placed over the tip of the radius, the latter to act very much as does a Smith-Petersen cup in a hip joint arthroplasty. Recently the author has had success in correcting two cases of synostosis by covering the

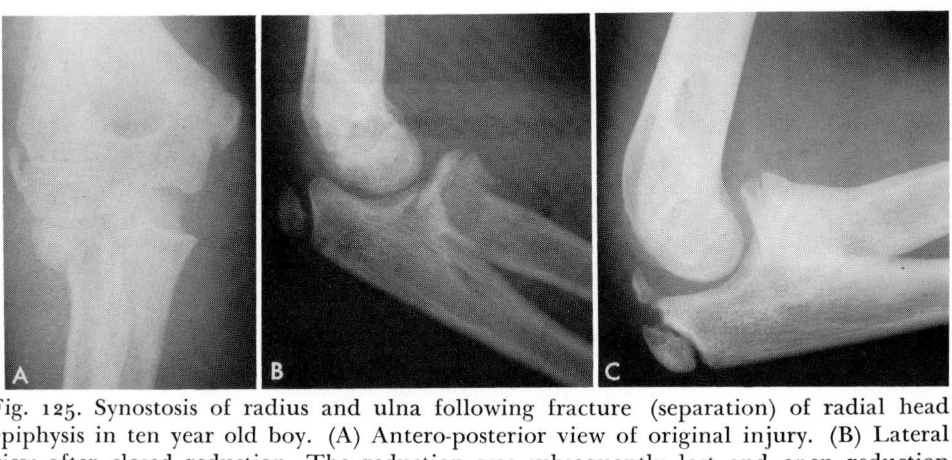

Fig. 125. Synostosis of radius and ulna following fracture (separation) of radial head epiphysis in ten year old boy. (A) Antero-posterior view of original injury. (B) Lateral view after closed reduction. The reduction was subsequently lost and open reduction was then performed on the seventh day after injury. (C) Lateral view six and one-half months later showing synostosis between radius and ulna. (The mistake in this case was not performing the open reduction within the first two days after the original injury.)

raw bone surfaces with several layers of oxidized cellulose (Oxycel). No recurrence of the synostosis followed and the return of active pronation and supination was excellent in both cases. Following such operative correction it is of the utmost importance to obtain the patient's cooperation in performing frequent pronation and supination exercises. These should be carried out always within pain limits so as not to cause further damage or bleeding which would almost certainly aid recurrence of a synostosis.

ANKYLOSIS

Fortunately today ankylosis is not common following fracture or dislocation in the region of the elbow. This is largely because present day treatment is directed towards early restoration of joint function rather than making an attempt to restore and preserve the anatomy without regard to function as was formerly the case. Ankylosis may occur following severe crushing or shattering injuries where it has been necessary to give a certain amount of immobilization and where it has been impossible to get the patient to begin early function. It is also seen following compound fractures that have become infected and result in bony ankylosis of the joint. Ankylosis may occur between the humerus and the ulna only, leaving the superior radio-ulnar joint completely free to pronate and supinate. Such an elbow may be a very useful one with its rotary function preserved and there may be no definite indication for operating upon and attempting to correct the stiffness of the humero-ulnar joint. This of course will depend entirely upon the position

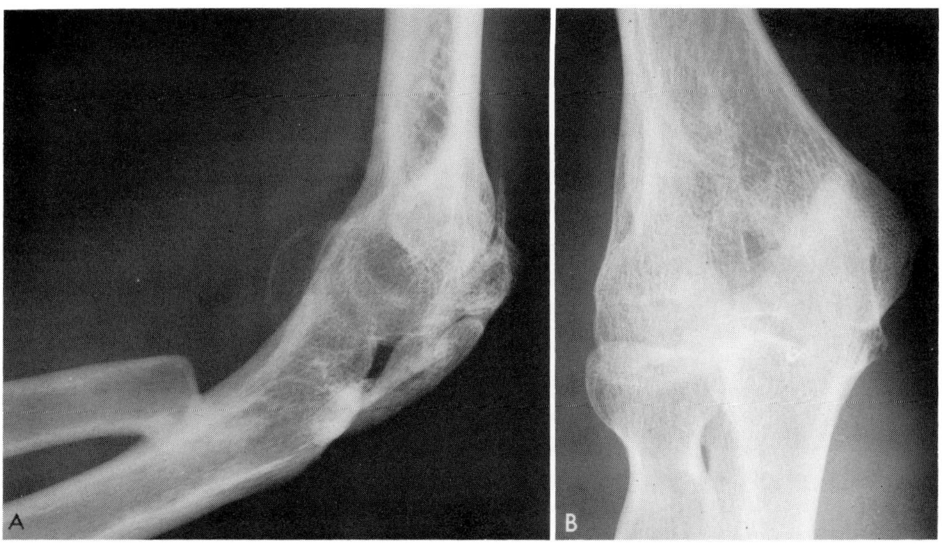

Fig. 126. Bony ankylosis of the elbow. (A) In partial flexion. This was in a 29 year old man who had received an open (compound) fracture of the radial head and olecranon four years previously. (B) In extension. This patient was 22 years old and his elbow had been ankylosed for 12 years following fracture, operation, infection and manipulation.

of the ankylosis and what particular function the patient has to perform with this arm in his daily routine. More serious, however, is complete bony ankylosis where the radius, humerus and ulna are entirely ankylosed as one bone. This may leave the elbow (or even the entire arm) completely useless because it is ankylosed in complete extension or in so much flexion that the patient is unable to reach with it. If both elbows by chance should become ankylosed which, of course, is an extremely rare condition following trauma (though not so rare following rheumatoid arthritis), one elbow should be in a position of moderate extension and the other should be in a position where the patient can get his hand to his face and mouth. If it is deemed advisable and the patient demands operation for improving motion in the joint, several types of arthroplasty may be offered him.

Before arthroplasty is undertaken on any such joint the surgeon must give careful consideration to the occupation of the patient, his desire for a movable elbow and, most of all, he should try to determine whether he believes this particular patient is one who will cooperate thoroughly in carrying out elbow exercises following an arthroplasty procedure. If he is not the type of individual who will continue to exercise his elbow for at least six months to one year, there is very little use in attempting an arthroplasty operation. Some patients seem to get the impression that they have to do nothing for

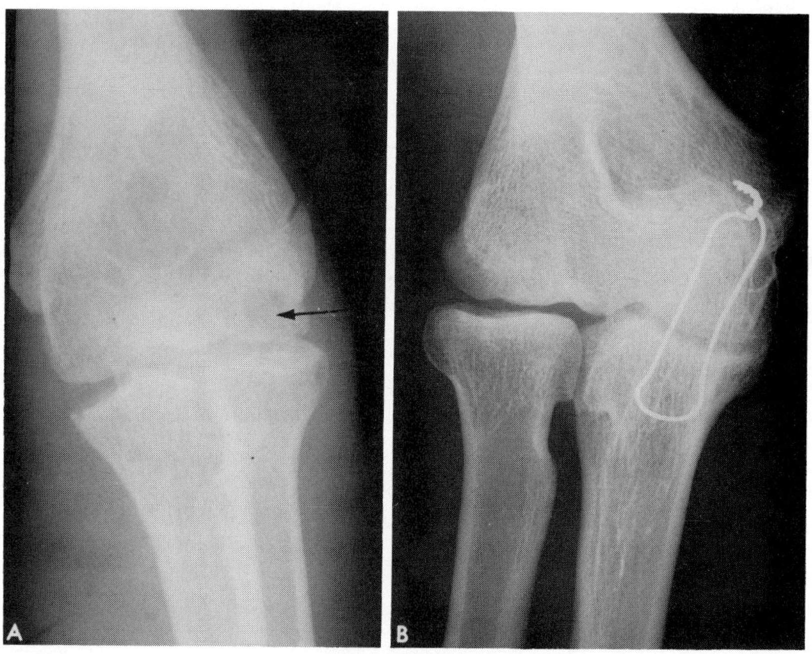

Fig. 127. Osteochondritis dissecans (Panner's disease) of the capitellum. (A) Original antero-posterior view in 14 year old boy complaining of pain on motion. The degenerated cartilage on capitellum was removed with sharp scalpel and a loose body was removed. (B) Same elbow five years after operation. (Print reversed.) The wire loop was used to repair the olecranon which was transected for exposure of the joint. *Result:* excellent.

themselves and that the operation will accomplish the entire purpose. These patients are not only a disappointment to themselves, but to the surgeon as well and cause him to perform what is essentially an unnecessary operation. There are in general two types of elbow joint arthroplasties, the functional type as advocated by Haas and the anatomical type as described by MacAusland. (For details of arthroplastic procedures the reader is referred to the Chapter XXIV.)

OSTEOCHONDRITIS DISSECANS

Osteochondritis dissecans in the elbow joint usually follows trauma and may even be seen following repeated small traumas without actual fracture or dislocation. The lesion consists of a degeneration of the articular cartilage of the humerus mainly in the capitellar region or in the radial head. Occasionally a fragment of articular cartilage becomes loose and acts as a loose body within the joint. This is sometimes seen in baseball pitchers where it is often called a "chipped elbow." It usually causes pain, limited motion and disability. The treatment at the beginning is rest and heat. If this does not bring about sufficient relief and return of function, operation is indicated for the purpose of removing loose bodies and shaving off degenerated, soft fissured articular cartilage that may interfere with perfectly smooth motion within the joint. If the condition is allowed to progress too far, synovitis or even traumatic arthritis may develop in which the prognosis for continued strenuous activities is poor following any form of treatment.

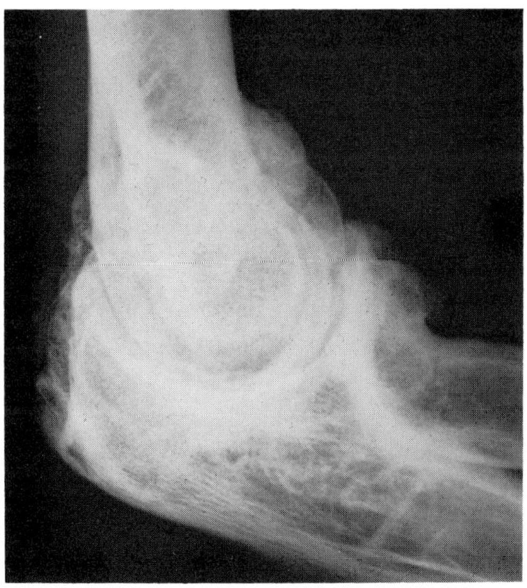

Fig. 128. Post-traumatic arthritis of the elbow joint.

TRAUMATIC ARTHRITIS

Traumatic arthritis results from long standing irritation in the elbow joint following injury which causes roughening of the joint surfaces, lipping of their margins, thinning of the joint space and marked thickening of the synovial lining. Conservative treatment consists of rest and heat, and if the patient cannot return to his usual work following moderate rest, operation may be indicated. The operation usually consists of a modified "house-cleaning" of the joint, such as is sometimes necessary in the knee joint. It may be necessary only to remove the radial head, provided the offending pathology is limited to this bone. Frequently, the synovial lining is edematous and thrown up into thick, long, villus-like folds which are extremely hyperemic. It may be necessary to excise a considerable portion of this redundant and edematous synovial tissue. If an extensive operation is necessary such as a "house-cleaning" of the joint, the probable best exposure is via a trans-olecranon approach, repairing the olecranon at the end of operation by means of a sturdy wire loop (No. 22 gauge) or by means of a long screw. After such a thorough cleaning-out of the joint, it is often advisable to permit only limited activities, otherwise the patient is extremely likely to develop further symptoms and disability within the joint.

VOLKMANN'S CONTRACTURE

Volkmann's contracture is the result of ischaemia usually following a supracondylar fracture or occasionally following an elbow joint dislocation in which there has been marked interference with the blood supply to the forearm. (The reader is referred to the Chapter XIV for discussion as to the treatment of this particular serious complication.)

Chapter XXII

Conditions in the Elbow Region Due to Trauma Other than Fracture or Dislocation

LOOSE BODIES

LOOSE BODIES in the elbow joint composed of bone and cartilage may form as a result of minor repeated traumas or as a result of osteochondritis dissecans. These by constant irritation may set up a synovitis causing continued formation of loose bodies which may bring about the condition known as osteochondromatosis. If such occurs, the elbow presents a rather bizarre picture of multiple loose bodies and very little joint space. The usual presenting symptoms are disability from limited motion and pain on certain motions preventing the individual from carrying out his usual work. Treatment consists of operative removal of the loose bodies and removal also of arthritic spurs and redundant, edematous synovial tissue. The prognosis in such cases should always be guarded since loose bodies may be over-looked at the time of the operative procedure or there may be further formation of these bodies following operation.

CHRONIC SYNOVITIS

The elbow may become the site of chronic irritation with effusion into the joint oftentimes showing limited motion and pain. It is difficult to differentiate this from such conditions as tuberculosis except by aspiration of joint fluid, inoculation into a guinea pig and by skin testing with tuberculin. At times it may be necessary even to perform biopsy of the synovial lining to rule out tuberculosis. The physical signs usually are a mildly swollen elbow with generalized thickening of the synovial lining plus some excess fluid within the joint and with limited flexion and extension. Tenderness is rarely very marked. The joint may show repeated collections of fluid with interim phases of appearance and disappearance of the symptoms as well. If repeated attacks do not respond completely to rest and the milder forms of physiotherapy, it may be advisable to explore the joint for the possibility of non-opaque loose bodies and redundant synovial tissue that may be getting pinched from joint motion. The surgeon should be guarded in his prognosis and not guarantee any real success from such an operative procedure. The advantages of operation must also be weighed of course against the risks, such as possible infection, however slight this may be.

CHRONIC BURSITIS OF THE OLECRANON BURSA
(Miner's Elbow)

Chronic bursitis of the olecranon bursa (formerly known as miner's elbow) results usually from one or more attacks of acute bursitis which in turn is the result of contusion. The initial trauma causes a collection of blood or synovial fluid within the bursa, which may respond to aspiration and compression dressings without recurrence. If the presence of fluid persists in the bursa, the sac usually becomes thick-walled and chronically inflamed. This leaves an enlarged bursa over the point of the olecranon which gives an unsightly prominence. It rarely causes pain or loss of function.

The treatment of chronic olecranon bursitis is not so simple as it might seem. Several forms of treatment are frequently tried, some of which are not without danger from the standpoint of causing infection within the bursal sac and possibly within the bone beneath the floor of the bursa. The types of treatment that may cause such infection are (1) aspiration which may intro-

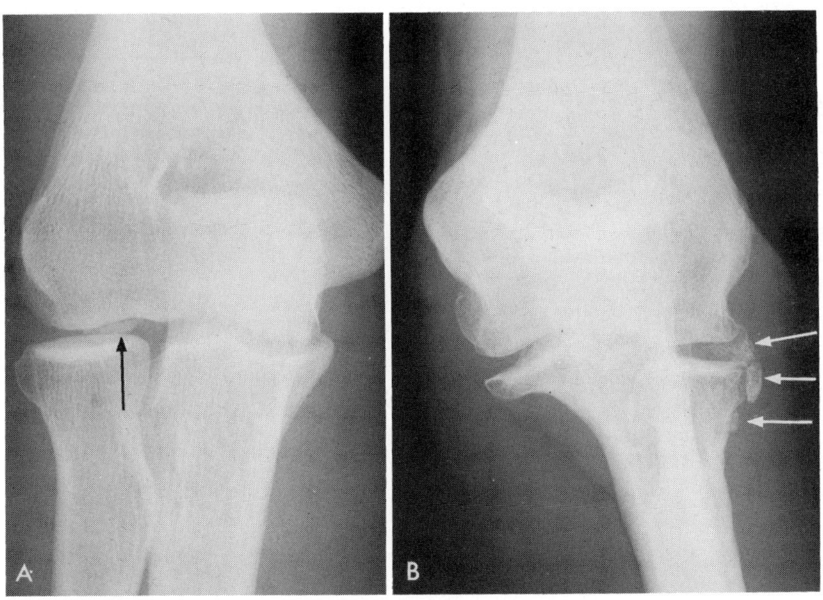

Fig. 129. Loose bodies in elbow joint. (A) Single loose body in joint between capitellum and radial head. No known trauma in this patient. (B) Three loose bodies at margin of radial head causing locking. This latter patient 20 years previously had sustained a marginal fracture of the radial head at the age of 22 years. Operation had been performed and the broken off fragment had been removed, but the main portion of the head was left in situ. She was free from symptoms for 20 years when the locking suddenly occurred. Operation was required to remove the loose bodies and radial head.

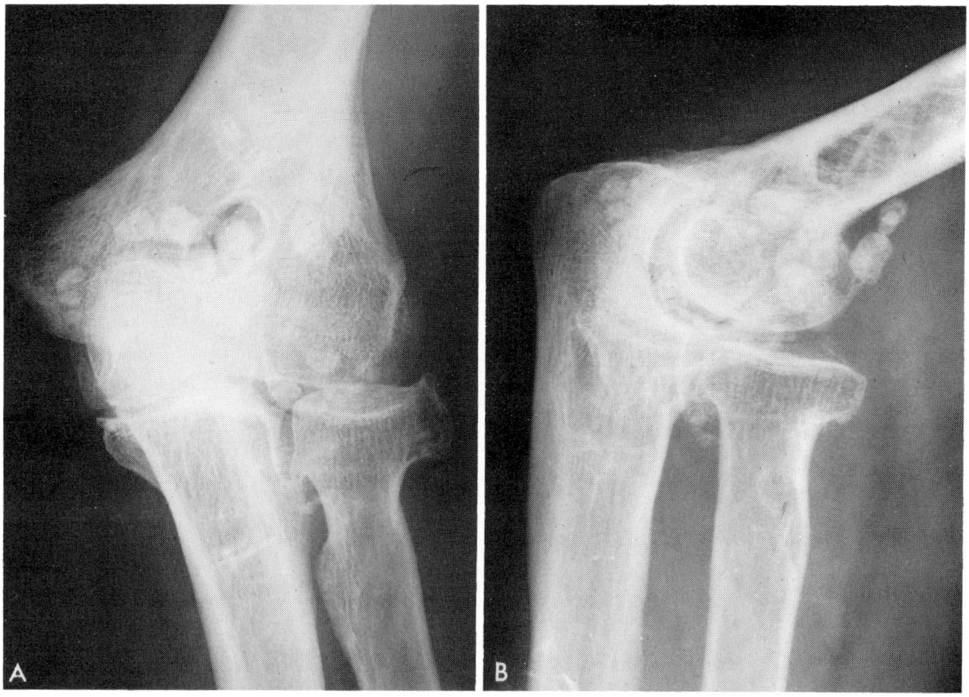

Fig. 130. Osteochondromatosis (multiple loose bodies) of elbow joint. (A) and (B) Antero-posterior and lateral views of elbow joint. Flexion and extension of joint limited and painful at the extremes.

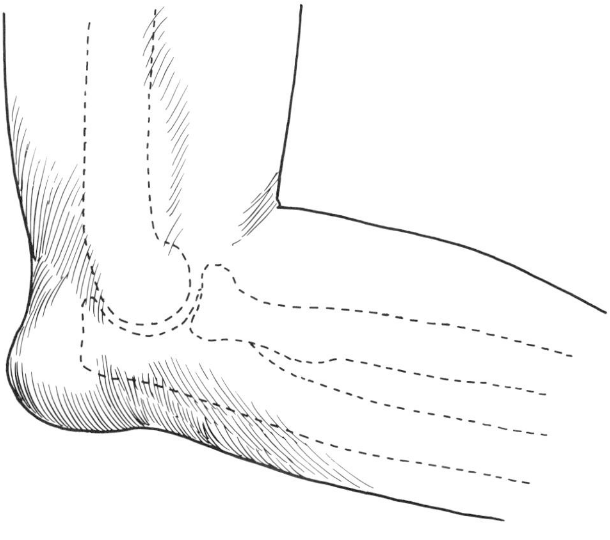

Fig. 131. Sketch of olecranon bursa distended with fluid over-lying the point of the olecranon process. This is often called "miner's elbow."

duce a few organisms into the bursal sac; (2) injection of sclerosing fluids which may cause necrosis of the skin over-lying the bursa; or (3) injudicious attempts at excision which, if without splint protection against extension of the elbow joint, may allow separation of the skin edges with the introduction of organisms into the deeper tissues.

It is the author's belief that the surest and safest way of relieving the patient of a chronically infected olecranon bursa is by operative removal. This must not be done as an office procedure. It should be performed in a completely equipped operating room where all facilities are available and where asepsis is complete. If the bursa is large, an ellipse of skin should be excised with it. A transverse incision is better than a longitudinal one and it may be planned to include an ellipse of skin. The reason for removing the ellipse is partly to remove extra skin and partly to remove skin that may be thinned out, attenuated, have a poor blood supply and be subject to poor healing after closure. The bursa itself should be dissected cleanly; all bleeders should be clamped and ligated and hemostasis should be perfect. The bursal wall is very often adherent to periosteum and bone over-lying the tip of the olecranon, and, if necessary, the periosteum should be removed from the olecranon with a sharp bone elevator. Hemostasis of the bone itself may be achieved by hot compresses or by cellulose gauze, or even by electrocautery. Closure of the skin with subcutaneous tissue should be accomplished with interrupted silk sutures and a compression dressing should be applied to the elbow and the joint kept in partial extension to enhance wound healing. It is wise to forbid more acute flexion of the elbow than a right angle for a period of ten days to two weeks until wound healing is perfect.

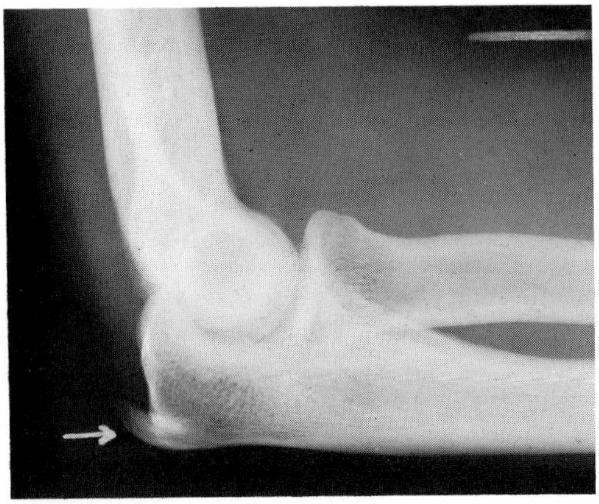

Fig. 132. Olecranon spur (exostosis). These sometimes become fractured and cause pain by the constant pull of the triceps tendon in which they lie.

EPICONDYLITIS (TENNIS ELBOW)

The condition commonly called "tennis elbow" is an inflammatory reaction in the periosteum over-lying the lateral epicondyle and in the conjoined tendon of the extensor muscles attached to this epicondyle. This apparently results from constant trauma and tension of this tendon upon its attachment to the epicondyle. It is manifested by pain, which is more or less constant, and aggravated by any motions which tend to increase the tension of this group of muscles at its source of origin from the epicondyle. The physical signs are tenderness directly over or below the lateral epicondyle and increased pain on such motions as resisted extension and supination of the wrist. Roentgen examination is frequently negative. Occasionally a small deposit of calcium is seen just distal to the summit of the lateral epicondyle.

Treatment is usually conservative and best carried out by some form of heat and rest. Heat may be applied to the elbow in any one of the usual forms, such as moist hot compresses, hot water bags, soaks in hot water, diathermy, radiant heat, etc. Massage may also be given with benefit. Occasionally it may be necessary to resort to the injection of the area with one percent procaine hydrochloride solution. This, however, is usually not advisable unless the condition does not clear up following other conservative forms of therapy. If this is not sufficient, it may even be necessary to operate and release the tendinous attachment from this epicondyle. The rationale of this form of treatment apparently is to change the status of the pull of the tendon on the periosteum and also to change the status of the local circulation. This does more actual good than the excision of any collection of calcium in the neighborhood of this tendon.

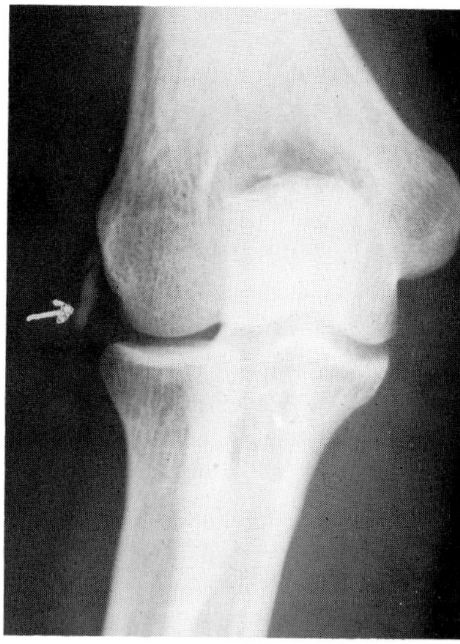

Fig. 133. Acute "bursitis" of radiohumeral bursa with calcium deposit. This patient was treated with radiotherapy, but the pain was aggravated and she was unable to sleep for three days. The calcium was then washed out through aspirating needles, employing 1 per cent procaine hydrochloride with immediate and lasting relief of pain and without recurrence in more than six years.

Whatever form of conservative therapy is carried out, however, the most important part of the treatment seems to be rest, and rest is not sufficiently obtained without the use of a cock-up splint for the wrist. A cock-up splint may be built of a plaster-of-Paris molded splint or it may be obtained through the use of one of the commercial metal or plastic cock-up splints. The purpose of the splint is to put the extensor muscles of the wrist and hand in relaxation which thereby relieves the tension of these tendons at their attachment to the lateral epicondyle. Cases treated with the wrist cocked-up in this fashion seem to recover much more quickly and much more completely than those treated by physiotherapy without such relaxation of the wrist muscles.

RADIO-HUMERAL BURSITIS

A condition frequently mistaken for epicondylitis or "tennis-elbow" but much more acute in form is a true bursitis in the region of the radio-humeral joint on the lateral aspect. Although it is extremely rare to find a bursa at this anatomical site, we frequently see patients with pain in the outer aspect of the elbow and becoming very acute within twelve to twenty-four hours and not necessarily following any specific trauma. The pain becomes so acute the condition may behave exactly as does the shoulder with an acute sub-deltoid bursitis. Examination reveals marked spasm, limitation of motion, and acute tenderness. The point of maximum tenderness is lower than the lateral epicondyle and is more likely to be at the level of the radio-humeral joint. The pain is so exquisite that the patient is unable to sleep and unable to move or rotate the arm without increasing his discomfort. Roentgen examination may show a small, rather circumscribed soft deposit of calcium with not quite the same appearance as that seen in "tennis elbow." It is more like that seen in the cases of acute sub-deltoid bursitis.

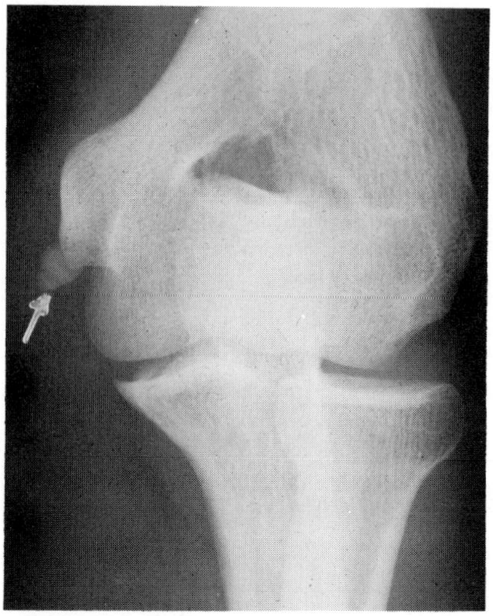

Fig. 134. Medial epicondylar "bursitis" with calcium deposit. This is not actually a bursitis, but is an acutely inflamed calcium deposit in the common tendon of origin of the flexor-pronator group of muscles. It behaves exactly like similar deposits situated below the lateral epicondyle of the humerus or in the supra-spinatus tendon. Aspiration under local anesthesia gives complete and immediate relief if performed properly in these *acutely* painful deposits.

The treatment consists either of aspiration of the bursa under local procaine infiltration or by actual operative incision and drainage. If the bursa is successfully aspirated and the patient put on a regime of frequent active exercises his relief should be almost immediate and complete. If relief is not thus obtained, incision and drainage is probably the method of choice rather than attempts at re-aspiration. Whether an actual bursa is located in this situation or not is not of particular importance; the main point is that there is a collection of soft, calcified material, visible roentgenologically, and this is either in a bursa or in a cavity in the tendon of origin of the extensor muscles and in either case it is under tension. This is the cause of the acute pain; if the tension is released, the patient is immediately relieved of his pain and disability.

MEDIAL EPICONDYLE "BURSITIS"

A condition similar to radio-humeral bursitis is very infrequently seen on the medial aspect of the elbow joint. It consists of a collection of soft calcified material just distal to the medial epicondyle of the humerus. It is doubtful that this is in a bursa. It is probably in the tendon of origin of the flexor-pronator group of muscles. The symptoms are identical to those in radio-humeral bursitis, namely, acute pain, distress, disability, and marked loss of function. The *treatment* is identical, i. e., either aspiration under procaine anesthesia or operative incision and drainage. The former is preferable and usually successful since it completely decompresses the area and gives the patient complete and instant relief.

RUPTURE OF THE BICEPS TENDON

The biceps tendon occasionally becomes ruptured near its insertion into the bicipital tuberosity of the radius or it may even be completely avulsed from its insertion into this tuberosity. In either case the cause is from a sudden jerk applied to the forearm while the patient is caught off guard. In addition to the main tear in the biceps tendon, there is usually a tear on either side of the overlying fascia. The main belly of the biceps retracts in a proximal direction with the torn or avulsed tendon surrounded by extravasated blood. Flexion of the arm is weak as is also supination of the forearm.

If the patient seeks relief early following injury, the best treatment is operative repair of the avulsed or torn tendon. If the tendon is avulsed from the bicipital tuberosity, it may be extremely difficult to re-insert this into the bone. It is possible to accomplish this by sutures applied through the tendon and through drill-holes in the tuberosity. Drill-holes may be made at right angles to each other in the tuberosity while the radius is held first in pronation and secondarily in supination and the tendon sutures may be drawn through these holes by means of a wire loop bent to pass through them. If it is too difficult to perform re-insertion of the tendon into the tuberosity, it may be best merely to attach the biceps tendon to the tendon of the brachialis anticus muscle. This will help in recovering full strength of flexion at the elbow, but, of course, will not assist in recovery of full strength of supination. It is probably advisable for the surgeon to make his decision as to whether or not he should attempt to re-insert the avulsed tendon to its original attachment or not after he has studied the existing pathology. If the patient comes late after injury, treatment is probably best carried out by suturing the biceps to the brachialis anticus tendon. Following operative repair, it is necessary to keep the tendon protected from any forced motion for a period of at least four weeks. Mild active motion and motion not against gravity or resistance may be carried out within one week after operative repair.

SPRAIN OF THE ELBOW JOINT

A sprain of the elbow joint is a very *rare* condition. It is much more likely that a fracture has occurred, such as of the radial head or of the coronoid process with or without displacement, or of the olecranon process without displacement. The patient may think that his condition is a sprain. The history of the injury plus bony tenderness, evidence of hemarthrosis or loss of function should make the examining surgeon suspicious of one of these fractures and cause him to have a roentgenological examination made. Owing to swelling it may be difficult to determine definite linear bony tenderness or to palpate bony landmarks readily without causing the patient too much distress. Should it be impossible to determine the nature of the injury readily from clinical examination, roentgen examination is definitely indicated. If no fracture is found and there is no hemarthrosis worthy of aspiration, it may be wise to treat the injured elbow by rest in a sling alternating with active motion and hot soaks at frequent intervals. Such patients should be seen once or twice a week at first to recheck for further physical signs and for improvement in joint function. If further signs develop or function does not improve, it may be advisable to try some other form of treatment such as rest in a splint for a short period to overcome muscle spasm.

In children one should *never* make the diagnosis of sprain of the elbow without first ruling out all possible epiphyseal injuries, since it is almost impossible to sprain a child's elbow without causing harm to one of the epiphyseal plates. The elbow of a child, which may have had made upon it the erroneous diagnosis of sprain, if not protected properly, may develop subsequent growth disturbance and serious deformity. This can occur since epiphyseal injuries may be present without roentgenological evidence of the same appearing on the films. Unless the surgeon or physician examining the child originally is aware that epiphyseal injuries are common and looks for them by testing for linear tenderness along the epiphyseal lines, he may fall into one of these pitfalls and not splint the epiphyseal injury properly and for a long enough period. It is far safer, if an epiphyseal injury is suspected even though not definitely known, to splint the elbow in a posterior molded splint in moderate flexion. If a recheck by clinical means reveals that the tenderness has disappeared completely within five to seven days it may be assumed that the diagnosis is a sprain and the splint may be discarded and early active motion instituted. If, on the other hand, tenderness persists for seven days or longer, it must be assumed that an epiphyseal injury has occurred and the splint should be kept in place for a period of two to three weeks or until epiphyseal tenderness disappears. This is the only safe way to treat possible epiphyseal injuries in the region of the elbow. In other words it should be assumed that the injury is more likely to be one of the epiphysis than one of the ligaments. If subsequent events disprove the epiphyseal injury, the splint may be removed and no harm will have been done, whereas the opposite may be true if the original treatment was directed as for a sprain and insufficient protection and rest given to the epiphysis.

Chapter XXIII

Non-Traumatic Conditions of the Elbow

INFECTIONS

TRUE INFECTION within the elbow joint may be classed as acute or chronic.

Acute (non-pyogenic) elbow joint infections result from the pneumococcus, gonococcus, meningococcus, B. typhosus, etc., all of which are blood-borne and not true surgical infections. They are usually treated by rest (splinting) and by antibiotic therapy (local instillation into the joint after aspiration and by the general administration of the drug). These infections formerly resulted in frequent bony ankylosis of the joint and still may do so. If the infection is not combatted properly and early, it would be highly advisable to splint the elbow for rest in a useful position, i. e., the most optimum one for ankylosis should such stiffening seem probable.

Suppurative arthritis occurs in this as in other joints and is serious from the standpoint of destroying function in the joint. This type of infection may be blood-borne, but more probably results from external contamination due to a compound fracture, compound dislocation, puncture or bullet wound. The organisms commonly causing this type of infection are the staphylococcus aureus, hemolytic streptococcus, and B. pyocyaneus. Infection by any of these leads to pus formation, early destruction of the joint cartilages, severe pain, distention of the joint capsule and the likelihood of fibrous or bony ankylosis. Surgical measures must be instituted early to save the joint from complete destruction. Aspiration of joint fluid for smear and culture not only permit determination of the infective organism, but will lead to proper antibiotic therapy should the organism prove to be sensitive to one of the drugs. Such therapy may be administered locally by instillation of the drug into the joint or by its general administration. Rest (splinting and/or traction) will help to diminish articular cartilage destruction. Elevation will assist venous and lymphatic drainage and thereby improve the circulation locally and in general to the infected part.

If, in spite of all these measures, pain, distention, fever and leucocytosis continue, it must be assumed that additional measures of treatment are necessary. This would best be carried out by performing adequate surgical drainage of the joint by opening it on both the medial and posterolateral aspects, especial care being taken to avoid damage to the ulnar nerve. Drains may be placed down to, but never into the joint. The wounds and joint may

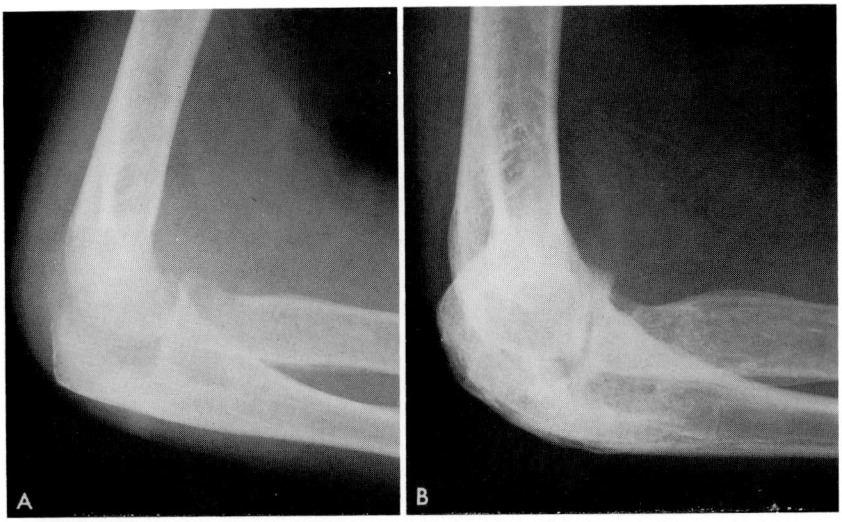

Fig. 135. Tuberculosis of the elbow joint. Note destruction of the bone adjacent to the greater sigmoid notch of the ulna in (A) original lateral film. (B) Lateral view 16 months after operative arthrodesis of the elbow (Hallock type). The disease has been arrested clinically and roentgenologically. The use of anti-tuberculosis drugs is at the present time indicated in addition to bony fusion.

be irrigated at the time of drainage and daily thereafter with a solution of penicillin (5000 units per cc.) or any other antibiotic to which the infective organisms are sensitive until the infection is well under control. Mild active motion every few hours will assist drainage of this joint. Care must be employed to prevent too early closure of the drainage incisions as long as residual exudate can be washed out of the joint at the time of dressing. Chemotherapy or antibiotic therapy, however, should minimize this time, thereby lessening joint destruction, morbidity and disability time and offering a very much better prognosis than without its use.

Chronic infection in this joint is usually of one or two varieties: tuberculous and rheumatoid arthritis.

Tuberculosis of the elbow joint as with other joints is fortunately much less common than it was twenty-five or more years ago in the United States. However, in countries where dairy control by tuberculin testing of cattle and pasteurization of milk is either absent, or not well regulated, there will continue to be found a high incidence of bone and joint tuberculosis.

The symptoms and signs of elbow joint *tuberculosis* are pain, limitation of flexion and extension, spasm at the extremes of these motions when tested passively, swelling, increased warmth over the joint, and atrophy of the arm and forearm muscles. The swelling consists of thickening in the periarticular tissues as well as increase in the joint fluid. It often appears greater than it actually is owing to muscular atrophy above and below the joint which tends to accentuate its size. The onset is often slow and insidious and sinus formation may develop. In present day practice assisted by roentgen examination there should be no great delay in establishing the diagnosis. Roentgen films in the early case may show nothing other than mild local decalcification of the bone ends forming the joint. Later there will appear increased decalcification of these bones and very likely partial destruction of the joint surfaces or loss of surface distinction of these bones.

To assist in making the diagnosis of tuberculosis, the history is of importance in respect to infection in other members of the family or infection of this nature in the patient himself (pulmonary, lymph node, or other joint). The patient should be given a Mantoux test and observed at 48 hours. This may not be of great importance in adults if positive, but if negative, active tuberculous joint infection is highly improbable. In early cases with negative roentgenologic findings it is advisable to aspirate the joint, make a smear of some of centrifuged fluid obtained and stain and examine for acid-fast organisms. Some of this same fluid, if negative for growth on ordinary culture media, should be tested by inoculation into a guinea pig. Any distended joint resulting from trauma should have its fluid injected into a guinea pig if the aspiration yields turbid yellow rather than bloody fluid, so that there will not result needless delay in establishing the diagnosis and instituting proper therapy.

There may still result insufficient evidence to establish the diagnosis as definitely tuberculous and it may be necessary to perform operative biopsy of the synovial membrane. In hospitals with well equipped pathological laboratories and experienced pathologists a quick-frozen section may be made. If the diagnosis is definite for tuberculosis, operative fusion of the joint may be carried out. If any doubt in the diagnosis exists on examination of the biopsy specimen, or if the pathologists prefer to examine permanent paraffin sections, then the wound should be closed and further operative treatment reserved for a later date.

The **treatment** of tuberculosis of the elbow joint, once the diagnosis has been definitely established, is preferably operative fusion. This is the only means by which definite cure of the local disease can be expected since this method alone puts the joint at *complete* rest. The future may see cures of tuberculous joint disease by means of immobilization in plaster plus the intensive use of streptomycin or other antibiotic. When it becomes necessary to ankylose the joint surgically, due consideration must be given as to whether it is the patient's right or left elbow, to his occupation, and to his other needs with this arm. The joint must therefore be arthrodesed in the optimum position for the particular patient (see Chapter XXIV).

ARTHRITIS

Five types of arthritis affect the elbow joint:—rheumatoid, osteo-arthritis, post-traumatic arthritis, non-specific arthritis, osteochondritis dissecans.

1. **Rheumatoid** arthritis may affect one or both elbows and other joints

at the same time. It is due to infection usually from the hemolytic streptococcus. The primary focus cannot always be found, but teeth and tonsils may be at fault.

It is beyond the scope of this work to go into the course and treatment of this disease in general, but certain surgical aspects must be considered.

Owing to pain and spasm from the inflammatory reaction in the subsynovial tissues these patients rest their elbows by flexing them acutely. There may thus result either partial (fibrous) or complete (bony) ankylosis of the joint, since the inflammatory reaction may last for many months during which time the patient moves his elbow as little as possible. Subsequent active exercises and other rehabilitating measures will do but little or nothing to assist him in regaining motion. Since bi-lateral involvement of the elbow is not uncommon in this disease, patients so afflicted become severely disabled through loss of elbow extension and their inability to reach. It is with such patients that surgical measures may be carried out and the treatment may be considered here.

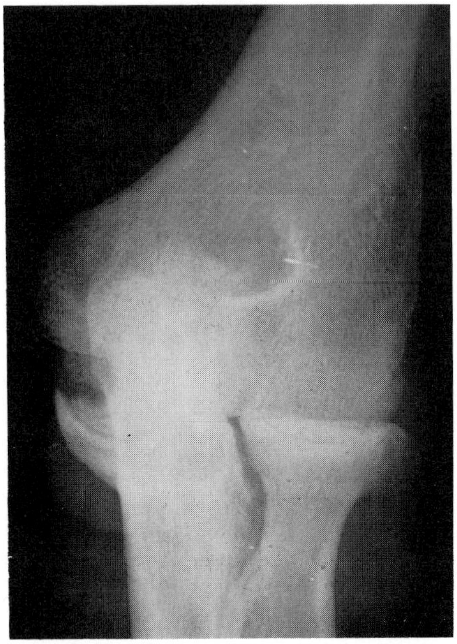

Fig. 136. Rheumatoid arthritis of the elbow joint. Antero-posterior roentgenogram showing narrowed joint space.

The treatment of bi-lateral ankylosis of the elbow must be directed to overcoming the flexed position in one of these joints. With both joints ankylosed it is important to have one in such a position that the patient may get his hand to his face for eating, washing, shaving, etc., but the other must be in a position of some extension (roughly 135 degrees) for reaching, carrying, caring for toilet necessities, etc. The flexed and ankylosed joint (if it lacks active rotation) must be in a position of mid-rotation or slight pronation. One method of securing extension is to osteotomize the site of ankylosis and place the bones in a position of optimum extension and permit it to become re-ankylosed. The other method of treatment for such a joint (and probably the better) would be to perform an arthroplasty after the method of MacAusland (Chapter XXIV). This of course must *not* be performed while the disease is still locally active as evidenced by pain, fever, local tenderness and elevated sedimentation rate. If performed after the inflammatory process has subsided, the prognosis for a movable, useful, and painless joint is good. Following such operative procedure it will be necessary for the patient to practice active exercises for a prolonged period of time (six months minimum) in order to regain motion range, strength, and stability.

At any time during the first two or three months if it becomes evident that the inflammatory process has become re-activated, care should be taken to prevent subsequent renewal of the flexion contracture. Splint must be applied to keep the elbow extended as long as there is a possibility of ankylosis recurring.

2. **Osteoarthritis** of the elbow joint is not a common condition. It probably follows trauma (fracture into the joint, dislocation, repeated strains, and hard usage). It may also occur as a late result following osteochondritis dissecans. The joint surfaces become roughened and irregular, their margins showing proliferative lipping and overhanging edges, and the joint space as seen on the roentgenogram is greatly narrowed (see Fig. 128). A certain amount of chronic synovitis accompanies the bony and cartilaginous changes and gives rise to periarticular thickening and excess fluid formation within the joint. The entire joint may become involved in the process. However, the bony and cartilaginous changes may be limited largely to the head of the radius and to the capitellar process of the humerus. This type is usually the result of an old fracture of the radial head which was permitted to heal in a position of mal-union and which became a constant source of irritation as it moved upon the capitellum. Such mal-union and irritation result in irregular and eccentric enlargement of the radial head. Adhesions of a fibrous nature may also form between the radial head and a portion of the joint lining. This pathology will therefore give rise to a limited range of motion, pain on motion or on the extremes of motion (including rotation).

Should the arthritic process be limited to the radial head and lateral half of the articular surface of the humerus, the treatment is simple and satisfactory, namely excision of the radial head (see Chapter XXI). Where the osteoarthritic process involves a considerable portion of the joint, treatment may consist of rest (sling and curtailment of activity), heat, gentle massage, and mild sedation. Should these measures fail to relieve pain and should disability continue, operative exploration may be carried out and a "house-cleaning" of the joint performed.

A painful joint with limited motion may often thus be rendered painless, useable, and strong. Were the results successful for a period of only five years, it would still be a useful procedure. It could always be followed by an arthroplasty in an individual occupied in a skilled trade requiring elbow motion.

3. **Post-traumatic** arthritis of the elbow joint is similar in its nature, symptomatology and treatment to osteoarthritis (see above).

4. **Non-specific** arthritis may occur in this joint as in other joints. It is usually manifested by gradual onset of chronic swelling (synovial tissue thickening and excess fluid formation in the joint), little or no limitation of flexion or extension, mild pain, lack of increased heat and lack of tenderness. There is usually no spasm or atrophy. Other acute or chronic infectious processes and foci must be ruled out. Gout and allergic conditions must also

be found lacking. Roentgen examination reveals no characteristic changes in the bones or the joint surfaces. The pathology consists mainly of a synovitis.

Treatment should be directed towards rest, gentle compression with elastic bandage, the milder forms of heat and massage, and repeated aspirations to remove the excess fluid within the joint. Should this fail to relieve the condition, it would be highly advisable to explore the joint, obtain biopsy of the synovial lining, subsynovial tissues, and even to perform a partial synovectomy.

5. **Osteochondritis dissecans** in the elbow joint is a form of arthritis caused by trauma or the result of embolic obstruction in the terminal vessels of one of the humeral condyles (see Fig. 127). It occurs more commonly upon the anterior or antero-inferior aspect of the articular surface of the capitellum, but it may occur on the trochlear process. An irregular shallow crater caused by a defect in the articular cartilage extends down to the underlying bone. The detached and degenerated articular cartilage may give rise to one or more loose bodies within the joint and cause episodes of locking and pain.

Should symptoms be sufficiently severe, operative exploration will be warranted with correction of the offending pathology. A trans-olecranon approach (Chapter XVII) is a wise one here since it is necessary to view the front and back of the joint thoroughly to rid it of loose bits of cartilage as well as to smooth off the edges of any crater on the articular surface of the capitellum. The olecranon fragment and divided triceps expansion and periosteum should be repaired as described.

NEUROTROPHIC JOINT

The elbow, though not commonly affected by neurotrophic disturbances as are the weight-bearing joints, is still subject to this condition. Briefly, a neurotrophic joint may result when certain nerve innervation of the joint is cut off as a result of disease such as in syphilis or syringomyelia. The joint presents swelling of the periarticular structures, excess fluid, weakness, instability, usually with absence of heat, tenderness or pain. (About twenty percent of Charcot joints are accompanied by pain.) Roentgenograms reveal early loss of joint architecture and this may go on to multiple loose body formation and even to extreme disintegration of all the joint surfaces. The syphilitic, neurotrophic (Charcot) joint must have its diagnosis confirmed by the history of positive serology. The spirocheata pallida is not present in the joint fluid or capsular structures on microscopic examination. The neurotrophic joint due to syringomyelia must have its diagnosis confirmed by such characteristic neurologic findings as lack of pain and temperature sensation resulting from degenerative lesions of the spino-thalmic tracts in the spinal cord.

Treatment of the neurotrophic elbow joint does not have to take into consideration the problem of weight-bearing. The treatment problem would thereby have to consider mainly disability due to weakness, lifting power, and stability of the joint in pushing or on lifting the arm over-head. Rarely is pain a problem. This type of joint is most often seen in persons of middle-age or older. If the patient has to use his elbow to a considerable extent in his work and needs a strong extremity, one of two things may be done. The conservative form of treatment should consist of support by a brace hinged at the elbow joint and fitted with leather cuffs to be laced on to the arm and forearm. The purpose of the brace is purely to lend stability to the joint to permit the patient to utilize his muscular strength for flexion and extension. Should this support fail to give adequate stability and strength to permit work and should pain likewise be present, one might be justified in performing an operative arthrodesis of the joint. Such an arthrodesis is accompanied by considerable risk of failure and should never be attempted in this particular type of joint except as a procedure of last resort.

OSTEOMYELITIS

Acute suppurative osteomyelitis of the bones in the region of the elbow most commonly results from open (compound) fractures ("truck swipe" injury, gun-shot wounds or fracture of the olecranon). Emergency treatment which is inadequate from the standpoint of complete debridement, irrigation, etc. in compound fractures, may permit infective organisms to establish a foot-hold in the traumatized tissues. Inadequate drainage and inadequate sequestrectomy (once infection has occurred) may permit its spread and allow it to get into a chronic stage.

Adequate surgery is the best means of avoiding infection following an open fracture in any region of the body (Chapter XV). Chemotherapy may be utilized as soon as there is a suggestion of infection and to greater advantage than as a prophylactic measure. It should *never* be used as a substitute for adequate surgical toilet of the contaminated wound, but only as an adjunct to this if used in connection with it, always realizing that its benefit is frequently greater to the surgeon's conscience than to the patient's wound. When the time arrives to treat an infection, one must *never* overlook the fact that wide open surgical drainage still remains a sound surgical principle in spite of the availability of all chemotherapeutic agents. This may prevent an acute suppurative osteomyelitis from passing into a chronic scarred and sclerosed osteomyelitis which is so difficult to cure except by very radical surgical measures. Scarred and sclerosed bone and surrounding soft parts may harbor infectious organisms that no amount of chemotherapy will clear up because the blood supply is so poor that no drug can be brought into adequate contact with the organisms.

Dead or sclerosed bone should be removed where possible and all pockets containing infected granulation tissue must be opened widely and eradicated, permitting soft parts to fall into and obliterate them. With the use of penicillin or some other antibiotic it may be possible to obtain primary

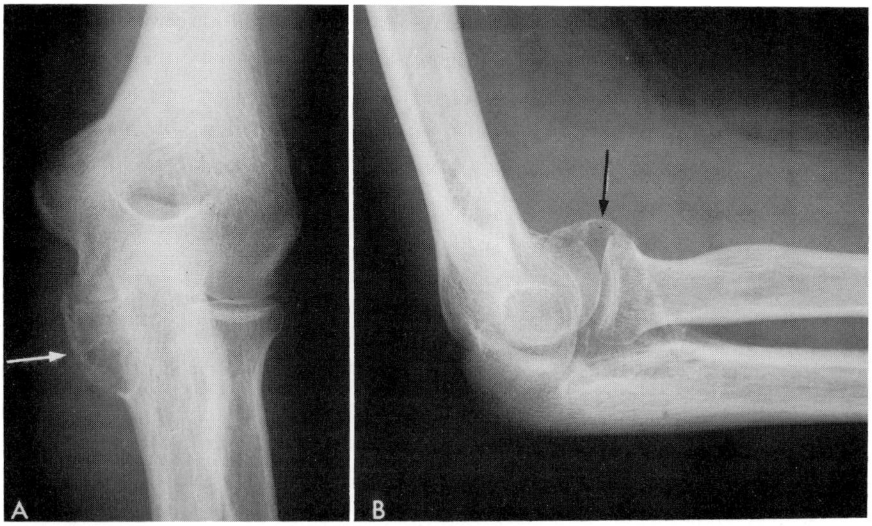

Fig. 137. Giant cell tumor of coronoid process of ulna. Biopsy and pathological examination confirmed the diagnosis. This patient, a male aged 24 years, was improved following roentgen-therapy.

(loose) closure of the wound after removal of such chronically infected bone. It is not to be considered advisable to attempt primary closure in the presence of acute infection.

Chemotherapy or other antibiotics may be used at any time in conjunction with adequate surgery in definitely infected cases. The author would strongly advise its use in such cases.

The most direct approach to the bones adjacent to the elbow must be carried out for the purposes of incision and drainage, for sequestrectomy or for removal of other dead bone and scar tissue, especial care being taken to avoid harming the radial, ulnar and median nerves, and the brachial vessels. Any one of these may be masked by scar tissue. If the incision is in the neighborhood of any one of them, the structure should be identified early and protected to avoid injury.

OSTEOID OSTEOMA

The condition known as osteoid osteoma has been observed to occur in the lower aspect of the humerus in either the medial or the lateral condyle. It is characterized by pain and subsequently by progressive sclerosis of the bone in the affected condyle, with perhaps some overlying thickening. Eventually a small cavity develops within the sclerosed area and within this a tiny nidus.

The treatment once the diagnosis has been established is wide surgical removal of the sclerosed bone, cleaning out of the granulation tissue and sequestrum within the cavity. The prognosis is excellent when surgical treatment is adequate.

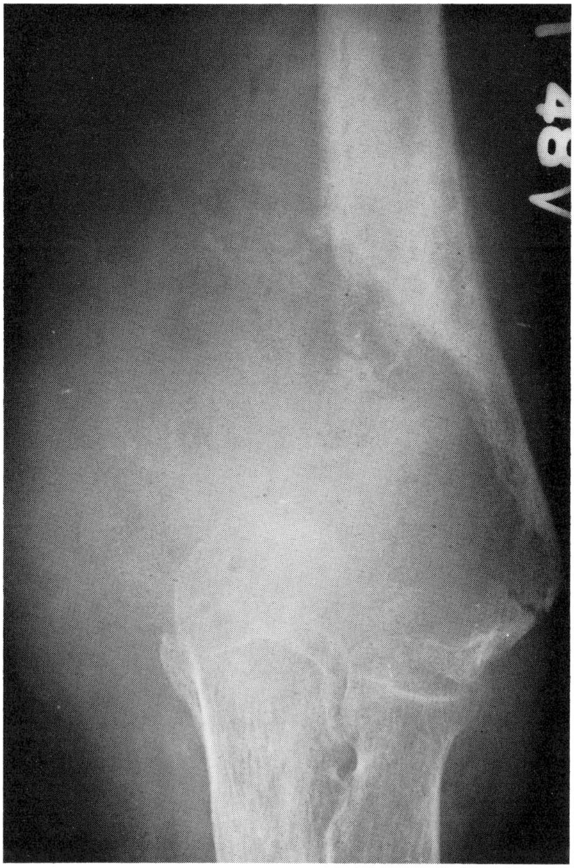

Fig. 138. Plasma cell myeloma of lower extremity of humerus. Antero-posterior roentgenogram showing marked destruction and a pathological fracture through lateral condyle.

NEOPLASMS

The elbow is not a common site for primary neoplasms, benign or malignant. Most tumefactions at this site are not neoplastic, but the result of chronic inflammation of the joint lining or of the olecranon bursa. The benign neoplasms of bony origin occurring here are osteochondromas and giant cell tumors. The latter is more common. It can involve the entire upper extremity of the ulna, but it may involve only the coronoid process of this bone. The diagnosis of this tumor can be made by characteristic roentgen findings, or, if these are not present, by biopsy. The treatment is with radiotherapy. It is practically never advisable to attempt excision of such a tumor, and it is considered bad surgery to curette and cauterize them. The treatment of osteochondromata or exostoses should be by local excision.

Primary malignant neoplasms in the region of the elbow are very *rare*. Osteogenic sarcomata or Ewing tumors may occur as tumors of bony origin. Synoviomata are highly malignant tumors arising from the synovial lining

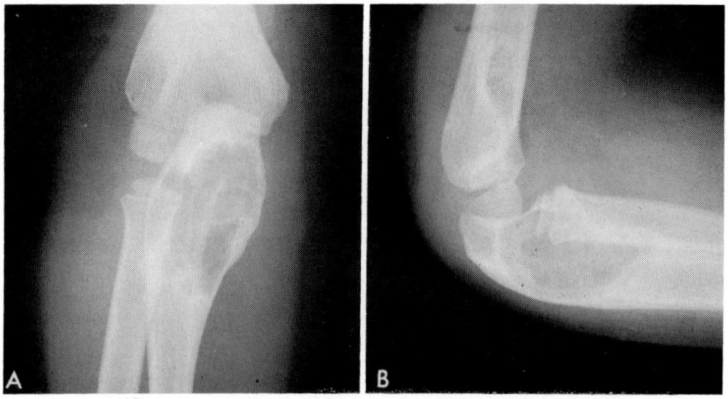

Fig. 139. Benign solitary bone cyst of upper shaft of ulna. (A) Antero-posterior, and (B) lateral roentgenograms in eight year old patient.

cells of the joint and like bone sarcomata they commonly metastasize to the lungs. The treatment except for Ewing's tumor is amputation of the arm. The treatment for Ewing's tumor is still controversial, but radiotherapy gives fair to good results considering that the over-all prognosis for any of these malignant bone tumors is none too good.

Metastatic involvement can occur from other primary tumor sites, such as the mammary gland, prostate, lung, kidney, etc. The first intimation of such skeletal metastasis may come as a result of a pathological fracture through one of these areas. Pain may precede the fracture and lead to the discovery of the lesion on roentgen examination. Such lesions if recognized as secondary lesions may be given palliative radiotherapy, but should not be operated upon. Should pathological fracture result, the arm and fragments must be given rest and quiet in order to minimize pain. This may be accomplished by splints, plaster casings or traction and suspension.

True bone cysts (osteitis fibrosa cystica) or areas of fibrous dysplasia are extremely rare in the region of the elbow. The surgeon would rarely have opportunity to diagnose one of these conditions unless his or another physician's attention were drawn to it by a roentgenogram taken because the patient had complained of pain resulting from trauma or other causes. The diagnosis would have to be based mainly upon roentgen findings, blood studies and possibly surgical biopsy. The treatment of choice is thorough curettage, cauterization of the cyst lining with phenol followed by absolute alcohol, and implantation of bone chips into the cavity.

METABOLIC DISORDERS

Gout. Enlargement of the olecranon bursa occasionally occurs due to deposits of mono-sodium urates in its wall. Such a bursa is moderately firm and in general, spherical. It is non-tender and its deep surface is firmly fixed to the underlying periosteum. The overlying skin is not inflamed and lacks the characteristic yellowish appearance of tophi seen elsewhere. The diagnosis is usually not difficult since by the time the deposit becomes large enough to cause the patient to question its presence, it is known that he has

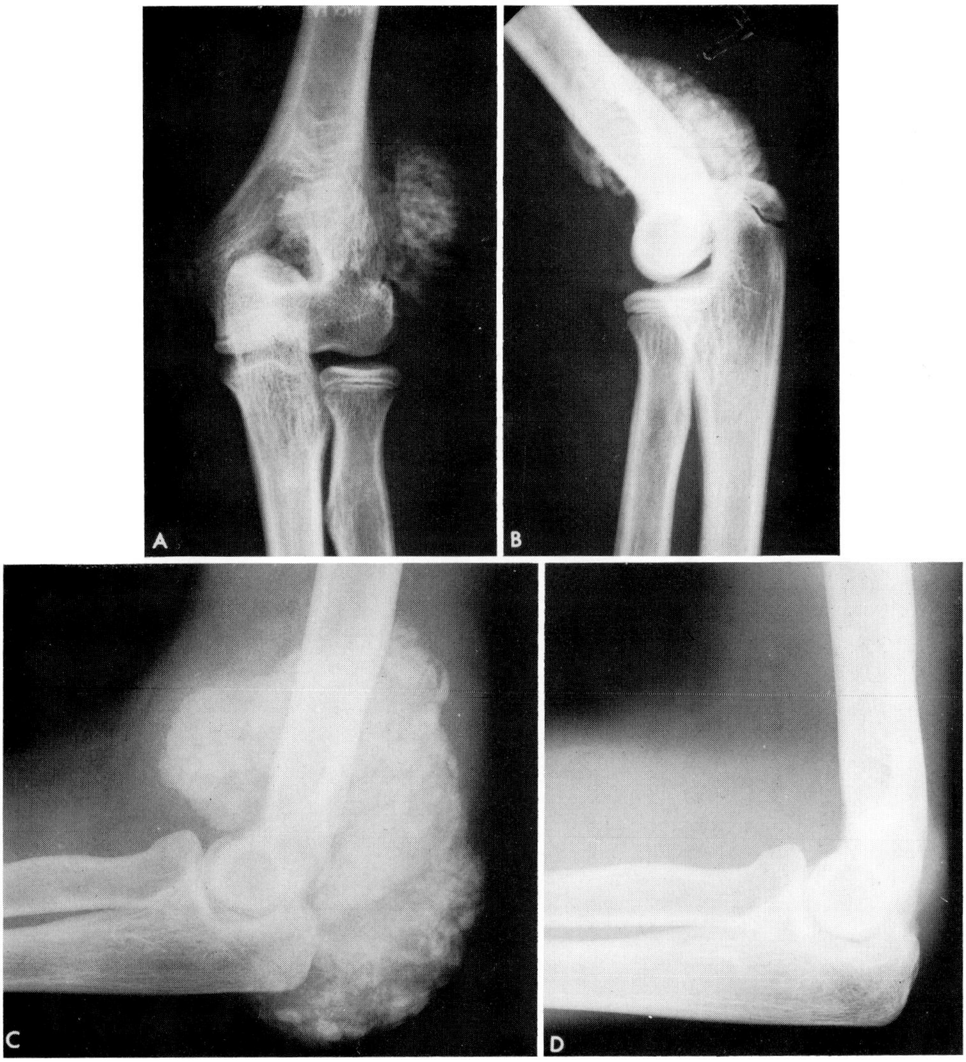

Fig. 140. Tumoral Calcinosis in an 11-year-old boy. (A) and (B) Antero-posterior and lateral roentgenograms of left elbow at age of 11 years. This patient had similar deposits in the right elbow, both trochanteric regions, one wrist and one shoulder. (C) Lateral view of left elbow at age of 16 years. Operative removal of this deposit and of those in the right elbow and both lateral hip regions was performed, because all were becoming progressively larger and unsightly. (D) Lateral view of left elbow two years after excision of the deposit. No recurrence had occurred.

gout. Some of these bursae become as large as a medium-sized plum. The treatment, if the condition fails to respond to conservative measures (purine free diet, colchicine, allopurinol) and the patient is bothered enough by the bursal enlargement, is excision. Some surgeons advise putting the patient on a course of colchicine for twenty-four hours before and following operation to forestall the possibility of an acute attack of gout.

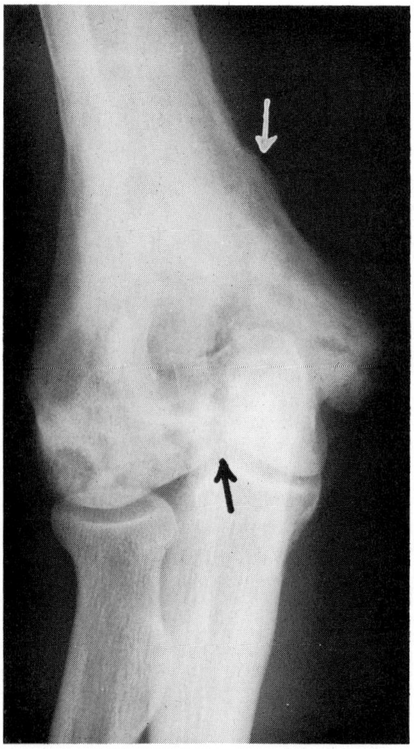

Fig. 141. Paget's disease (osteitis deformans) of lower humerus and fracture of medial condyle (healed). Arrows point to site of the old fracture line. The medial condyle fragment was essentially undisplaced. Paget's disease of bone does not interfere per se with the healing of fractures.

Xanthomatosis. Certain metabolic disturbances in which the patient has a high serum cholesterol content may give rise to deposits of cholesterol crystals in the olecranon bursa. These deposits involving part of the triceps tendon and periosteum are firmer, less freely movable and have a yellowish appearance if the overlying skin has become sufficiently thinned. The deposits often take the form of fibromas with deposits of cholesterol crystals scattered throughout. Such cholesterol deposits have a predilection for the posterior aspect of the elbow and the region of insertion of the Achilles tendon and are often symmetrical. General careful metabolic studies should be made. The treatment consists of surgical excision if the deposit bothers the patient sufficiently.

Calcinosis. Aside from deposits of calcium in the extensor tendon origin often associated with lateral epicondylitis (tennis elbow) there may occasionally appear deposits in the olecranon bursa or in a portion of the joint capsule deep to the triceps tendon and muscle called Tumoral Calcinosis by Thomson and Tanner. These may become extremely large and bizarre in clinical as well as in roentgenologic appearance since they are readily visible on films. They occur in other regions besides the elbow. The underlying metabolic condition causing them is little understood. The deposits are medical and surgical curiosities, and, after thorough metabolic studies, it may be justified in excising one or more of these masses in toto for pathological study as well as to remove them for cosmetic and functional reasons.

Paget's Disease (Osteitis Deformans). This condition may involve one or more of the bones making up the elbow joint (most commonly the humerus). It tends to involve the shaft of the bone first. Its presence is usually detected only because of pain due to fracture or other trauma. There is no particular treatment for this condition other than radiotherapy for pain. Should a fracture be present, it should be treated as any other similar fracture without particular concern for the presence of Paget's disease.

HEMOPHILIA

Persons suffering from hemophilia are subject to repeated episodes of bleeding (hemarthrosis) into one or more joints as a result of minor traumata such as contusions and sprains. The joint becomes tensely distended from the continued bleeding into it and associated with this there is severe pain. With recurrent hemarthrosis these joints are subject to partial ankylosis as a result of incomplete absorption of blood and the formation of fibrous adhesions. Roentgenologic changes occur in the bone ends of the frequently involved joints and are characterized mainly by the appearance of small cyst-like areas beneath the articular cartilage.

Treatment. *Local* treatment of a hemophilic joint consists of rest, cold compresses, and elevation to diminish the bleeding. Adequate rest and relief from pain can sometimes be obtained only by splinting. Elevation not only helps to diminish bleeding, but also lessens subsequent inflammatory swelling. As soon as pain ceases to be a factor, it is important for the patient to carry out active joint exercises in order to lessen the formation of adhesions. The unfortunate part of this type of therapy is the delay in starting exercises due to pain and to the length of time it takes to absorb the blood, which in turn permits the initiation of adhesion formation.

Hemophilia was formerly considered the one cause of hemarthrosis in which surgical aspiration of the joint for the relief of pain was contraindicated. More recently, however, it has been demonstrated conclusively by Gartland and Mac Ausland that relief of pain and absorption of the blood from the distended joint can be greatly hastened by partial aspiration in conjunction with the instillation of the enzyme *hyaluronidase.* This rids the patient of pain in hours rather than days and permits him to start exercises in days rather than after a week or two. Morbidity and hospitalization are likewise reduced by the increased permeability of the joint capsule brought about by action of this enzyme. The tendency to fibrous ankylosis is similarly reduced.

The technique of aspiration is as described in Chapter XIII. It is not necessary in these cases to remove all of the blood from the joint. A small amount (5 to 10 cubic centimeters) is removed and 1500 turbidity reducing units of hyaluronidase is dissolved in a quantity of one percent procaine hydrochloride equal to the blood removed and the whole is instilled into the joint. The aspirating needle is removed, the wound covered with a sterile dressing and the joint is wrapped with an elastic bandage. The compression afforded by this bandage is of particular importance in assisting diffusion of the blood through the joint capsule. It may be necessary to re-wrap the elastic bandage once or even twice within the first day after instillation of the enzyme owing to the rapid absorption of fluid and blood in order to maintain a constant external positive pressure.

General treatment of hemophilia and associated joints is primarily a medical and not a surgical problem, so will not be discussed in great detail. Recently there has been developed an antihemophilic globulin (Cohen's Fraction I) which has been found definitely helpful in the arrest of bleeding due to hemophilia. If this is not available, repeated whole blood transfusions are indicated.

AFFECTIONS OF THE NERVOUS SYSTEM

Flexor Power

Paralysis or weakness of the flexor muscles of the elbow (biceps, brachialis anticus and brachioradialis) may call for surgical procedures designed to substitute other muscles for those affected, such as (1) transference of the flexor-pronator muscle group origin as advocated by Steindler; (2) a modification of Steindler's method; (3) transfer of the triceps muscle; (4) of the pectoralis major muscle, or (5) of the sternocleido-mastoid muscle; or to prevent complete paralysis by over-stretching of the already weakened muscles by the bone block technique of Putti and Scaglietti.

Steindler's technique, advocated for paralysis or weakness of the flexors at the elbow, consists of transplantation of the common origin of the flexor-pronator group of the forearm from the medial epicondyle to a site about five centimeters more proximal upon the humerus. This may be performed by removing a block of bone with muscles attached and placing it in a hole made to receive it. It is fastened here with a wire loop or heavy silk suture. Before the operation is carried out the operator should be certain that a pronator muscle contracture is not already present. He should also be certain that it is possible to obtain passive supination after having thus transplanted the muscle, otherwise a pronation contracture will result. Care must be used to isolate and protect the ulnar nerve during this procedure.

The **after-treatment** consists of immobilization of the acutely flexed elbow in plaster splints or casing, with the forearm held in mid-rotation. After two weeks the splints may be discarded and heat and mild active exercises may be permitted to improve the circulation and muscular strength.

The **modification** of Steindler's method as advocated by Bunnell is for the purpose of lessening the tendency to pronation following transfer of the flexor-pronator group upwards upon the medial border of the humerus. It is useful when the flexor carpi ulnaris muscle is not available (because of paralysis) to transfer around the back of the forearm to the lower extremity of the radius. The method consists of utilizing a free graft of fascia lata to prolong the flexor-pronator origin and transfer this to a point two inches upwards upon the lateral rather than the medial border of the humerus.

Transfer of the triceps muscle to the biceps tuberosity of the radius has been advocated by Bunnell as a means of furnishing flexion power to the forearm. In general the power of elbow flexion is of greater importance than that of extension. In order to make the triceps reach the tuberosity of the radius it is necessary to prolong it by means of a free tendon or fascia lata graft which is attached to the tuberosity by means of a No. 30 stainless steel wire suture braided through the tendon and passed through a drill hole in the bone and out through the posterior aspect of the forearm where it is tied over a button while the elbow is held flexed. A pull-out wire is utilized for the purpose of removing this wire suture at the end of one month.

Transfer of pectoralis major muscle (Clark's method) utilizes the lower part of this muscle which retains a nerve supply separate from that of the main bulk of the muscle. He separates a strip of this muscle two and one-half inches wide from its origin on the ribs and raises this strip with its blood

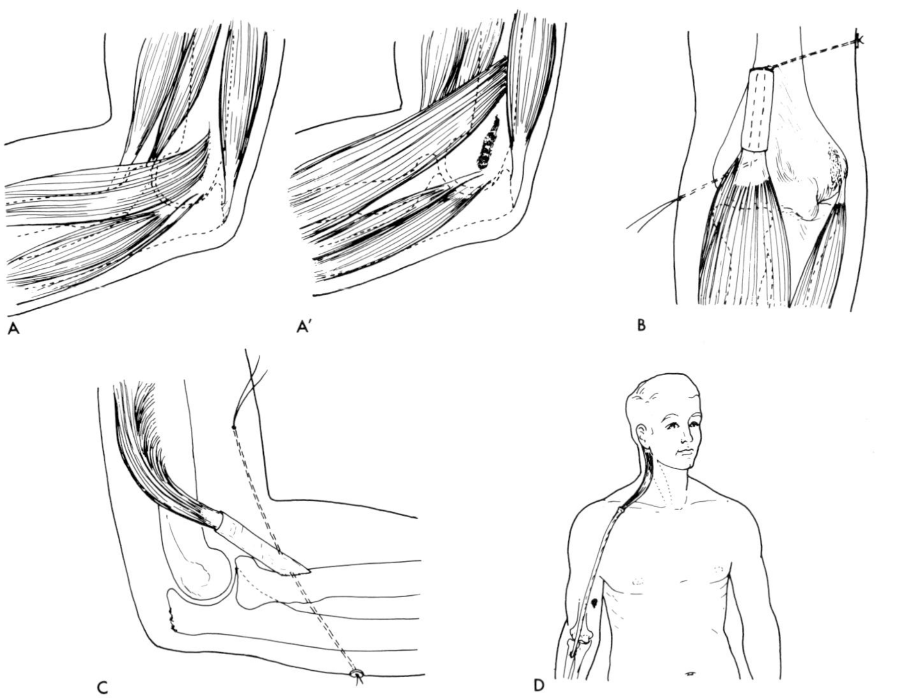

Fig. 142. Methods of restoring flexion power to the paralyzed elbow by flexorplasty operation. (A and (A') Method of Steindler which transfers the origin of the flexor-pronator group of muscles attached to the medial epicondyle to a point two inches higher up on the humerus. (B) Bunnell's modification of Steindler's method utilizing a free fascial graft to attach the flexor-pronator group origin upwards and to the lateral side of humerus. (This method may be used when it is not feasible to pass the flexor carpi ulnaris tendon around the posterior aspect of the forearm and insert it in the lower radius to act as a supinator.) (C) Bunnell's method of utilizing the triceps muscle as a supinator by inserting its prolongation with a free fascial graft into the bicipital tuberosity of the radius with a pull-out wire suture. (D) Transfer of the sternocleidomastoid muscle and prolongation of it by a free fascial graft to insert into the bicipital tuberosity. (Redrawn from Bunnell: *J. Bone & Joint Surg.*, *33-A*:566, 1951.)

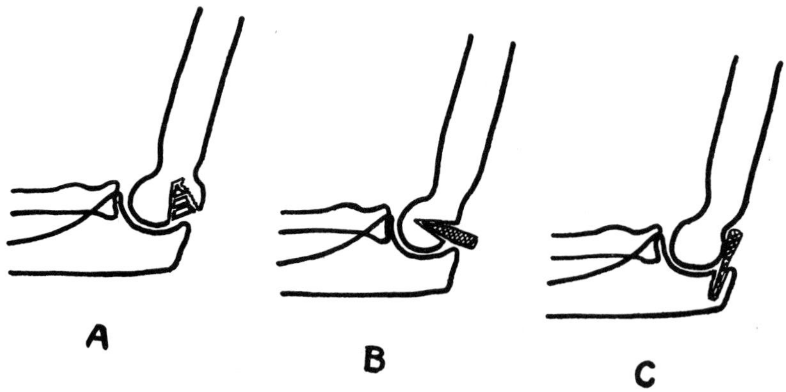

Fig. 143. Posterior bone block technique of Putti and Scaglietti to limit extension of the elbow. Three variations are shown. (A) The preferred technique in which a small osseous flap is raised from the posterior articular surface of the humerus and the defect thus created is packed with chips from the adjacent area. (B) and (C) Methods of creating a similar bone block with the introduction into the humerus and olecranon respectively of a small peg from the tibia (after Campbell).

and nerve supply intact and in turn passes it downward and sutures it to the paralyzed biceps muscle close to the musculotendinous junction.

Transfer of the sternocleidomastoid muscle may be accomplished by detaching the lower end of this muscle from clavicle and sternum and passing it distally in the subcutaneous tissues by means of a free graft of fascia lata to prolong it down the arm where it is re-attached to the biceps tuberosity of the radius by a pull-out wire suture. The pull-out wire and suture are removed at the end of one month.

The last two methods present somewhat difficult techniques, but are useful in patients without available forearm flexors.

The bone block technique of **Putti and Scaglietti** is designed to prevent over-stretching of a weakened biceps muscle and in turn complete loss of its power. A postero-lateral incision is employed to expose the posterior aspect of the elbow joint. By means of a sharp osteotome a small bony shelf is raised on the posterior articular surface of the trochlea, of the humerus and bone chips are packed into the defect beneath the shelf. This will thus act as a block to the olecranon, preventing extension of the forearm to beyond 90 or 100 degrees. The *after-treatment* consists of plaster immobilization for three weeks, followed by warm soaks and active exercises in flexion to increase the range and strength of the flexor muscles.

EXTENSOR POWER

Although gravity assists elbow extension and operations to increase the power of the triceps muscle are rarely indicated, it may sometimes be advisable to transpose muscles to improve weakness of this muscle.

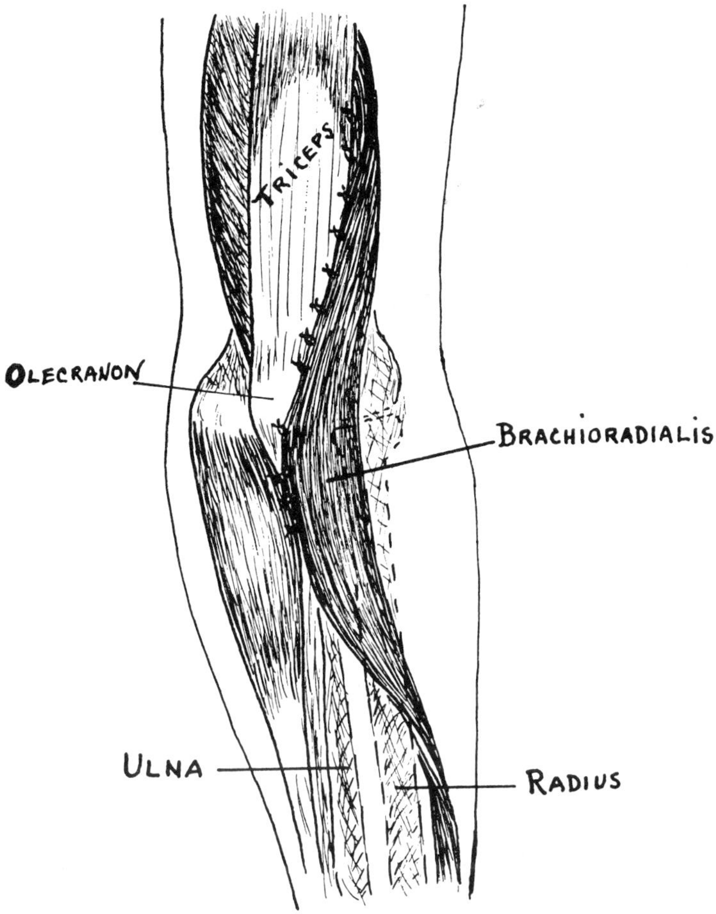

Fig. 144. Brachioradialis muscle transposition for triceps paralysis after the method of Ober and Barr. The anterior margin of the muscle is freed by dissection and rolled laterally and posteriorly and sutured to fascia and periosteum along the posterior margin of the ulna, olecranon, and to the tendon of the triceps. The nerve supply which enters the muscle high up is left intact. The schematic sketch shows the muscle after transposition, the deeper muscles having been omitted for clarity.

The technique of **Ober and Barr** utilizes the brachioradialis muscle, dissecting its anterior margin proximally and distally for a distance of ten centimeters each and isolating and saving its blood and nerve supply (radial recurrent artery and muscular branch from radial nerve). Leaving the muscle origin intact, the freed anterior margin is rolled posteriorly and laterally and sutured to the periosteum and fascia attached to the subcutaneous border of the olecranon and ulnar shaft and to the tendon of the triceps muscle.

The **after-treatment** consists of plaster immobilization with the elbow in full supination and extension. Active exercises should be started ten days after operation and kept up as long as power to extend the elbow continues to increase.

Chapter XXIV

Special Operations upon the Elbow Joint

ARTHRODESIS

ARTHRODESIS (surgical stiffening) of the elbow joint is a procedure chiefly employed for the treatment of tuberculosis. Many orthopedic surgeons consider arthrodesis of this joint the only acceptable treatment for tuberculosis; there are others who advocate excision of the joint as the preferred treatment for this disease. Although bony arthrodesis is desired if the disease is to be completely arrested, there remains a stiff joint. The disadvantage of stiffness may be quite considerable; the advantage is cure of the disease without recurrence in a very high proportion of the cases.

Technique of Arthrodesis

The following techniques for performing arthrodesis of the elbow are given along with their indications as described by the individual authors:

Campbell. This author feels that arthrodesis of the elbow is seldom advisable as treatment for tuberculous or non-tuberculous affections of this joint.

The articular surfaces are disturbed as little as possible in his operation, the technique of which he describes as follows: "An incision is made over the posterior aspect of the elbow joint, extending three inches distal and proximal to the olecranon process. Dissection is carried through the triceps muscle to the posterior surface of the humerus and the olecranon process of the ulna. Bone shavings are chiseled from the cortices of these areas. While this procedure is being carried out, an osteoperiosteal graft of suitable dimensions is removed from the tibia. The osseous surface of the graft is placed over the denuded portions of the humerus and olecranon process and maintained in close approximation by sutures or autogenous bone nails" (Fig. 145).

After-treatment. The elbow is immobilized at a right angle and in midrotation in a plaster cast from the axilla to the palm (bivalved to allow for postoperative swelling). Skin sutures are removed at two weeks and a fresh snug-fitting plaster is applied. At the end of eight weeks following operation the plaster is replaced by a leather laced corset reinforced with steel strips and worn until bony union has taken place.

Hallock. His method of elbow fusion for tuberculosis is similar to the Hibb's type of hip fusion, i. e., utilizing a mass of cancellous bone from the olecranon with tissues attached to bridge the gap between the ulna and humerus.

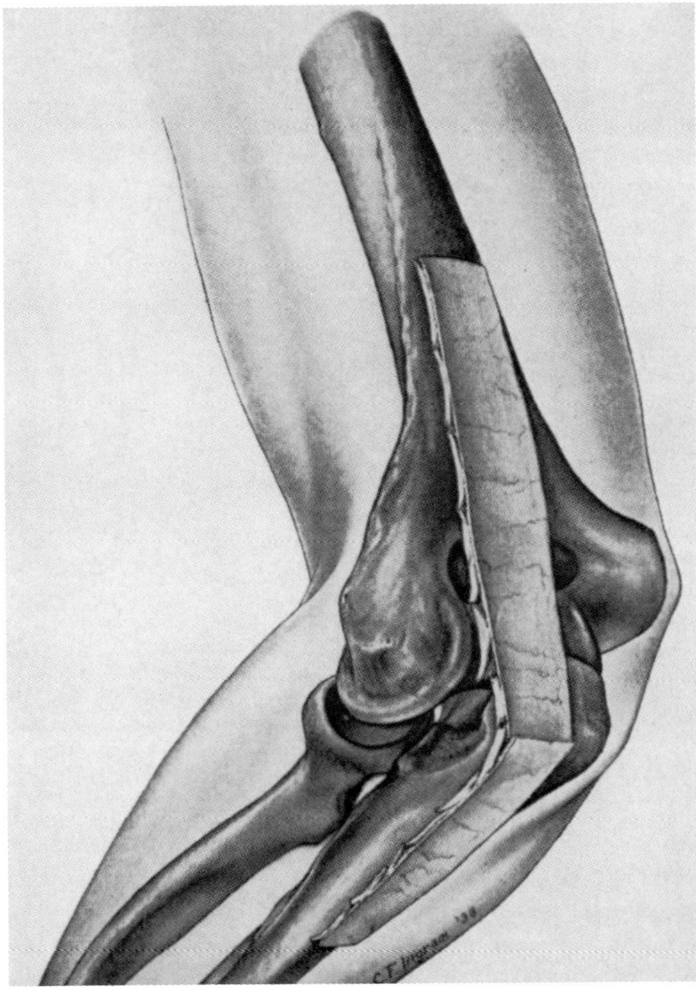

Fig. 145. Arthrodesis of elbow after method of Campbell. An osteoperiosteal graft from tibia is layed on the exposed posterior surface of humerus and upper ulna. (Campbell, W. L.: *Operative Orthopedics.* St. Louis, Mosby, 1939.)

The patient is operated upon in the prone position with the elbow flexed. The joint is exposed through a posterior midline incision and the periosteum is stripped from both sides of the olecranon and upper ulnar shaft. By means of a chisel the olecranon process with intact triceps tendon is removed obliquely from the ulna (Fig. 146) and reflected proximally. Just above the olecranon fossa a slot is cut obliquely upward into the humerus and the detached olecranon process is rotated one hundred eighty degrees and its tip driven into the slot in the humerus. Additional bone chips may be placed alongside this olecranon bone-graft which is anchored with interrupted sutures of chromic catgut.

After-treatment. Similar to that of Campbell.

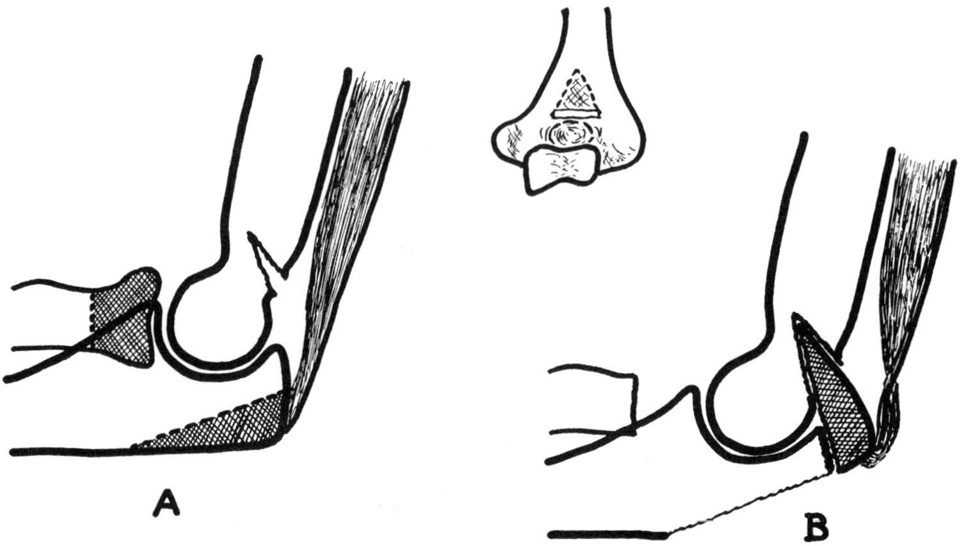

Fig. 146. Hallock's method of arthrodesis for the elbow. This utilizes a wedge-shaped portion of olecranon with triceps tendon attached which is rotated and driven into the lower posterior humerus into a hole previously made with a chisel. The radial head is excised.

Steindler. This author gives as indications for arthrodesis of this joint: the flail elbow, tuberculosis of the joint, osteoarthritis, and painful elbow where it is inadvisable to perform arthroplasty. He believes it is the operation of choice for elbow joint tuberculosis. He feels that arthroplasty is more frequently indicated in traumatic and arthritic conditions of the elbow, but where not feasible, arthrodesis must be performed.

The technique of operation utilizes the posterior longitudinal incision of Langenbeck or Ollier over the triceps, olecranon, and posterior edge of the ulna (Chapter XVII). The olecranon with attached triceps is temporarily resected and the posterior aspect of the joint is dissected. The joint is strongly flexed and the articular cartilage of the capitellum, trochlea, and greater sigmoid fossa of the ulna is removed. The anterior aspect of the capitellum and trochlea is reached and denuded of cartilage by stripping the soft tissues away from the lateral and medial sides of the lower humerus. Following this the arthrodesis is further reinforced by a graft from the tibia placed in a prepared bed on the posterior humerus and driven down into a hole properly cut in the upper ulna. The wound is closed in layers and the elbow is immobilized at a right angle in a plaster casing. (Extreme care must be exercised in identifying and retracting the ulnar nerve to avoid injuring it during the operative procedure.)

Scuderi. This author has described a technique of arthrodesis extremely useful in severe war (gun-shot) wounds of the elbow with extensive loss of bony substance of the humerus, ulna, and radius. This gives a stable, stiff elbow instead of a completely flail, weak joint. It is assumed that extensive nerve damage has not occurred to make the hand useless before such an arthrodesis is considered.

The technique in general is to bridge the gap between the humerus and the forearm bones by means of a long bone graft taken from the fibula or tibia, preferably the latter, and fastened securely in place with screws (Fig. 148). Immobilization at a right angle in plaster is advisable until revascularization and bony union is complete. Before this procedure is contemplated following a severely damaged and infected area three important pre-operative requirements must be met: (1) no drainage should be present in the area for at least three months prior to bone grafting; (2) good vascular skin and subcutaneous tissue must be present to cover the bone graft; otherwise it will not survive. It can only obtain its blood supply from the surrounding tissues and must become revascularized before it can unite with the host bone. It may therefore be necessary to fill large defects or replace dense scar tissue by pedicle-flap plastic operations to prepare the field for bone graft surgery. (3) Chemotherapy in adequate amounts must be administered before and two weeks following operation to minimize the risk of infection and certain failure if it occurred.

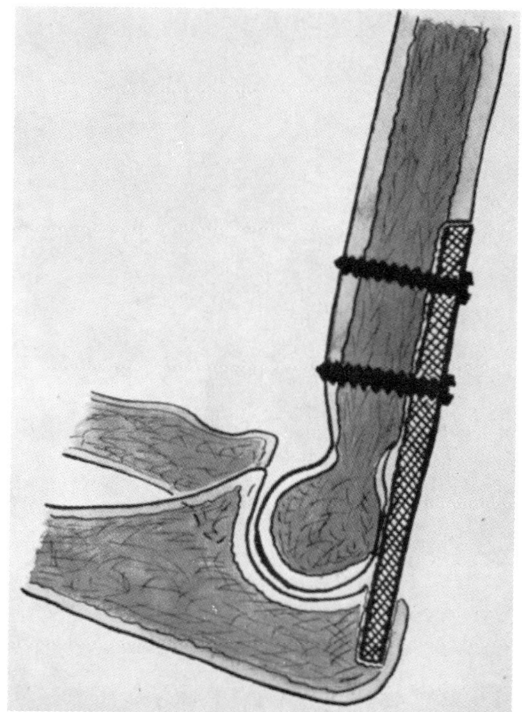

Fig. 147. Steindler's method of arthrodesis of elbow joint utilizing tibial graft counter-sunk into posterior surface of humerus where it is anchored with screws. The lower end of graft is driven into a previously made cut in olecranon. As much cartilage as possible is removed from the articular surfaces of the humerus and ulna before the graft is applied. Plaster fixation is used to immobilize the joint after operation.

ARTHROPLASTY

The procedure of arthroplasty is fairly well established for the correction of complete ankylosis of the elbow joint. For a joint with malunion following a fracture in which there is marked restriction of motion arthroplasty may also be employed.

The elbow joint may become completely ankylosed because of trauma, infection or a combination of both of these causes. Infection may be blood

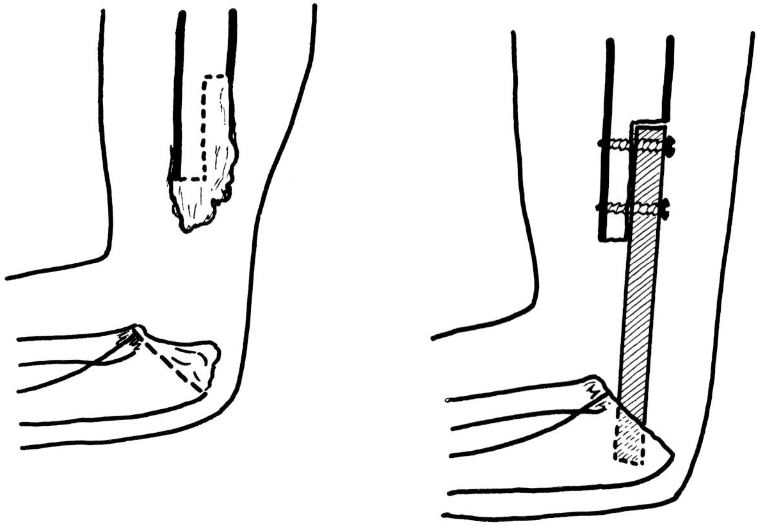

Fig. 148. Scuderi's method of arthrodesis advocated to stabilize the elbow where there has been extensive loss of bony substance. This utilizes a free tibial graft which is countersunk into the freshened humerus and ulna and fastened internally with screws. Additional plaster fixation is advisable. This method may be excellent in old cases, but presupposes a useful hand.

borne or introduced through an open (compound) wound. It may be due to gonococcus, to rheumatoid arthritis, or even to tuberculosis. Arthroplasty is more likely to be successful where the stiffness has been the result purely of trauma not associated with infection. Ankylosis following gonorrheal infection is the type most amenable for arthroplasty and the least likely to show recurrence of the infection after operation. Elbow joints that have become fused as a result of tuberculosis or have been fused operatively in order to cure tuberculosis of the joint, should never have arthroplasty attempted. Any joint the site of previous sepsis should not have arthroplasty performed upon it prior to one year following the last evidence of infection, and operation should be accompanied by the use of penicillin or other suitable antibiotics prior to and after the operative procedure in order to minimize any flare-up of infection.

Several conditions must be present before arthroplasty of the elbow is to be seriously considered: first, it is best done between the ages of twenty and fifty years; second, the bone must not be excessively sclerosed or atrophied; third, the muscles must not be completely fibrotic in the region of the elbow; and fourth, the skin and subcutaneous tissues must not be completely adherent to the underlying bone. It is extremely important that the patient's general health be good and that he is the type of patient that will cooperate thoroughly in the after-care period in attempting to recover his motion by frequent active exercises. It is of utmost importance that patients of foreign nationalities, who do not speak the language, should not be operated upon

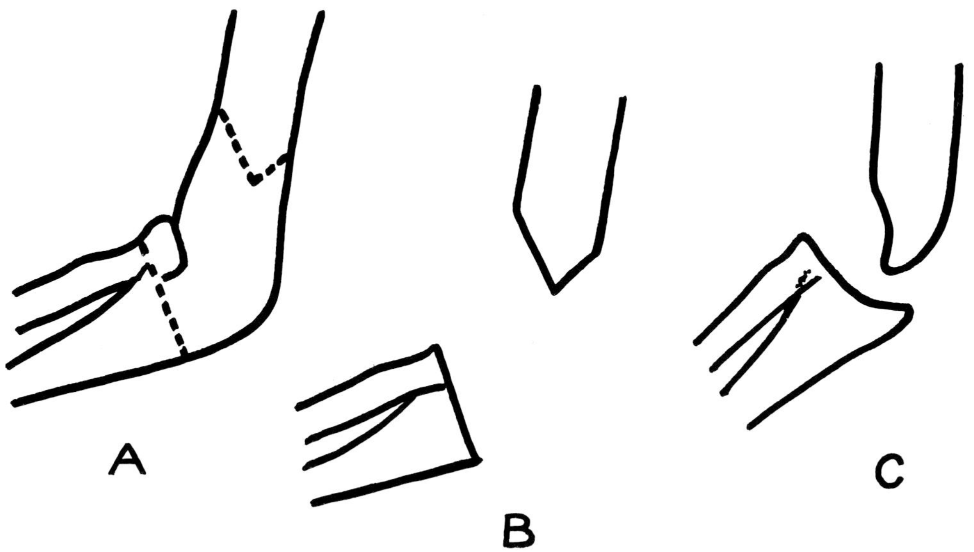

Fig. 149. Haas' type of elbow arthroplasty. A generous resection of the lower humerus is made with the long arm of the point on the flexor side. The ulna is transected at the level of the radial head (unless there is synostosis between radius and ulna when it is removed at the lower margin of the radial head). (A) Line of resection. (B) The defect. (C) The attempt of nature to partially re-shape the bone ends after prolonged exercise and function.

until it is possible to make them understand explicitly verbal instructions that must be given them from day to day. An arthroplasty to be successful must furnish a useful range of motion in the elbow. It must give a stable elbow and one that the patient can control well. It must also be painless.

There are in general two types of arthroplasties that may be performed in the elbow region. The first is the **functional type** as described by Haas. The technique of this consists mainly of a resection of the ankylosed elbow joint, taking out a large section of the lower humerus, upper ulna, and, if necessary, the radial head. The lower humerus is cut across in a V-shape on lateral view with the long arm of the V on the anterior (flexor) surface. The upper ulna is cut straight across. All of this is performed sub-periosteally. Following operation the arm is placed in traction straight-out and the patient is prevented from bending the elbow for at least two to three weeks. Following removal of traction, which has been for the purpose of separating the raw bone ends and of preventing the growth of new bone across the gap created by operation, the patient is allowed up and started on gradual flexion exercises with the arm dependant at his side for five minutes every hour during the daytime. When first starting these exercises, he may obtain little or no active flexion, but he must persevere. It may be at least two to three months before he shows as much as 45 or 50 degrees of active flexion from the full position of extension.

The second type of elbow arthroplasty, known as the **anatomical type,** is that described by MacAusland.

Operative Technique. "The elbow joint is approached by a semi-circular incision that curves over the olecranon and extends from one condyle to the other. The skin and subcutaneous tissues are dissected, and the flap is retracted. The ulnar nerve is retracted to the ulnar side. A transverse incision is made through the deep fascia, ligaments and capsule down to the periosteum. The olecranon is chiseled through transversely at the joint line.

"The joint is then ready to be broken open. This step is more easily carried out when the joint line is still visible and the joint surfaces can be separated by means of curved chisels. When the joint cavity is entirely obliterated in a bony bridge, the site of the old joint line is determined as closely as possible and then chiseled or sawed through. The forearm is flexed, the olecranon segment freed, and the flap dissected back in toto. The flap is preserved for a subsequent covering of the joint.

"In the remodeling of the articular surfaces, the normal contours of the joint are followed as closely as possible. The articular ends should fit together accurately. Care should be taken to remove only enough bone to permit free motion. An electric burr is used to remodel the condyles of the humerus. The olecranon fossa is deepened, care being taken to preserve the olecranon ridge, which is an aid in maintaining the lateral stability of the joint. It may be necessary to deepen the radial and ulnar surfaces somewhat

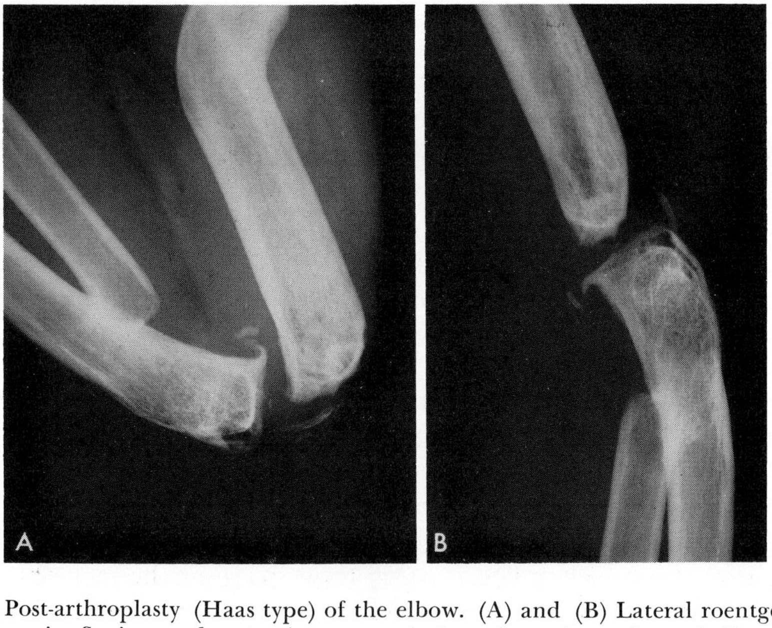

Fig. 150. Post-arthroplasty (Haas type) of the elbow. (A) and (B) Lateral roentgenograms with elbow in flexion and extension respectively, taken six and one-half years after operation. (For pre-operative roentgenogram of this patient see Fig. 126A.)

with an electric burr, so that they will conform to the humeral surfaces. The ulnar ridge, which articulates with the intercondylar notch, should not be disturbed.

"A flap of fascia lata is removed from the outer part of the thigh. After the flap has been freed of all fat, it is wrapped around the newly formed humeral condyles and attached anteriorly and posteriorly to the capsule. No. 2 chromic catgut is wound tightly around the base of the fascial flap and firmly tied.

"The articular ends are brought into apposition. A screw is driven through the olecranon and into the ulna. The capsule is closed with interrupted sutures of catgut, the skin is closed with interrupted sutures of silk. A small compression dressing is applied and the arm is immobilized in a neck and wrist sling, with the foream flexed just above the right angle."

The **postoperative treatment** is an essential part of the arthroplastic procedure, and the success of the operation depends to a great extent on the cooperation of the patient in this after-care. The patient should practise contraction exercises of the arm and forearm muscles hourly, to maintain their tone and to improve the circulation. The dressing is changed in a week. Passive motions are carried out in about ten days after the operation. Gentle

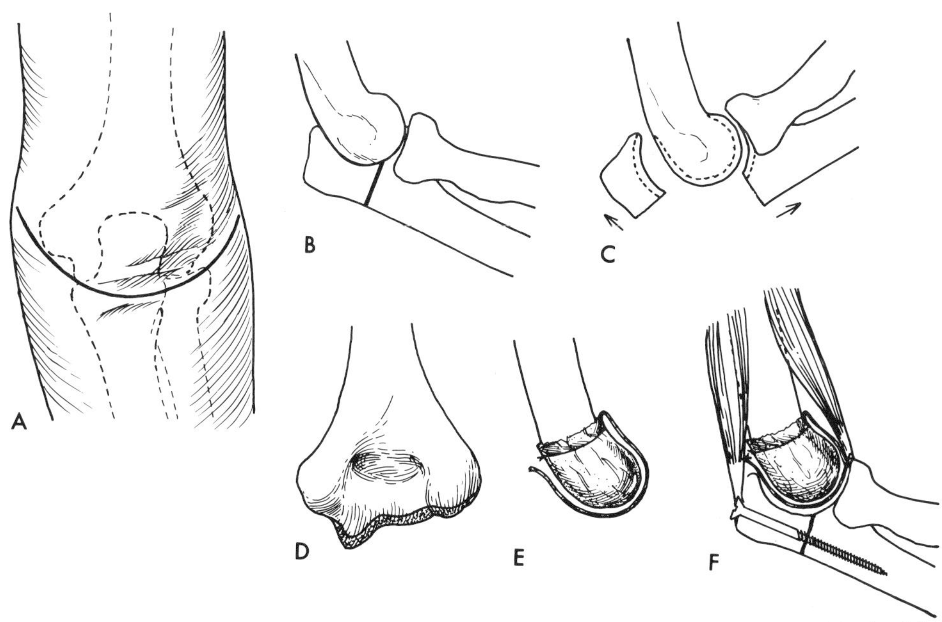

Fig. 151. MacAusland's arthroplasty of the elbow. (A) Posterior U-shaped skin incision. (B) Line of transection of olecranon which is then retracted in a proximal direction. (C) and (D) Joint is broken open widely and dotted lines show amount of bone removed as humerus and ulna are remodeled with chisels and gouges. (E) Double layer of fascia lata is fastened in place over lower end of humerus. (F) The olecranon is replaced and fastened in position with a single wood-type screw. The remainder of the periosteum, deep fascia and skin are closed as usual with interrupted sutures.

massage may be given in three weeks. The patient also begins to use the arm after the third week, returning it to the sling only for rest.

Prognosis

The prognosis following arthroplasty of the elbow joint naturally depends mostly upon the patient and very little upon the actual operative procedure. The surgeon, however, should use some judgment in selecting cases for arthroplasty and should not attempt to perform this operation upon an elbow unless the patient has a completely or nearly completely useful hand on the same extremity.

Articular Replacement

The substitution of an artificial joint surface as devised by Hudack offers an entirely new type of arthroplasty for partially or wholly stiff elbow joints and one that should give good stability and little or no pain. The procedure consists of resection of the lower extremity of the humerus, re-shaping of the articular surfaces of the upper radius and ulna if necessary, preservation of the medial and lateral epicondyles with their muscular attachments and replacement of the trochlea and capitellum by a lucite replica anchored to the lower shaft of the humerus by means of an intramedullary rod of stainless steel.

The plastic internal prosthesis furnishes a smooth gliding surface for the forearm bones to move upon, and, being shaped to resemble the original articular surface of the humerus, it therefore permits free motion while maintaining stability, since the lateral muscular and periosteal attachment are preserved. The lucite and stainless steel replacement is inert in the tissues and should therefore cause no inflammatory reaction.

Although articular replacement has been employed successfully in a few cases of elbow joint ankylosis, it is not the type of operative procedure that should be undertaken lightly. For all practical purposes at the present time it must be considered as still in the experimental stage. An arthroplasty of this type should be performed only by a surgeon who has had experience with the method and who can depend as well upon the materials and workmanship that go into the prosthesis.

Resection (Excision) of the Elbow Joint

This procedure consists of excision of the ends of the bones forming the joint. It is most commonly employed for tuberculosis, but occasionally may be performed for recent injury with overwhelming destruction of the joint surfaces, either as a primary or a secondary procedure. It is an especially helpful procedure in severe war wounds when no reconstruction is possible. It may also be performed as a secondary procedure in: (1) acute arthritis not yielding to incision and drainage after injury when ankylosis is the best

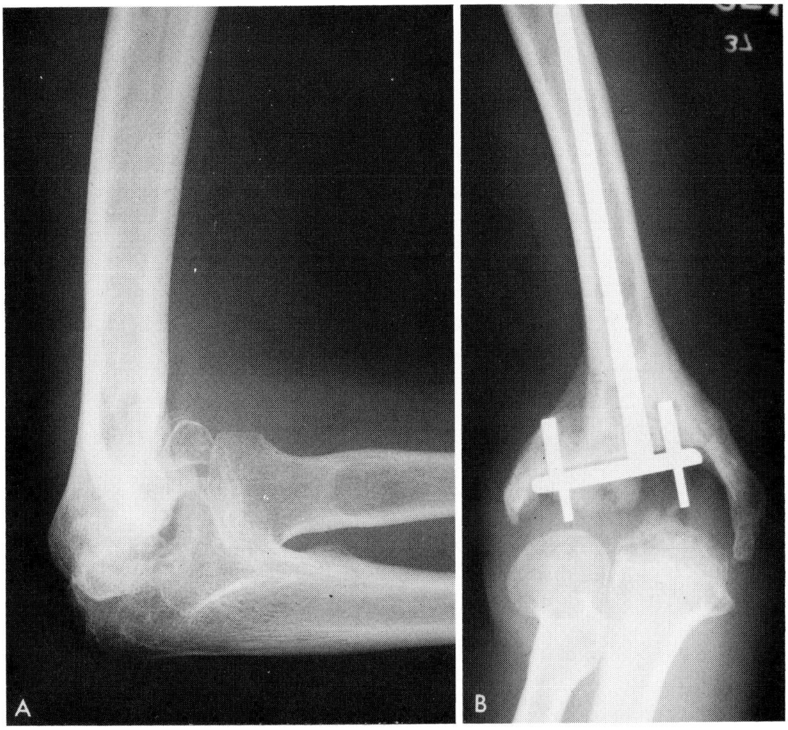

Fig. 152. Articular replacement arthroplasty of elbow joint for fibrous ankylosis. (A) Lateral roentgenogram prior to operation. (B) Antero-posterior view five months after operation. The articular surface of the replacement is of plastic material shaped to conform to that of the humerus. An intramedullary element of stainless steel was used to lend stability, prevent rotation, and distribute pressure. The epicondyles were left intact as muscular attachments. This 24-year-old man was able to move his elbow through a range of 60 to 150 degrees five months after operation and had a strong, stable elbow (case of Dr. S. S. Hudack).

result that can be expected; (2) for an old injury to the elbow joint in preference to a strict arthroplastic procedure; (3) where the elbow is ankylosed in faulty position; or (4) in a disorganizing arthritis due to pyemia, rheumatic fever or to old osteo-arthritis.

Ordinarily, for tuberculosis of the elbow joint excision is not considered a good procedure in children. It is much better to treat these conservatively by means of plaster immobilization plus streptomycin therapy. In adults operative arthrodesis has been considered a better type of procedure since it puts the joint at complete rest and thereby assists in arresting the disease. It is possible that motion in a number of tuberculous joints may be preserved by excision assisted with the use of anti-biotic (streptomycin) therapy whereas formerly, without the use of streptomycin, a high percentage of recurrence of the tuberculous infection was to be expected.

Points to be considered in a case where excision of the joint is contemplated are: (1) age—this is usually best done before the age of thirty-five; (2) complications such as other tuberculous joints; (3) value of preserving the periosteum at the time of excision (since preservation of this helps to cut down on the amount of hemorrhage from the procedure and removal of the periosteum leads to less lateral stability following operation). If the periosteum is retained, the bones must be more freely resected than otherwise since motion may be impaired.

Technique of Excision of Elbow. Operation may be performed through a single posterior vertical incision, two lateral incisions, or a bayonet-shaped incision. The center of the incision should be just lateral to the tip of the olecranon. The muscles are peeled off the bone subperiosteally, care being taken to protect the ulnar nerve. The ulna is resected just below the lesser sigmoid notch, the radius just below its head and the humerus at the upper margin of the medial epicondyle. It is usually wise to leave a gap of approximately two to two and one-half inches between the humerus above and the radius and ulna below. The operative area is thoroughly irrigated with saline and drains may be placed in the wound for twenty-four hours for evacuation of possible hematoma. Following closure the elbow should be splinted either in a straight line or at a right angle, preferably in the latter position because the patient can exercise it either in flexion or extension and this also offers a better chance for the elbow to become stabilized in a more useful position.

Finger exercises should be started the day after operation. Gentle passive motion of the joint may be begun in seven to ten days and active elbow motion may be started at the end of four weeks. If the bones tend to pull together, light weight-carrying may be permitted. It may be necessary to tie up the good arm in order to get the patient to use the operated arm. Special attention must be paid to exercises to increase pronation and supination; and at a later date systematic exercise must be carried out for strengthening of the arm muscles. Twelve months must elapse before full benefit of the operation can be expected, i. e., complete combination of mobility and stability. It may even be necessary to wear a brace after four weeks if a flail joint seems likely, provided temporary immobilization for one month in plaster does not tend to stabilize it.

Partial excision of the elbow joint is definitely *not* indicated in tuberculosis or ankylosis. It may be used for excision of a radial head (in toto) or of a medial epicondyle fractured and displaced into the joint. (See Chapters X and XII on these specific fractures.)

Unfavorable Results and Sequelae of Elbow Joint Excision. Excision of the joint is not always successful and may result in: persistence of tuberculous disease, caries and chronic osteomyelitis, ankylosis, flail-like joint, infection of the wound, useless limb, injury to the ulnar nerve, and adherent scar.

Erasion of the Elbow Joint

The procedure of erasion of a joint consists of removal of the diseased portions by scraping away with a curette or by a chisel. This is a procedure formerly used in elbow joint tuberculosis in children, but would now be considered *obsolete*. It was a poor procedure for removal of diseased tissue and frequently ended in fibrous ankylosis, or in recurrence of the disease. Since better procedures are at hand no further description will be given of this obsolete procedure.

Arthrotomy of the Elbow Joint

An arthrotomy consists of an opening into the joint. The indications for this are: (1) drainage for acute suppurative arthritis resulting from puncture wound into the joint or due to blood-borne infection; (2) for removal of loose bodies; (3) correction of malunion of fracture of articular surface; (4) removal of bone or fragment (radial head, capitellum, medial epicondyle); and (5) biopsy.

For incision and drainage of the elbow joint, two lateral incisions, one on either side of the olecranon, are to be preferred. No drain should be inserted into the joint cavity, but one may be inserted down to the joint lining.

Amputation

Amputation in the region of the elbow is an operation that should be avoided except in great necessity as in severe crush injuries or in extensive gun-shot wounds of the upper forearm with laceration of the arterial blood

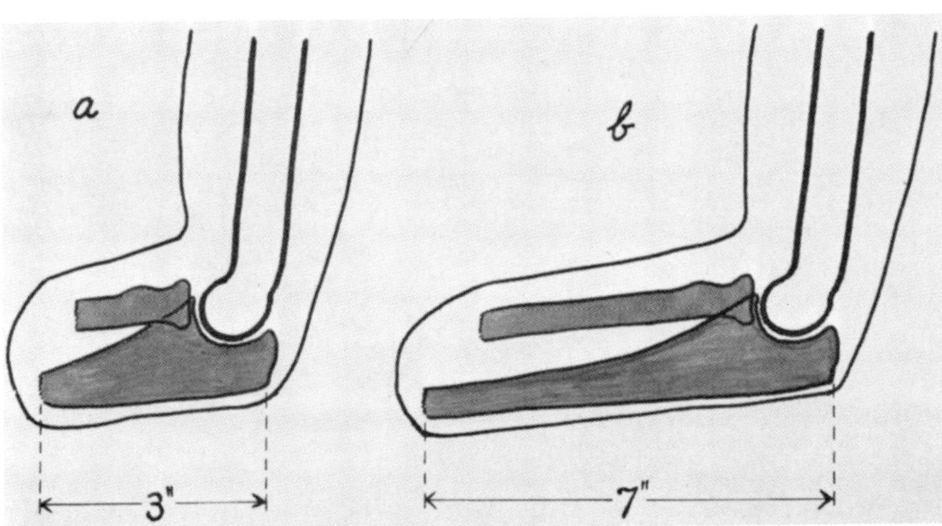

Fig. 153. Amputation sites for upper forearm (below elbow). (a) Shortest possible. (b) Optimum. (After Watson-Jones.)

supply. Where it is thus imperative to amputate at this level, it should be performed with the idea of probable revision of the stump being necessary at a later date. A stump of at least three inches of ulna must be left to make a forearm amputation of any functional benefit. It is for this reason that amputation or disarticulation at the level of the elbow joint should be frowned upon. The disadvantages of amputation near the joint level are that it leaves an expanded stump; (1) difficult to be fitted with a prosthesis, (2) which is poor cosmetically, and (3) which is useless from the standpoint of applying a cineplastic prosthesis. It would therefore be preferable to amputate at a slightly higher level, i. e., just above the humeral condyles.

The following types of skin flaps may be employed if amputation (or disarticulation) must be performed: (1) long anterior flap; (2) long posterior flap; (3) large anteromedial and short posterolateral flap; (4) long anterior and short posterior; (5) lateral flap (single and double); (6) guillotine (circular) method.

The flaps should be so arranged that the longest extends three inches distal to the articular surface or resected end of the lower humerus in order that there will be adequate soft parts to cover it. In disarticulation the joint is opened on the lateral side between the capitellum and head of the radius. The bones are thus separated and divided. The bleeders are clamped and ligated and the brachialis and triceps muscles are sutured to each other, thus covering the bone ends. The skin and subcutaneous tissue is closed with deep through-and-through sutures of silk. A drain may be inserted for twenty-four hours and a compression dressing is applied.

Bibliography

Fractures of the Elbow – General

Armitage, H. M. and Armitage, G. L., Jr.: Treatment of Injuries in the Vicinity of the Elbow-Joint. *Ann. Surg., 63:*598, 1916.
Ashhurst, A. P. C.: *Fractures of the Elbow.* Philadelphia, Lea and Febiger, 1910.
Babcock, W. W.: *Textbook of Surgery.* Philadelphia, W. B. Saunders Co., 1935.
Beekman, F. and Sullivan, J. E.: Some Observations on Fractures of Long Bones in Children. *Am. J. Surg., 51:*722, 1941.
Bennett, G. E.: Shoulder and Elbow Lesions of the Professional Baseball Pitcher. *J.A.M.A., 117:*510, 1941.
Blount, W. P., Schulz, I. and Cassidy, R. H.: Fractures of the Elbow in Children. *J.A.M.A., 146:*699, 1951.
Blount, W. P.: *Fractures in Children.* Baltimore, Williams and Wilkins Co., 1955.
Böhler, L.: *The Treatment of Fractures.* Vienna, Wilhelm Maudrich, 1929.
Böhler, L.: *Medullary Nailing of Küntscher.* 1st English Ed. Baltimore, Williams and Wilkins Co., 1948.
Bonnin, J. G.: *A Complete Outline of Fractures.* London, William Heinemann (Medical Books) LTD., 1941.
Bontrous, T. A., Blain, A. and Chipman, W. A.: Non-Splinting Treatment of Elbow Joint Injuries (Report of Its Use in 20 Cases). *Am. J. Surg., 68:*212, 1945.
Boyd, H. B. and Altenberg, A. R.: Fractures About the Elbow in Children. *Arch. Surg., 49:* 213, 1944.
Brewster, A. H. and Karp, M.: Fractures in the Region of the Elbow in Children (An End-Result Study). *Surg., Gynec. & Obst., 71:*643, 1940.
Campbell, W. C.: Malunited Fractures and Unreduced Dislocations About the Elbow. *J.A.M.A., 92:*122, 1929.
Campbell, W. C.: *Operative Orthopedics.* St. Louis, C. V. Mosby Co., 1939.
Casagrande, P. A. and Frost, H. M., Jr.: *Fractures About the Elbow; Sprains and Dislocations of the Elbow.* New York, Grune and Stratton, 1953.
Charnley, J.: *The Closed Treatment of Common Fractures.* Edinburgh, E. & S. Livingstone, LTD., 1950.
Clough, F. E.: Stumbling Blocks in Treatment of Fractures. *J.-Lancet (Minneapolis), 68:*100, 1948.
Cohn, I.: Fractures of the Elbow. *Am. J. Surg., 55:*210, 1942.
Cole, W. H. and Evans, E. T.: Fractures in Children. *Staff Meeting Bulletin—Hospitals of the Univ. of Minnesota, 9:*329, 1938.
Colp, R. and Mage, S.: The Treatment of Joint Fractures. *Ann. Surg., 97:*177, 1933.
Compere, E. L. and Banks, S. W.: *Pictorial Handbook of Fracture Treatment.* 2nd Ed., Chicago, Year Book Medical Publishers, Inc., 1947.
Conn, J. and Wade, P. A.: Injuries of the Elbow: A Ten Year Review, *J. Trauma, 1:*248, 1961.
Cox, F. J., Hurley, M. T. and Compton, R. B.: Fractures About the Elbow in Children. *California Med., 76:*13, 1952.
Curry, G. J.: Excision of the Elbow for Multiple Compound Comminuted Fractures. *Am. J. Surg., 70:*243, 1945.
Davis, L.: *Christopher's Textbook of Surgery.* 9th Ed. Philadelphia, W. B. Saunders Co., 1968.
Devine, J.: Shattering Gunshot Wound of the Elbow. *Australian & New Zealand J. Surg., 13:* 208, 1944.
Eliason, Eldridge L.: *Fractures of the Humerus, Radius and Ulna.* New York, D. Appleton and Company, 1925.
Fairbanks, H. A. T.: Prognosis in Injuries of the Elbow Joint. *Lancet, 227:*263, 1934.
Farr, R. S.: Fractures of the Elbow. *New York State J. Med., 40:*1288, 1940.

FITTS, W. T., JR.: Fractures of the Upper Extremity. (A Review of Experience in World War II.) *Am. J. Surg., 72*:393, 1946.

GARTLAND, J. J., JR.: *Fundamentals of Orthopaedics.* Philadelphia, W. B. Saunders Co., 1965.

GECKELER, E. O.: *Fractures and Dislocations for Practitioners.* 2nd Ed. Baltimore, Williams and Wilkins Co., 1940.

GODFREY, J. D.: Trauma in Children. *J. Bone & Joint Surg., 46-A*:422, 1964.

GOULD, A. L.: A Neglected Danger in the Treatment of Elbow Fractures. *Maine Med. J., 27*:116, 1936.

GREEN, W. T.: Fractures of the Elbow in Children. *Chicago Med. Soc. Bull.,* Jan. 26, 1952.

HAMPTON, O. P. and FITTS, W. T., JR.: *Fractures and Dislocations of the Upper Extremity. Principles and Practice of Surgery.* 2nd Ed. (Harkins, Moyer, Rhoads and Allen). Philadelphia, J. B. Lippincott Co., 1961.

HENDERSON, M. S.: Fractures of Hip, Ankle and Elbow. *Ann. Surg., 93*:968, 1931.

HEYGROVES, E. W.: Direct Skeletal Traction in the Treatment of Fractures. *Brit. J. Surg., 16*:149, 1928.

HOWORTH, M. B.: *Textbook of Orthopedics.* Philadelphia, W. B. Saunders Co., 1952.

JONES, R.: A Note on the Treatment of Injuries About the Elbow. *Prov. Med. J., 14*:28, 1895.

JONES, R.: Injuries About the Elbow in Children. *Brit. Med. J., 1*:739, 1932.

JUDET, J. and JUDET, R.: Treatment of Epiphyseal Fractures by Temporary Transarticular (Pegs) Wires. *Sem. Hôp. Paris, 24*:2423, 1948.

KEY, J. A. and CONWELL, H. E.: *Fractures, Dislocations and Sprains.* 4th Ed. St. Louis, C. V. Mosby Co., 1946.

KNAPP, M. E.: Physical Therapy in Fractures About the Elbow Joint. *Arch. Phys. Therap., 21*:709, 1940.

KULOWSKI, J.: Fractures of the Elbow Joint. *Am. J. Roentgenol., 79*:692, 1958.

LORTHIOR, P., SMETS, W. and PARISEL, F.: Treatment of Fresh Fractures of the Elbow in Children. *Acta Orthop. Belgica, 12*:165, 1946.

MACLENNAN, A.: Common Fractures About the Elbow Joint in Children. *Surg., Gynec. & Obst., 64*:447, 1937.

MAGNUSON, P. B. and STACK, J. K.: *Fractures.* 5th Ed. Philadelphia, J. B. Lippincott Co., 1949.

MCLAUGHLIN, H. L. and STIMSON, B. B.: Injuries of the Elbow. *In* McLaughlin, H. L.: *Trauma.* Philadelphia, W. B. Saunders Co., 1959.

MOORHEAD, J. J.: *Clinical Traumatic Surgery.* Philadelphia, W. B. Saunders Co., 1945.

MOORHEAD, J. J.: *Traumatotherapy.* Philadelphia, W. B. Saunders Co., 1931.

MURRAY, C. R.: The Early Use of Physical Therapy in the Treatment of Injury. *New York State J. Med., 41*:1052, 1941.

MURRAY, C. R.: The Status of Fracture Treatment in the Field of Surgery. *Surg., Gynec. & Obst., 62*:433, 1936.

MURRAY, C. R.: *Treatment of Injury by the General Practitioner.* New York, Harper & Bros., 1931.

MURRAY, D. A.: An Unusual Condition of the Elbow Joint—(Case Report). *J. Bone & Joint Surg., 11*:395, 1929.

MURRAY, J. M.: Traumatic Flail Elbow. *J.A.M.A., 106*:282, 1936.

NEUWIRTH, A. A.: Non-splinting Treatment of Fractures of the Elbow Joint. *J.A.M.A., 118*:971, 1942.

NICHOLSON, J. T.: Compound Comminuted Fractures Involving the Elbow Joint. (Treatment by Resection of the Fragments). *J. Bone & Joint Surg., 28*:565, 1946.

PERKINS, G.: *Fractures.* London, Oxford University Press, 1940.

PHILIPPEDES, D.: Reduction of Fractures by Traction. *Der Chirurg, 9*:409, 1937.

SANDISON, C.: Management of Injuries of the Elbow Joint. *J. M. A. Georgia, 37*:121, 1948.

SHANDS, A. R., JR.: *Handbook of Orthopaedic Surgery.* St. Louis, C. V. Mosby Co., 1952.

SHARKE, H. B.: Car Window Elbows. *South. M. J., 34*:372, 1941.

SIRIS, I. E.: Elbow Fractures and Dislocations. *Surg., Gynec. & Obst., 40*:665, 1925.

SMITH, F. M.: Children's Elbow Injuries: Fractures and Dislocations. *Clin. Orthop., 50*:7, 1967.

SMITH, F. M.: Fractures and Dislocations Involving the Elbow Joint. Chapter 32 in BANCROFT, F. W. & MARBLE, H. C., *Surgery of the Motor Skeletal System.* 2nd Ed. Philadelphia, J. B. Lippincott Co., 1951.

SMITH, F. M.: Traction and Suspension in the Treatment of Fractures. *Surg. Clin. North America, 31*:545, 1951.

SNEDECOR, S. T. and GRAHAM, W. C.: Severe War Injuries of the Elbow. *J. Bone & Joint Surg., 27*:623, 1945.

SPEED, J. S. and BOYD, H. B.: Fractures About the Elbow. *Am. J. Surg., 38*:727, 1937.

Speed, J. S. and Macey, H. B.: Fractures of the Humeral Condyles in Children. *J. Bone & Joint Surg., 15*:903, 1933.

Speed, J. S. and Smith, H.: *Campbell's Operative Orthopedics.* 2nd Ed. St. Louis, C. V. Mosby Co., 1949.

Speed, K.: *Fractures and Dislocations.* 4th Ed. Philadelphia, Lea and Febiger, 1942.

Steindler, A.: *The Traumatic Deformities and Disabilities of the Upper Extremity.* Springfield, Illinois, Charles C Thomas, Publisher, 1946.

Stimson, B. B.: *A Manual of Fractures and Dislocations.* 2nd Ed. Philadelphia, Lea and Febiger, 1947.

Stimson, L. A.: *Fractures and Dislocations.* Philadelphia, Lea Bros., 1900.

Thomas, A.: Fractures About the Elbow in Children. *J. Oklahoma State M. A.,* Dec., 1950.

Thomas, T. T.: A Contribution to the Mechanism of Fractures and Dislocations in the Elbow Region. *Ann. Surg., 89*:108, 1929.

Thorndike, A., Jr. and Dimmler, C. L., Jr.: Fractures of the Forearm and Elbow in Children. *New England J. Med., 225*:475, 1941.

Van Gorder, G. W.: *Dislocations and Fractures of the Elbow.* Chicago, Year Book Medical Publishers, Inc., 1958.

Venable, C. S., and Stuck, W. G.: *The Internal Fixation of Fractures.* Springfield, Illinois, Charles C Thomas, Publisher, 1947.

Villagrana, J. C.: Advantages of Operative Treatment of Fractures of the Elbow. *J. Bone & Joint Surg., 14*:65, 1932.

Waring, T. L.: *Surgical Lesions of the Elbow.* Lectures on Regional Orthop. Surg. & Fundamental Orthop. Problems No. II. Ann Arbor, J. W. Edwards, Inc., 1948.

Watson-Jones, Sir Reginald: *Fractures and Joint Injuries.* 3rd Ed. Baltimore, Williams and Wilkins Company, 1946.

Wilson, P. D.: Fractures and Dislocations in the Region of the Elbow. *Surg., Gynec. & Obst., 56*:335, 1933.

Wilson, P. D.: *Management of Fractures and Dislocations.* Philadelphia, J. B. Lippincott Co., 1938.

Yancey, D. L.: Fractures About the Elbow Joint. *J. Mo. Med. Ass., 44*:262, 1947.

Fractures of the Humerus

Adams, J. D.: A Report on Six Cases of Supracondylar Fractures of the Elbow. *New England J. Med., 216*:837, 1937.

Aitken, A. P. and Blackett, C. W.: Supracondylar Fractures in Children. *Am. J. Surg., 59*: 161, 1943.

Aitken, A. P. and Childress, H. M.: Intra-Articular Displacement of the Internal Epicondyle Following Dislocation. *J. Bone & Joint Surg., 20*:161, 1938.

Allen, P. D. and Gramse, A. E.: Transcondylar Fractures of the Humerus Treated by Dunlop Traction. *Am. J. Surg., 57*:217, 1945.

Anderson, R.: Fractures of the Humerus. *Surg., Gynec. & Obst., 64*:919, 1937.

Baumgartner, M. J.: Traction for Supracondylar Fractures of Humerus in Children. *Rev. Méd. Suisse Rom., 41*:201, 1921.

Bickel, W. H. and Perry, R. E.: Comminuted Fractures of the Distal Humerus. *J.A.M.A., 184*:553, 1963.

Böhler, J.: Closed Wire Fixation of Supracondylar Fractures in Children. *Chir. Praxis.,* p. 397, 1959.

Böhler, J.: Percutaneous Internal Fixation Utilizing the X-ray Image Amplifier. *J. Trauma, 5*:150, 1965.

Borsky, V. L.: Reposition of Fragments with the Aid of the CITO Clamp in Transcondylar Fractures of the Humerus in Children. *Ortop. Travma. Protez., 8*:20, 1969.

Büttner, A. and Vorwerk, A.: Fractures of the Humerus Near the Elbow in Children. (Supracondylar). *Beitr. zur Klinischen Chirurgie, Berlin, 177*:51, 1948.

Cassebaum, W.: Open Reduction of T- and Y-Fractures of the Lower End of the Humerus. *J. Trauma, 9*:915, 1969.

Cassebaum, W. H.: Operative Treatment of T and Y Fractures of the Lower End of the Humerus. *Am. J. Surg., 83*:265, 1952.

Chacha, P. B.: Fracture of the Medial Condyle of the Humerus with Rotational Displacement. *J. Bone & Joint Surg., 52-A*:1453, 1970.

Christopher, F. and Bushnell, L. F.: Conservative Treatment of Fracture of the Capitellum. *J. Bone & Joint Surg., 17*:489, 1935.

Connor, A. N. and Smith, M. G. H.: Displaced Fractures of the Lateral Humeral Condyle in Children. *J. Bone & Joint Surg., 52-B*:46, 1970.

Crane, L.: Fractures of the Elbow in Children. *J. Maine Med. Ass.,* Jan., 1959.

DARRACH, W.: Open Reduction of Fractured External Condyle of Humerus. *Ann. Surg., 63:* 486, 1916.
DARRACH, W.: Open Reduction of Fracture of Capitellum. *Ann. Surg., 63:*487, 1916.
DONCHESS, J. C.: Treatment of Supracondylar Fracture of the Humerus. *J. Indiana Med. Ass., 42:*217, 1949.
DUNLOP, J.: Transcondylar Fractures of the Humerus in Childhood. *J. Bone & Joint Surg., 21:* 59, 1939.
DUNLOP, J.: Traumatic Separation of the Medial Epicondyle of the Humerus in Adolescence. *J. Bone & Joint Surg., 17:*577, 1935.
DUNN, N.: Supracondylar Fracture of the Elbow. *Brit. Med. J., 2:*633, 1936.
EASTWOOD, W. J.: The T-shaped Fracture of the Lower End of the Humerus. *J. Bone & Joint Surg., 19:*364, 1937.
FAHEY, J. J. and O'BRIEN, E. T.: Fracture-Separation of the Medial Humeral Condyle in a Child Confused with Fracture of the Medial Epicondyle. *J. Bone & Joint Surg., 53-A:*1102, 1971.
FLYNN, J. C. and RICHARDS, J. F.: Non-Union of Minimally Displaced Fractures of the Lateral Condyle of the Humerus in Children. *J. Bone & Joint Surg., 53-A:*1096, 1971.
FRENCH, P. A.: Varus Deformity of the Elbow Following Supracondylar Fractures of the Humerus in Children. *Lancet, 2:*439, 1959.
GARCEAU, G. J.: Fractures of the Lower End of the Humerus. *J.A.M.A., 112:*623, 1939.
GENNER, CAPT. B. A., III: Fracture of the Supracondylar Process (Case Report). *J. Bone & Joint Surg., 41-A:*1333, 1959.
HAMMOND, G.: Management of Supracondylar Fractures of the Humerus in Children. *Surg. Clin. North America, 32:*747, 1952.
HAMMOND, G., SPONSEL, K. H. and HOPKINS, G. S.: Supracondylar Fractures of the Humerus in Children Treated by Skeletal Suspension Traction. *Bull. Guthrie Clinic, 19:*5, 1949.
HARDACRE, J. A., NAHIGIAN, S. H., FROIMSON, A. I. and BROWN, J. E.: Fractures of the Lateral Condyle of the Humerus in Children. *J. Bone & Joint Surg., 53-A:*1083, 1971.
HART, V. L.: Reduction of Supracondylar Fractures in Children. *Surgery, 11:*33, 1942.
HASNER, E. and HUSBY, J.: Fracture of Epicondyle and Condyle of Humerus. *Acta Chir. Scand., 101:*195, 1951.
HEYL, J. H.: Fracture of the External Condyle of the Humerus in Children. *Ann. Surg., 101:* 1069, 1935.
HIGGS, S. L.: Fractures of the Internal Epicondyle of the Humerus. *Brit. Med. J., 2:*666, 1936.
HITZROT, J. M.: Fractures at the Lower End of the Humerus in Adults. *Surg. Clin. North America, 12:*291, 1932.
HOLMBERG, L.: Fractures of the Distal End of the Humerus in Children. *Acta Chir. Scand. (Suppl. 103), 92:*1, 1945.
HOYER, A.: Treatment of Supracondylar Fracture of the Humerus by Skeletal Traction in an Abduction Splint. *J. Bone & Joint Surg., 34-A:*623, 1952.
JUDET, J. and R.: Treatment of Epiphyseal Fractures by Temporary Transarticular Pegs. *Sem. Hôp. Paris, 24:*2423, 1948.
KAPLAN, S. S. and RECKLING, F. W.: Fracture-Separation of the Lower Humeral Epiphysis with Medial Displacement. *J. Bone & Joint Surg., 53-A:*1105, 1971.
KELLY, R. P. and TAYLOR, W. G.: Open Reduction of T-condylar Fractures of the Humerus Through an Anterior Approach. *J. Trauma, 9:*901, 1969.
KUKSOV, V. F.: Intra-articular Fractures of the Distal Humerus in Children. *Ortop. Travma. Protez., 8:*16, 1969.
LADD, W. E.: Fractures of the Lower End of the Humerus. *Boston Med. & Surg. J., 175:*220, 1916.
LEE, H. G.: Fractures of the Humeral Condyles in Children. *Surg., Gynec. & Obst., 75:*97, 1942.
LEE, W. E. and SUMMEY, T. J.: Fracture of the Capitellum of the Humerus. *Ann. Surg., 99:* 497, 1934.
MCDONNELL, D. P. and WILSON, J. C.: Fractures of the Lower End of the Humerus in Children. *J. Bone & Joint Surg., 30-A:*347, 1948.
MAZEL, M. S.: Fracture of the Capitellum. *J. Bone & Joint Surg., 17:*483, 1935.
MILCH, H.: Fractures of the External Humeral Condyle. *J.A.M.A., 160:*641, 1956.
MILCH, H.: Fractures and Fracture-Dislocations of the Humeral Condyles. *J. Trauma, 4:*592, 1964.
MILLER, E. M., FELL, E. H., BROCK, C., TODD, M. D. and REQUARTH, W. H.: Progress in the Management of Severe Supracondylar Fractures of the Elbow. *Ann. Surg., 113:*1098, 1941.
MILLER, O. L.: Blind Nailing of the T Fracture of the Lower End of the Humerus which Involves the Joint. *J. Bone & Joint Surg., 21:*933, 1939.

MITCHELL, W. J. and ADAMS, J. P.: Effective Management for Supracondylar Fractures of the Humerus in Children. *Clin. Orthop., 23:*197, 1962.

MITCHELL, W. J. and ADAMS, J. P.: Supracondylar Fracture of the Humerus in Children. *J.A.M.A., 175:*119, 1961.

MIYAGI, S. and MAEDA, T.: A Method of Non-Operative Reduction of Fractured Lateral Condyle of the Humerus. *Kurume Med. J., 2:*180, 1955.

NOHRMAN, B. A.: Fractures in the Elbow with Particular Regard to the Distal Humerus End (A Survey). *Acta Radiol., 27:*409, 1946.

PATRICK, J.: Fracture of the Medial Epicondyle with Displacement into the Elbow Joint. *J. Bone & Joint Surg., 28:*143, 1946.

PATTERSON, R. F.: A Method of Applying Traction in T and Y Fractures of the Humerus. *J. Bone & Joint Surg., 17:*476, 1935.

PERSSON, M.: Treatment of Supracondylar Fractures of the Humerus. *Nord. Med. Tidshr., 15:* 457, 1938.

PERSSON, M.: Treatment of Supracondylar Fractures of the Humerus. *Der Chirurg., 10:*650, 1938.

RANEY, R. B.: Fractures of the Lower End of the Humerus in Children. *N. C. Med. J., 11:*192, 1950.

RHODIN, R.: On the Treatment of Fracture of the Capitellum. *Acta Chir. Scand., 86:*475, 1942.

ROBERTS, N. W.: Displacement of the Internal Epicondyle into the Elbow Joint. *Lancet, 227:* 78, 1934.

ROBERTSON, R. C. and BOGART, F. B.: Fracture of the Capitellum and Trochlea, Combined with Fracture of the External Humeral Condyle. *J. Bone & Joint Surg., 15:*206, 1933.

ROTH, PAUL B.: Transverse (Supracondylar) Fracture of the Lower End of the Humerus. *Brit. Med. J., 2:*1215, 1923.

SCHMIER, A. A.: Fracture Dislocation of the Elbow with Displacement of the Internal Epicondyle into the Joint. *Am. J. Surg., 45:*116, 1939.

SCHMIER, A. A.: Fracture-Dislocation of the Elbow with Ulnar Nerve Involvement. *J. Bone & Joint Surg., 18:*1030, 1936.

SCHMIER, A. A.: The Internal Epicondylar Epiphysis and Elbow Injuries. *Surg., Gynec. & Obst., 80:*416, 1945.

SIFFERT, R. S.: Displacement of the Distal Humeral Epiphysis in the Newborn Infant. *J. Bone & Joint Surg., 45-A:*165, 1963.

SIRIS, I. E.: Supracondylar Fracture of the Humerus (An Analysis of 330 Cases). *Surg., Gynec. & Obst., 68:*201, 1939.

SMITH, E. J. R.: Detachment of the Medial Epicondyle of the Humerus with Displacement into the Elbow Joint. *Brit. J. Surg., 26:*785, 1939.

SMITH, F. M.: Displacement of Medial Epicondyle of Humerus into the Elbow Joint. *Ann. Surg., 124:*410, 1946.

SMITH, F. M.: Kirschner Wire Traction in Elbow and Upper Arm Injuries. *Am J. Surg., 74:*770, 1947.

SMITH, F. M.: Medial Epicondyle Injuries. *J.A.M.A., 142:*396, 1950.

SMITH, L.: Deformity Following Supracondylar Fractures of the Humerus. *J. Bone & Joint Surg., 42-A:*235, 1960.

SOEUR, R.: Fractures of the True Condyle of the Humerus. *Acta Orthop. Belgica, 12:*235, 1946.

SPEED, J. S. and MACEY, H. B.: Fractures of the Humeral Condyles in Children. *J. Bone & Joint Surg., 15:*903, 1933.

STAPLES, O. S.: Supracondylar Fractures of the Humerus in Children. *J.A.M.A., 168:*730, 1958.

SUIRE, P., HAKIM, H. and DESROUFFET, D.: Treatment of Displaced Supracondylar Fractures in Children. *Ann. Chir., 23(11-12):*619.

SWENSON, A. L.: The Treatment of Supracondylar Fractures of the Humerus by Kirschner-Wire Transfixion. *J. Bone & Joint Surg., 30-A:*993, 1948.

THORNTON, L.: Fractures of the Humerus Treated by Means of the Hoke Plaster Traction Apparatus. *J. Bone & Joint Surg., 12:*911, 1930.

TYLER, G. T., JR.: Malunion in Supracondylar Fracture of Humerus—Result 15 Years after Operation. *Am. J. Surg., 39:*652, 1938.

TRYNIN, A. H.: Intercondylar T-Fracture of Elbow. *J. Bone & Joint Surg., 23:*709, 1911.

VALLS, J. and OTTOLENGHI, C. E.: Fracture of the Medial Epicondyle with Intra-articular Displacement and Paralysis of the Ulnar Nerve. *Rev. Ortop. Traum., 3:*209, 1933.

VOSHELL, A. F. and TAYLOR, K. P. A.: Regeneration of the Lateral Condyle of the Humerus after Excision. *J. Bone & Joint Surg., 21:*421, 1939.

WADE, F. V. and BATDORF, J.: Supracondylar Fractures of the Humerus: A Twelve Year Review with Follow-up. *J. Trauma, 1:*269, 1961.

WADSWORTH, T. G.: Premature Epiphyseal Fusion after Injury of the Capitellum. *J. Bone & Joint Surg., 46-B:*46, 1964.
WATSON-JONES, R.: Primary Nerve Lesions in Injuries of the Elbow and Wrist. *J. Bone & Joint Surg., 12:*121, 1930.
WILSON, J. N.: The Treatment of Fractures of the Medial Epicondyle of the Humerus. *J. Bone & Joint Surg., 42-B:*778, 1960.
WILSON, P. D.: Fracture of the Lateral Condyle of the Humerus in Childhood. *J. Bone & Joint Surg., 81:*301, 1936.
ZENO, L. O.: Supracondylar Fractures of the Humerus. *Rev. Ortop. Traum., 3:*452, 1934.

Fractures of the Radius

ADLER, J. B. and SHAFTAN, G. W.: Radial Head Fractures, Is Excision Necessary? *J. Trauma, 4:*115, 1964.
BOHRER, J. V.: Fractures of the Head and Neck of the Radius. *Ann. Surg., 97:*204, 1933.
BUFFINGTON, C. B.: The Treatment of Simple and Comminuted Fractures of the Head of the Radius. *W. Va. M. J., 43:*198, 1947.
BURTON, A. E.: Fractures of the Head of the Radius. *Proc. Roy. Soc. Med., 35:*764, 1942.
BUXTON, ST. J. D.: Fractures of the Head of the Radius and Capitellum Including External Condylar Fractures of Childhood. *Brit. Med. J., 2:*665, 1936.
CUTLER, C. W.: Fractures of the Head and Neck of the Radius. *Ann. Surg., 83:*267, 1926.
DICKSON, F. D.: Fractures of the Upper End of the Radius and Ulna. *Surg., Gynec. & Obst., 88:*69, 1949.
FLEMMING, C. W.: Fractures of the Head of the Radius. *Proc. Roy. Soc. Med., 25:*1011, 1932.
GASTON, S. R., SMITH, F. M. and BAAB, O. D.: Adult Injuries of the Radial Head and Neck (Importance of Time Element in Treatment). *Am. J. Surg., 78:*631, 1949.
GASTON, S. R., SMITH, F. M. and BAAB, O. D.: Epiphyseal Injuries of the Radial Head and Neck. *Am. J. Surg., 85:*266, 1953.
GOLDENBERG, R. R.: Closed Manipulation for the Reduction of Fractures of the Neck of the Radius in Children. *J. Bone & Joint Surg., 27:*267, 1945.
JACOBS, J. C. and KERNODLE, H. B.: Fractures of the Head of the Radius. *J. Bone & Joint Surg., 28:*616, 1946.
JEFFERY, C. C.: Fractures of the Head of the Radius in Children. *J. Bone & Joint Surg., 32-B:* 314, 1950.
JONES, E. R. L. and ESAH, M.: Displaced Fracture of the Neck of the Radius in Children. *J. Bone & Joint Surg., 53-B:*429, 1971.
KEY, J. A.: Treatment of Fractures of the Head and Neck of the Radius. *J.A.M.A., 96:*101, 1931.
KEY, J. A.: Survival of the Head of the Radius in a Child after Removal and Replacement. *J. Bone & Joint Surg., 28:*148, 1946.
KEY, J. A.: Survival and Growth of an Epiphysis after Removal and Replacement. *J. Bone & Joint Surg., 31-A:*150, 1949.
KING, B. B.: Resection of the Radial Head and Neck (An end-result study of 13 cases). *J. Bone & Joint Surg., 21:*839, 1939.
LEWIS, R. W. and THIBODEAU, A. A.: Deformity of the Wrist Following Resection of the Radial Head. *Surg., Gynec. & Obst., 64:*1079, 1937.
MASON, J. A. and SHUTKIN, N. M.: Immediate Active Motion Treatment of Fractures of the Head and Neck of the Radius. *Surg., Gynec. & Obst., 76:*731, 1943.
MEEKISON, D. M.: Some Remarks on Three Common Fractures. (Carpal Scaphoid, Head of Radius, and Medial Malleolus.) *J. Bone & Joint Surg., 27:*80, 1945.
MURRAY, R. C.: Fractures of the Head and Neck of the Radius. *Brit. J. S., 28:*106, 1940.
POSTLETHWAIT, R. W.: Modified Treatment for Fracture of the Head of the Radius. *Am. J. Surg., 67:*77, 1945.
REIDY, J. A. and VAN GORDER, G. W.: Treatment of Displacement of the Proximal Radial Epiphysis. *J. Bone & Joint Surg., 45-A:*1355, 1963.
RIETH, PAUL L.: Fractures of the Radial Head. (Associated with Chip Fracture of the Capitellum in Adults: Surgical Considerations.) *Sth. Surg., 14:*154, 1948.
SCHWARTZ, R. P. and YOUNG, F.: Treatment of Fractures of the Head and Neck of the Radius and Slipped Radial Epiphysis in Children. *Surg., Gynec. & Obst., 57:*528, 1933.
SPEED, K.: Ferrule Caps for the Head of the Radius. *Surg., Gynec. & Obst., 73:*845, 1941.
SUTRO, C. J.: Regrowth of Bone at the Proximal End of the Radius Following Resection in this Region. *J. Bone & Joint Surg., 17:*867, 1935.
THOMPSON, C. F. and KALAYJIAN, B.: Madelung's Deformity and Associated Deformity at Elbow. *Surg., Gynec. & Obst., 69:*221, 1939.

Fractures of the Ulna

DALAND, E. M.: Fractures of the Olecranon. *J. Bone & Joint Surg., 15*:601, 1933.
ERIKSSON, E., SAHLIN, O. and SANDHAHL, U.: Late Results of Conservative and Surgical Treatment of Fracture of the Olecranon. *Acta Chir. Scand., 113*:153, 1957.
FLACK, K.: Management and Results of Fractures of the Olecranon in Adults. *Arch. Orthop. Unfall-Chir., 65*:173, 1969.
HARMON, P. H.: Treatment of Fractures of the Olecranon by Fixation with Stainless-Steel Screws. *J. Bone & Joint Surg., 27*:328, 1945.
HEINMAN, D,, SCHLACHETZKI, J. and BOMMERT, E.: Conservative Management of Fractures of the Olecranon. *Mschr. Unfallheilk., 73*:325, 1970.
McKEEVER, F. M. and BUCK, R. M.: Fracture of the Olecranon Process of the Ulna. *J.A.M.A., 135*:1, 1947.
MACAUSLAND, W. R.: The Treatment of Fractures of the Olecranon by Longitudinal Screw or Nail Fixation. *Ann. Surg., 116*:293, 1942.
NONNEMAN, H. C.: Spring Osteosynthesis of Fractures of the Olecranon. *Mschr. Unfallheilk., 72-(10)*:437, 1969.
PERKINS, G.: Fractures of the Olecranon. *Brit. Med. J., 2*:668, 1936.
ROMBOLD, C.: A New Operative Treatment for Fracture of the Olecranon. *J. Bone & Joint Surg., 16*:947, 1934.
RUSH, L. V. and RUSH, H. L.: A Reconstruction Operation for Comminuted Fracture of Upper Third of the Ulna. *Am. J. Surg., 38*:332, 1937.
SCHEUBA, G. and UNGAR, F.: Classification and Management of Olecranon Fractures. *Mschr. Unfallheilk., 73*:200, 1970.
WAINWRIGHT, D.: Fractures of the Olecranon Process. *Brit. J. Surg., 29*:403, 1942.
WAXMAN, A. and GESHELIN, H.: Fracture of the Olecranon Process Due to Muscle Pull with the Forearm in Hyperextension. *California Med., 66*:358, 1947.

Monteggia Fractures

BEDDOW, F. H. and CORKERY, P. H.: Lateral Dislocation of the Radio-Humeral Joint with Greenstick Fracture of the Upper End of the Ulna. *J. Bone & Joint Surg., 42-B*:782, 1960.
CORBETT, C. H.: Anterior Dislocation of the Radius and Its Recurrence. *Brit. J. Surg., 19*: 155, 1931.
CUNNINGHAM, S. R.: Fracture of the Ulna with Dislocation of the Head of the Radius. *J. Bone & Joint Surg., 16*:351, 1934.
CURRY, G. J.: Monteggia Fracture. *Am. J. Surg., 73*:613, 1947.
EDWARDS, E. G.: The Posterior Monteggia Fracture. *Am. Surgeon, 18*:323, 1952.
EVANS, E. M.: Pronation Injuries of the Forearm (with special reference to the Anterior Monteggia Fracture) . *J. Bone & Joint Surg., 31-B*:578, 1949.
MAY, V. R. and MAUCK, W.: Dislocation of the Radial Head with Associated Fracture of the Ulna. Sth. Med. J., *54*:1255, 1961.
MOBLEY, J. E. and JONES, J. M.: Monteggia Fractures. *Proc. Mayo Clin., 30*:497, 1955.
MONTEGGIA, G. B.: *Institutzione Chirurgiche.* 2nd Ed. Milan, G. Masper 1813-1815.
NAYLOR, A.: Monteggia Fractures. *Brit. J. Surg., 29*:323, 1942.
PAVEL, A., PITMAN, J. M., LANCE, E. M. and WADE, P. A.: The Posterior Monteggia Fracture: A Clinical Study. *J. Trauma, 5*:185, 1965.
PENROSE, J. H.: The Monteggia Fracture with Posterior Dislocation of the Radial Head. *J. Bone & Joint Surg., 33-B*:65, 1951.
RAMSEY, R. H. and PEDERSEN, H. E.: The Monteggia Fracture-Dislocation in Children. *J.A.M.A., 182*:1091, 1962.
SMITH, F. M.: Monteggia Fractures. (An Analysis of Twenty-Five Consecutive Fresh Injuries.) *Surg., Gynec. & Obst., 58*:630, 1947.
SPEED, J. S. and BOYD, H. B.: Treatment of Fractures of Ulna with Dislocation of Head of Radius (Monteggia Fracture) . *J.A.M.A., 115*:1699, 1940.
THEODOROU, S. D.: Dislocation of the Head of the Radius Associated with Fracture of the Upper End of the Ulna in Children. *J. Bone & Joint Surg., 51-B*:700, 1969.
TOMPKINS, D. G.: The Anterior Monteggia Fracture. *J. Bone & Joint Surg., 53-A*:1109, 1971.
WEIS, J.: Monteggia Fractures. *Mschr. Unfallheilk., 73*:409, 1970.
WENZEL, K. P. and SANDER, E.: Late Functional Result of Operation in Monteggia Fractures. *Mschr. Unfallheilk., 72(2)*:66, 1969.
WISE, R. A.: Lateral Dislocation of the Head of the Radius with Fracture of the Ulna. *J. Bone & Joint Surg., 23*:379, 1941.

Dislocations

ALLENDE, G. and FREYTES, M.: Old Dislocations of the Elbow. *J. Bone & Joint Surg., 24:*691, 1944.

AUFRANC, O., JONES, W. N. and TURNER, R. H.: Dislocation of the Elbow with Brachial Artery Injury. *J.A.M.A., 197:*127, 1966.

BUXTON, ST. J.: Ossification in the Ligaments of the Elbow Joint. *J. Bone & Joint Surg., 20:* 709, 1938.

CALLAHAN, J. J.: Dislocations. *J.A.M.A., 132:*440, 1946.

CHERRY, J. C.: Dislocations of the Elbow. *The Practitioner, 160:*191, 1948.

CHRISTOPHER, F.: Radial Exostosis Complicating Anterior Dislocation of the Elbow. *J. Bone & Joint Surg., 14:*949, 1932.

COHN, I.: Forward Dislocation of Both Bones of the Forearm at the Elbow. *Surg., Gynec. & Obst., 35:*776, 1922.

ERBAN, W.: Atraumatic Reduction of Dislocation of the Elbow. *Chir. Praxis,* p. 401, 1959.

FRIEDMANN, E.: Simple Rupture of the Brachial Artery Sustained in Elbow Dislocation. *J.A.M.A., 177:*106, 1961.

GOSMAN, J. A.: Recurrent Dislocation of the Ulna at the Elbow. *J. Bone & Joint Surg., 25:*448, 1943.

HAMILTON, A. T.: Three Common Orthopedic Problems. (De Quervain's Disease, Pulled Elbow and Morton's Toe.) *N. C. Med. J., 10:*267, 1949.

HART, G. M.: Subluxation of the Head of the Radius in Young Children. *J.A.M.A., 169:*1734, 1959.

HENDERSON, R. S. and ROBERTSON, I. M.: Open Dislocation of the Elbow with Rupture of the Brachial Artery. *J. Bone & Joint Surg., 34-B:*636, 1952.

HOWARD, N. J.: Epiphyseal Fracture-Dislocation at the Elbow Joint. *J. Bone & Joint Surg., 17:*123, 1935.

HUME, A. C.: Anterior Dislocation of the Head of the Radius Associated with Undisplaced Fracture of the Olecranon in Children. *J. Bone & Joint Surg., 39-B:*508, 1957.

KAPEL, O.: Operation for Habitual Dislocation of the Elbow. *J. Bone & Joint Surg., 33-A:*707, 1951.

KERIN, R.: Elbow Dislocation and Its Association with Vascular Disruption. *J. Bone & Joint Surg., 51-A:*756, 1969.

KING, O. C.: Fractures and Dislocations About the Elbow. *Surg. Clin. North America, 20:*1645, 1940.

KINI, M. G.: Dislocation of the Elbow and Its Complications. *J. Bone & Joint Surg., 22:*107, 1940.

LINSCHEID, R. L. and WHEELER, D. K.: Elbow Dislocations. *J.A.M.A., 194:*113, 1965.

LOOMIS, J. K.: Reduction and After-Treatment of Posterior Dislocation of the Elbow. *Am. J. Surg., 63:*56, 1944.

MCVEAGH, T. C.: The"Slipped Elbow" of Young Children. *Calif. Med., 74:*260, 1951.

OUTLAND, T. and HANLON, C. R.: Posterior Dislocation of the Elbow Joint Complicated by Fracture of the Medial Epicondyle and Ulnar-Nerve Injury. *J. Bone & Joint Surg., 20:*750, 1938.

PAWLOWSKI, R. F., PALUMBO, F. C. and CALLAHAN, J. J.: Irreducible Posterolateral Elbow Dislocation: Report of a Rare Case. *J. Trauma, 10:*260, 1970.

RAILTON, S. V.: Compound Dislocation of Elbow Joint without Fracture. (Case Report.) *Canad. M. A. J., 59:*367, 1948.

ROCYN-JONES, A.: Fractures and Dislocations at the Elbow. *The Practitioner, 144:*589, 1940.

SPEED, J. S.: An Operation for Unreduced Posterior Dislocation of the Elbow. *Sth. M. J., 18:* 193, 1925.

STARKLOFF, G. B.: Posterior Dislocations at the Elbow. *J. Missouri State M. A., 45:*895, 1948.

STELLING, F. H. and COTE, R. H.: Traumatic Dislocation of the Head of the Radius in Children. *J.A.M.A., 160:*732, 1956.

STRUG, L. H.: Anterior Dislocation of the Elbow with Fracture of the Olecranon. *Am. J. Surg., 75:*700, 1948.

Volkmann's Ischaemia and Contracture

BALSAC, R. H. DE: Acute Ischemia of Limbs. *Revista Brasileira de Medicina, Rio de Janeiro, 6:*517, 1949.

BROOKS, B.: Pathological Changes in Muscle as a Result of Disturbances of Circulation. (An Experimental Study of Volkmann's Ischaemic Paralysis.) *Arch. Surg., 5:*188, 1922.

CREGAN, J. C. F.: Prolonged Traumatic Arterial Spasm After Supracondylar Fracture of the Humerus. *J. Bone & Joint Surg., 33-B:*363, 1951.

GARBER, J. N.: Volkmann's Contracture as a Complication of Fractures of the Forearm and Elbow. *J. Bone & Joint Surg., 21:*154, 1939.

GRIFFITHS, D. L.: The Management of Acute Circulatory Failure in an Injured Limb. *J. Bone & Joint Surg., 30-B:*280, 1948.
GRIFFITHS, D. L.: Volkmann's Ischaemic Contracture. *Brit. J. Surg., 28:*239, 1940.
HILL, R. L. and BROOKS, B.: Volkmann's Ischaemic Contracture in Hemophilia. *Ann. Surg., 103:*444, 1936.
HORN, J. S. and SEVITT, S.: Ischaemic Necrosis and Regeneration of the Tibialis Anterior Muscle After Rupture of the Popliteal Artery. *J. Bone & Joint Surg., 33-B:*348, 1951.
JONES, S. G.: Volkmann's Contracture. *Am. J. Surg., 43:*325, 1930.
JONES, S. G.: Volkmann's Contracture. *J. Bone & Joint Surg., 17:*649, 1935.
JONES, S. G. and COTTON, F. J.: Ischaemic Paralysis of Leg Simulating Volkmann's Contracture. *J. Bone & Joint Surg., 17:*659, 1935.
KULOWSKI, J.: Subfascial Tension Hematoma and Impending Ischemia Resulting from Contusion of the Forearm: Case Report. *Am. Surg., 24:*346, 1958.
MEYERDING, H. W.: Volkmann's Ischaemic Contracture. *J.A.M.A., 106:*1139, 1936.
MORRISON, G. M. and KENNARD, H. E.: Ischaemic Paralysis from Pressure of Hematoma. *J. Bone & Joint Surg., 17:*656, 1935.
NOBEL, W.: Impending Volkmann's Ischemia. *Am. J. Surg., 100:*635, 1960.
OCHSNER, A.: Indications for Sympathetic Nervous System Block. *Ochsner Clin., 10:*12, 1951.
PARKES, A.: The Treatment of Established Volkmann's Contracture by Tendon Transplantation. *J. Bone & Joint Surg., 33-B:*359, 1951.
PEDEMONTE, P. V.: Fundamental Concepts in the Treatment of Completely Arrested Volkmann Contracture. *Arch. Urug. Med., 33:*123, 1948.
SPEER, H. C. and JANES, J. M.: Rupture of the Brachial Artery Accompanying Dislocation of the Elbow or Supracondylar Fracture. *J. Bone & Joint Surg., 33-A:*889, 1951.
THOMSON, S. A. and MAHONEY, L. J.: Volkmann's Ischaemic Contracture and Its Relationship to Fracture of the Femur. *J. Bone & Joint Surg., 33-B:*336, 1951.

Nerve Lesions, etc.

BERGMAN, E.: Tardy Ulnar Palsy. *Am. J. Surg., 80:*371, 1950.
BURMAN, M. S. and SUTRO, C. J.: Recurrent Luxation of the Ulnar Nerve by Congenital Posterior Position of the Medial Epicondyle of the Humerus. *J. Bone & Joint Surg., 21:*958, 1939.
CONWAY, F. M.: Traumatic Ulnar Neuritis. *Ann. Surg., 97:*425, 1933.
COTTON, F. J.: Elbow Dislocation and Ulnar Nerve Injury. *J. Bone & Joint Surg., 11:*348, 1929.
DAVIDSON, A. J. and HORWITZ, M. T.: Late or Tardy Ulnar-Nerve Paralysis. *J. Bone & Joint Surg., 17:*844, 1935.
FEIDEL, W. and STRATFORD, J.: Cause of Progressive Ulnar Nerve Palsy. *Canad. J. Surg., 1:* 287, 1958.
GAY, J. R. and LOVE, J. G.: Diagnosis and Treatment of Tardy Paralysis of the Ulnar Nerve. *J. Bone & Joint Surg., 29:*1087, 1947.
GODSHALL, R. W. and HANSEN, C. A.: Traumatic Ulnar Neuropathy in Adolescent Baseball Pitchers. *J. Bone & Joint Surg., 53-A:*359, 1971.
GURDJIAN, E. S. and GOETZ, A. G.: Radial Paralysis Complicating Fracture and Dislocation in the Upper Limb. *Ann. Surg., 99:*487, 1934.
HOLSTEIN, A. and LEWIS, G. D.: Fractures of the Humerus with Radial Nerve Paralysis. *J. Bone & Joint Surg., 45-A:*1382, 1963.
KING, T.: The Treatment of Traumatic Ulnar Neuritis. *Australian & New Zealand J. Surg., 20:*33, 1950.
KOPELL, H. P. and THOMPSON, W. A. L.: *Peripheral Entrapment Neuropathies.* Baltimore, Williams and Wilkins Co., 1963.
LEARMOUTH, J. R.: A Technique for Transplanting the Ulnar Nerve. *Surg., Gynec. & Obst., 75:*792, 1942.
MAYER, J. H. and MAYFIELD, F. H.: Surgery of the Posterior Interosseus Branch of the Radial Nerve. *Surg., Gynec. & Obst., 84:*979, 1947.
MCGOWAN, A. J.: The Results of Transposition of the Ulnar Nerve for Traumatic Ulnar Neuritis. *J. Bone & Joint Surg., 32-B:*293, 1950.
REGAN, J. R.: The Surgical Treatment of Delayed Ulnar Neuritis. *Am. J. Surg., 41:*501, 1938.
SANDELL, D. H.: Late Ulnar Nerve Paralysis. *Brit. Med. J., 2:*969, 1936.
SEDDON, H. J.: Nerve Lesions Complicating Certain Closed Bone Injuries. *J.A.M.A., 135:*691, 1947.
STRACHAN, J. C. H. and ELLIS, B. W.: Vulnerability of the Posterior Interosseus Nerve During Radial Head Resection. *J. Bone & Joint Surg., 53-B:*320, 1971.
STRONG, O. S. and ELWYN, A.: *Human Neuroanatomy.* 2nd Ed. Baltimore, Williams and Wilkins Co., 1948.

Surgical Approaches

BOYD, H. B.: *Surgical Approaches to the Elbow Joint.* Lectures on Regional Orthopedic Surgery and Fundamental Orthopedic Problems, No. II, Ann Arbor, J. W. Edwards, Inc., 1948.

BOYD, H. B.: Surgical Exposure of the Ulna and Proximal Third of the Radius Through One Incision. *Surg., Gynec. & Obst., 71:*87, 1940.

DARRACH, W.: Surgical Approaches for Surgery of the Extremities. *Am. J. Surg., 67:*237, 1945.

HENRY, A. K.: *Extensile Exposure.* Baltimore, Williams and Wilkins Co., 1945.

KAPLAN, E. B.: Surgical Approach to the Proximal End of the Radius and Its Use in Fractures of the Head and Neck of the Radius. *J. Bone & Joint Surg., 23:*86, 1941.

NICOLA, T.: *Atlas of Surgical Approaches to Bone and Joints.* New York, Macmillan Co., 1945.

SPEED, J. S. and BOYD, H. B.: Treatment of Fractures of Ulna with Dislocation of Head of Radius (Monteggia Fracture). *J.A.M.A., 115:*1699, 1940.

VAN GORDER, G. W.: Surgical Approach in Old Posterior Dislocation of the Elbow. *J. Bone & Joint Surg., 14:*127, 1932.

VAN GORDER, G. W.: Surgical Approach in Supracondylar "T" Fractures of the Humerus Requiring Open Reduction. *J. Bone & Joint Surg., 22:*278, 1940.

Synostosis

BALDWIN, C. H.: Fusion of the Radio-Ulnar Joint. *J. Bone & Joint Surg., 11:*345, 1929.

BOTTING, T. D. J.: Post-Traumatic Radio-Ulna Cross Union. *J. Trauma, 10:*16, 1970.

COHN, B. N. E.: Congenital Bi-lateral Radio-Ulnar Synostosis. *J. Bone & Joint Surg., 14:*404, 1932.

DAWSON, H. G. W.: Congenital Deformity of Forearm and Operative Treatment. *Brit. Med. J., 2:*833, 1912.

FAHLSTROM, S.: Radio-Ulnar Synostosis. Historical Review and Case Report. *J. Bone & Joint Surg., 14:*395, 1932.

MEILLAND, G.: Congenital Superior-Radio-Ulnar Synostosis. *Chir. Praxis, 37:*907, 1948.

WILKIE, D. P. D.: Congenital Radio-Ulnar Synostosis. *Brit. J. Surg., 1:*366, 1913-14.

Epicondylitis; Tennis Elbow; Radio-Humeral Bursitis, etc.

CARP, L.: Tennis Elbow (Epicondylitis) Caused by Radiohumeral Bursitis. Anatomical, Clinical, Roentgenological, and Pathological Aspects, with a Suggestion as to Treatment. *Arch. Surg., 24:*905, 1932.

CYRIAX, J. H.: The Pathology and Treatment of Tennis Elbow. *J. Bone & Joint Surg., 18:*921, 1936.

FROIMSON, A. I.: Treatment of Tennis Elbow with Forearm Support Band. *J. Bone & Joint Surg., 53-A:*183, 1971.

HAMILTON, A. R.: A Case of Calcification in the Epicondylar Bursa at the Elbow. *Brit. J. Surg., 26:*446, 1938-39.

HOHL, M.: Treatment of Tennis Elbow. *Clin. Orthop., 19:*232, 1961.

HUGHES, E. S. R.: Acute Deposition of Calcium Near the Elbow. *J. Bone & Joint Surg., 32-B:* 30, 1950.

ILFELD, F. W. and FIELD, S. M.: Treatment of Tennis Elbow (Use of a Special Brace). *J.A.M.A., 195:*111, 1966.

MEHERIN, J. M. and COOPER, C. E.: Tennis Elbow. *Am. J. Surg., 80:*622, 1950.

MERCER, W.: Tennis Elbow. *Practitioner, 164:*293, 1950.

MICHELE, A. A. and KRUEGER, F. J.: Lateral Epicondylitis of the Elbow Treated by Fasciotomy. *Surgery, 39:*277, 1956.

MOORE, M.: Radiohumeral Synovitis. *Arch. Surg., 64:*501, 1952.

NORTH, J. P.: Tennis Elbow (Collective Review). *Internat. Abstr. Surg., 67:*176, 1938.

Arthroplasty

ALBEE, F. H.: Arthroplasty of the Elbow. *J. Bone & Joint Surg., 15:*979, 1933.

ARMSTRONG, A. C.: A Technique for Arthroplasty of the Elbow Joint. *Med. J. Australia, 8:*716, 1947.

BARR, J. S. and EATON, R. G.: Elbow Reconstruction with a New Prosthesis to Replace the Distal End of the Humerus (Case Report). *J. Bone & Joint Surg., 47-A:*1408, 1965.

BUZBY, B. F.: End-Results of Excision of the Elbow. *Ann. Surg., 103:*625, 1936.

HAAS, J.: Functional Arthroplasty. *J. Bone & Joint Surg., 26:*297, 1944.

JOHNSON, E. W. and SCHLEIN, A. P.: Vitallium Prosthesis for the Olecranon and Proximal Part of the Ulna (Case Report with 13 Year Follow-up). *J. Bone & Joint Surg., 52-A:*721, 1970.

KIRKALDY-WILLIS, W. H.: Excision of the Elbow Joint. *Lancet, 254:*53, 1948.

KNIGHT, R. A. and VAN ZANDT, I. L.: Arthroplasty of the Elbow (End Result Study). *J. Bone & Joint Surg., 34-A:*610, 1952.

MacAusland, W. R.: Arthroplasty of the Elbow. *New England J. Med., 236:*97, 1947.
Mellen, R. H. and Phalen, G. S.: Arthroplasty of the Elbow by Replacement of the Distal Portion of the Humerus with an Acrylic Prosthesis. *J. Bone & Joint Surg., 29:*348, 1947.
Pollock, W. J. and Parkes, J. C.: Early Reconstruction of the Elbow Following Severe Trauma. *J. Trauma, 10:*839, 1970.
Vogl, A.: Arthroplasty of the Elbow Joint. *Ztschr. Orthop., 78:*21, 1948.
Young, C., Jr.: Primary Elbow Arthroplasty. *Arch. Surg., 101:*78, 1970.

Miscellaneous

Aufranc, O. E., Jones, W. N. and Harris, W. H.: Sideswipe Injury to the Left Elbow. *J.A.M.A., 186:*855, 1963.
Bateman, J. E.: Denervation of the Elbow Joint for the Relief of Pain. *J. Bone & Joint Surg., 30-B:*635, 1948.
Bennett, G. E.: Shoulder and Elbow Lesions Distinctive of Baseball Players. *Ann. Surg., 126:* 107, 1947.
Birsner, J. W. and De Smet, D. H.: Patella Cubiti with Fracture. *Ann. West. Med. & Surg., 4:*744, 1950.
Blount, W. P.: Osteoclasis for Supination Deformities in Children. *J. Bone & Joint Surg., 22:*300, 1940.
Bowers, R. F.: Myositis Ossificans Traumatica. *J. Bone & Joint Surg., 19:*215, 1937.
Boyd, W.: *Surgical Pathology.* 4th Ed. Philadelphia, W. B. Saunders Co., 1938.
Bunnell, S.: Restoring Flexion to the Paralytic Elbow. *J. Bone & Joint Surg., 33-A:*566, 1951.
Bunnell, S.: *Surgery of the Hand.* 2nd Ed. Philadelphia, J. B. Lippincott Co., 1948.
Caffey, J.: *Pediatric X-ray Diagnosis.* 4th Ed. Chicago, Year Book Medical Publishers, Inc., 1961.
Callander, C. Latimer: *Surgical Anatomy.* 2nd Ed. Philadelphia, W. B. Saunders Co., 1939.
Carroll, R. E.: Restoration of Flexor Power to the Flail Elbow by Transplantation of the Triceps Tendon. *Surg., Gynec. & Obst., 95:*685, 1952.
Cave, E. F.: *Fractures and Other Injuries.* Chicago, Year Book Medical Publishers, Inc., 1958.
Compere, E. L.: *The 1950 Year Book of Orthopedics and Traumatic Surgery.* Chicago. Year Book Medical Publishers, Inc., 1951.
Cowan, I. I. and Stone, J. R.: Painful Periarticular Calcifications at Wrist and Elbow: Diagnosis and Treatment. *J.A.M.A., 149:*530, 1952.
Crenshaw, A. H.: *Campbell's Operative Orthopaedics.* 4th Ed. St. Louis, C. V. Mosby Co., 1963.
Davis, W. M. and Yassine, Z.: An Etiological Factor in Tear of the Distal Tendon of the Biceps Brachii. *J. Bone & Joint Surg., 38-A:*1365, 1956.
Dobbie, R. P.: Avulsion of the Lower Biceps Brachii Tendon (Analysis of Fifty-one Previously Unreported Cases). *Am. J. Surg., 51:*662, 1941.
Frantz, V. K. and Harvey, H. D.: *Introducton to Surgery.* New York, Oxford University Press, 1951.
Gellman, M.: Arthrodesis of the Elbow. *J. Bone & Joint Surg., 29:*851, 1947.
Glass, H. G. and Smith, E. T.: Incapacitating Contractures of the Elbow Following Intravenous Infusions. *Surgery, 37:*803, 1955.
Hait, G., Boswick, J. A. and Stone, N. H.: Heterotopic Formation Secondary to Trauma (Myositis Ossificans Traumatica). *J. Trauma, 10:*405, 1970.
Hallock, H.: Fusion of the Elbow Joint for Tuberculosis. *J. Bone & Joint Surg., 14:*145, 1932.
Hausmann, P. F. and Everett, H. H.: Wringer Injury. *Surgery, 28:*71, 1950.
Heller, C. J. and Wiltse, L. L.: Avascular Necrosis of the Capitellum Humeri (Panner's Disease). *J. Bone & Joint Surg., 42-A:*513, 1960.
Hodges, P. C., Phemister, D. B. and Brunschwig, A.: *The Roentgen-Ray Diagnosis of Diseases of the Bones and Joints.* New York, Thomas Nelson & Sons, 1938.
Holmes, G. W. and Ruggles, H. E.: *Roentgen Interpretation.* Philadelphia, Lea and Febiger, 1926.
Inclan, A.: Tumoral Calcinosis. *J.A.M.A., 121:*490, 1943.
Inglis, A. E., Ranawat, C. S. and Straub, L. R.: Synovectomy and Débridement of the Elbow in Rheumatoid Arthritis. *J. Bone & Joint Surg., 53-A:*652, 1971.
Jackson, C. M.: *Morris' Human Anatomy.* Philadelphia, P. Blakiston's Son & Co., 1923.
Kelly, P. J., Martin, W. S. and Coventry, M. B.: Bacterial (Suppurative) Arthritis in the Adult. *J. Bone & Joint Surg., 52-A:*1595, 1970.
Kessler, H. H.: Rehabilitation of the Arm Amputee. *New York State J. Med., 49:*1921, 1949.
King, D and Secor, C.: Bow Elbow (Cubitus Varus). *J. Bone & Joint Surg., 33-A:*572, 1951.
Kleinberg, S.: Osteochondromatosis of Elbow. *Ann. Surg., 99:*480, 1934.
Kulowski, J.: Segmental Arterial Spasm of the Brachial Artery. *Surgery, 38:*1087, 1955.

LASHER, W. W. and MATHEWSON, L. M.: Olecranon Bursitis. *J.A.M.A.*, *90*:1030, 1928.

LEVINE, M. A.: Patella Cubiti. *J. Bone & Joint Surg.*, *32-A*:686, 1950.

LIPSCOMB, P. R. and BURLESON, R. J.: Vascular and Neural Complications of Supracondylar Fractures of the Humerus in Children. *J. Bone & Joint Surg.*, *37-A*:487, 1955.

MACAUSLAND, W. R., JR. and GARTLAND, J. J.: The Treatment of Acute Hemophilic Hemarthrosis. (A Report on the Use of Hyaluronidase.) *New England J. Med.*, *247*:755, 1952.

MARMOR, L.: *Trauma to the Elbow and Forearm.* Clinical Orthopaedics and Related Research. Vol. 5. Philadelphia, J. B. Lippincott Co., 1967.

MATEV, I. B.: Symptomatic Enlargement of the Tuberosity of the Radius Causing Snapping in the Forearm. *J. Bone & Joint Surg.*, *52-A*:1661, 1970.

MCBRIDE, E. D.: *Disability Evaluation.* 4th Ed. Philadelphia, J. B. Lippincott Co., 1942.

MORTON, H. S. and CRYSLER, W. E.: Osteochondritis Dissecans of the Supratrochlear Septum. *J. Bone & Joint Surg.*, *27*:12, 1945.

MÜLLER, M. E., ALLGÖWER, M. and WILLENEGGER, H.: *Manual of Internal Fixation.* New York, Springer-Verlag, 1970.

NORELL, H. G.: Roentgenologic Visualization of the Extracapsular Fat: Its Importance in the Diagnosis of Traumatic Injury to the Elbow. *Acta Radiol.*, *42*:205, 1954.

O'DONOGHUE, D. H.: *Treatment of Injuries to Athletes.* 2nd Ed. Philadelphia, W. B. Saunders Co., 1970.

Orthopedic Subjects. (Military Surgical Manuals—National Research Council.) Philadelphia, W. B. Saunders Co., 1942.

PARNALL, E.: Reconstruction of the Elbow Joint. *J. Bone & Joint Surg.*, *30-A*:752, 1948.

PEREIRA, A. DE S.: Blocking of the Middle Cervical and Stellate Ganglions with Descending Infiltration Anesthesia. Technic, Accidents and Therapeutic Indications. *Arch. Surg.*, *50*: 152, 1945.

PIERSOL, G. A.: *Human Anatomy.* 8th Ed. Philadelphia, J. B. Lippincott Co., 1923.

RIETH, G. R.: Elbow Out of the Window Injuries: A Follow-up Study of 50 Cases. *J. La. Med. Soc.*, *111*:220, 1959.

ROB, C. and SMITH, R.: *Operative Surgery* (*Orthopaedics*). Philadelphia, J. B. Lippincott Co., 1969.

ROBERTS, N. and HUGHES, R.: Osteochondritis Dissecans of the Elbow Joint. (A Clinical Study.) *J. Bone & Joint Surg.*, *32-B*:348, 1950.

ROMBOLD, C.: Infection in a Simple Fracture. *J. Bone & Joint Surg.*, *17*:217, 1935.

ROSS, W. T.: Osteochondritis of the Supratrochlear Septum. *J. Bone & Joint Surg.*, *29*:514, 1947.

ROWLANDS, R. P. and TURNER, P.: *The Operations of Surgery.* 7th Ed. New York, Macmillan Co., 1927.

SACHS, J. and DEGENSHEIN, G.: Patella Cubiti. *Arch. Surg.*, *57*:675, 1948.

SCHLOSSBACH, T.: Avulsion of the Lower Biceps Tendon. *J. M. Soc. New Jersey*, *47*:166, 1950.

SCUDERI, C.: Restoration of Long Bone Defects with Massive Bone Grafts. *J.A.M.A.*, *127*:1116, 1948.

SHERBE, H. B.: Car Window Elbows. *Sth. M. J.* *34*:372, 1941.

SMITH, M. G. H.: Osteochondritis of the Humeral Capitellum. *J. Bone & Joint Surg.*, *46-B*: 50, 1964.

SPALTEHOLZ, W.: *Hand-Atlas of Human Anatomy.* 4th Ed., Philadelphia, J. B. Lippincott Co., 1923.

STAPLES, O. S.: Arthrodesis of the Elbow Joint. *J. Bone & Joint Surg.*, *34-A*:207, 1952.

STEINDLER, A.: *Orthopedic Operations.* Springfield, Illinois, Charles C Thomas, 1940.

SWENSON, S. A. and BISGARD, J. D.: Amputation of Extremities. *Am. J. Surg.*, *76*:461, 1948.

THOMSON, J. E. M. and TANNER, F. H.: Tumoral Calcinosis. *J. Bone & Joint Surg.*, *31-A*:132, 1949.

THORNDIKE, A., JR.: Myositis Ossificans Traumatica. *J. Bone & Joint Surg.*, *22*:315, 1940.

TORGERSON, W. B. and LEACH, R. E.: Synovectomy of the Elbow in Rheumatoid Arthritis (Report of Five Cases). *J. Bone & Joint Surg.*, *52-A*:371, 1970.

WIGHTMAN, J. A. K.: Clicking Elbow from a Torn Annular Ligament. *J. Bone & Joint Surg.*, *45-B*:380, 1963.

WILLNER, P.: Anterior Capsulectomy for Contractures of the Elbow. *J. Internat. Coll. Surg.*, *11*:359, 1948.

WILSON, P. D.: Capsulectomy for the Relief of Flexion Contractures of the Elbow Following Fracture. *J. Bone & Joint Surg.*, *26*:71, 1944.

YOUNG, H. H. and COVENTRY, M. B.: *Fractures. Lewis-Walter's Practice of Surgery.* Hagerstown, W. F. Prior Co., 1966.

ZEITLIN, A.: The Traumatic Origin of Accessory Bones at the Elbow. *J. Bone & Joint Surg.*, *17*:933, 1935.

Index